NURSING
Case Management

A Practical Guide to
Success in Managed Care

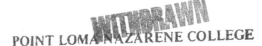

NURSING
Case Management

A Practical Guide to
Success in Managed Care

Suzanne K. Powell, RN, BSN, CCM

Director of Case Management
Health Services Advisory Group, Inc.
Phoenix, Arizona

In consultation with

Patty M. Wekell, RN, MS, CNAA

Director of Case and Quality Management
St. Joseph's Hospital and Medical Center
Mercy Healthcare Arizona
Phoenix, Arizona

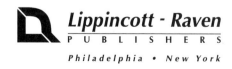
Lippincott - Raven
PUBLISHERS
Philadelphia • New York

Acquisitions Editor: Jennifer E. Brogan
Coordinating Editorial Assistant: Danielle J. DiPalma
Project Editor: Susan Deitch
Production Manager: Helen Ewan
Production Coordinator: Patricia McCloskey
Design Coordinator: Kathy Kelley-Luedtke

Library of Congress Cataloging in Publications Data

Powell, Suzanne K.
    Nursing case management: a practical guide to success in managed care/ Suzanne K. Powell, in consultation with
Patty M. Wekell.
       p.   cm.
    Includes bibliographical references and index.
    ISBN 0-397-55234-3 (alk. paper)
    1. Primary nursing. 2. Hospitals--Case management services. 3. Managed care plans (Medical care) 4. Nurse
practitioners.
    I. Wekell, Patty M.   II. Title.
    [DNLM: 1. Patient Care Planning--organization & administration. 2. Nurse Clinicians. 3. Managed Care
Programs--organization & administration. WY 100 P886n 1996]
    RT90.7.P68   1996
    362.1'0425--dc20
    DNLM/DLC
    for Library of Congress   95-32575
                                                                                                        CIP

⊚ This paper meets the requirements of ANSI/NISO 239.48-1992 (Permanence of Paper).

The material contained in this volume was submitted as previously unpublished material,
except in the instances in which credit has been given to the source from which some of
the illustrative material was derived.

Any procedure or practice described in this book should be applied by the healthcare practitioner under appropriate supervision in accordance with professional standards of care
used with regard to the unique circumstances that apply in each practice situation. Care has
been taken to confirm the accuracy of information presented and to describe generally
accepted practices. However, the author, editors, and publisher cannot accept any responsibility for errors or omissions or for any consequences from application of the information in
this book and make no warranty express or implied, with respect to the contents of this
book.

The author and publisher have exerted every effort to ensure that drug selection and
dosage set forth in this text are in accordance with current recommendations and practice at
the time of publication. However, in view of ongoing research, changes in government regulations and the constant flow of information relating to drug therapy and drug reactions,
the reader is urged to check the package insert for each drug for any change in indications
and dosage and for added warnings and precautions. This is particularly important when
the recommended agent is a new or infrequently employed drug.

Materials appearing in this book prepared by individuals as part of their official duties as
U.S. Government employees are not covered by the above-mentioned copyright.

9 8 7 6 5 4 3 2

*This book is dedicated
to my mother, Leah,
and
to the memory of my father,
Harry Kotlicky.*

Foreword

The 1990s are witness to great changes in the delivery of healthcare in the United States. Since colonial days, there has existed the concept of a medical practice; the physician opened an office, and patients arrived either by referral or by their own selection.

If the physician was diligent, worked well with patients, and satisfied their healthcare needs, an ongoing relationship was established. If the physician did not perform up to expectations, the patient could seek care elsewhere. Senior physicians proudly boasted of long-term practices; patients enjoyed being under the care of a certain doctor for many years.

The physician has traditionally been the patient advocate; primary responsibility was to provide appropriate care and to look out for the patient's best medical interest. In the healthcare universe (patient, physician, institution, and third party payor), the patient was the center. The conscientious physician would "go the extra mile," stay late in the office, return phone calls, or come into the hospital or emergency room setting at night. Normally, the quality of care and service delivered were far greater than was essential to satisfy the patient's basic medical concerns.

Patients engaged the services of a physician. Although they may have had insurance to assist with the payment of fees, they were responsible for the charges. The medical world appropriately "revolved" around the patient.

Now, the pendulum has shifted. The concept of a medical practice is becoming archaic; the patient is no longer the center of the healthcare universe. He or she is being superseded by the "Managed Care Entity" (MCE). The medical world revolves around this MCE, which has become the most important variable in the marketplace. The patient's role has been relegated to that of a "customer" (and an expensive one, too, because as the customer requires more services, the success of the MCE diminishes). The dissatisfied customer can move to another MCE during the next open enrollment period but otherwise for a given term must continue within the rules of his or her managed care organization.

Yielding to predetermined budgetary constraints, the MCE must provide the customer's total healthcare. It sets the standards, formulates treatment guidelines (mandates), and even determines what the needs will be by rationing available services and facilities to its perception of the greatest good.

The MCE must be responsive to the marketplace in order to remain competitive in the community. To accomplish this, it hires "providers" (previously called physicians) whose job security is predicated upon following the MCE's rules and keeping the customers satisfied. If the provider or the MCE becomes dissatisfied with the other, the mutual contract can be terminated. For the provider, such termination is often without recourse.

With these changes, the concept of a long-term doctor–patient relationship is no longer the most vital element. The key is now the survival of the entity. With the surplus of providers, the entity can even "bid out" its provider contracts or, in the staff model, can hire full-time salaried physicians. Unlike the traditional fee-for-service arrangements, in which patients are free to select physicians of their choice, cost containment will require them to choose a gatekeeper or primary care physician. That provider is often capitated, meaning that he or she will receive a set payment per month for each customer on his or her registry. The patient normally makes an additional nominal copayment (usually $5.00 to $15.00 depending on the MCE) at the time of the office visit. For further cost reduction, the primary care physician's role may be relegated to another professional (ie, nurse practitioner or physician's assistant) who effectively delivers the day to day outpatient care. Thus, the ultimate primary care giver may be a lesser credentialed individual than the physician.

In this scenario, much of the "hands on" benefit afforded by the traditional physician will be lost. Primary loyalty has been switched from the patient to the MCE. Similarly, patients no longer have a long-term commitment to a specific doctor–patient relationship. The employer may not renew the annual contract with the MCE, or provider physicians may be replaced. Because there is no guarantee of a long-term physician–patient relationship, the patient's and employer's concern is only which entity gives the most benefits for the premium dollar with the lowest copayment or deductible. From the provider's perspective, economics become a difficult constraint. With less reimbursement per patient, he or she must increase the patient load, translating into less time spent with a given patient, less time to return phone calls, and less enthusiasm to squeeze into an already overbooked schedule a patient who can probably be put off until the next day.

Into this new universe that has the MCE rather than the patient as the key player, thankfully emerges the nurse case manager (NCM). This individual has a difficult role to fill, needing to satisfy several demands.

First, he or she may be hired by the MCE (either as a full-time worker or an independent contractor) and is expected to demonstrate loyalty to the employer.

Secondly, the NCM has an ethical responsibility to ensure that high-quality care is appropriately rendered to the patient. This is an area in which the guidelines are a moving target. Current rules need continual modification. Traditionally, case management has been directed toward inpatient care. On admission, the NCM begins to monitor the course of treatment and simultaneously initiates the discharge planning process. To patients with chronic illness, outpatient management will open an entirely new dimension. For example, the diabetic will have more formal education to improve his or her understanding of the disease and to be more alert to the earliest signs of potential problems. While the primary care physician remains responsible for management of the patient's insulin and dietary needs, the NCM will assist with ancillary services, such as coordinating a diabetic education program and ensuring that appropriate patients have glucometers and keep outpatient appointments on schedule. Similarly, the emphysema patient will be assured of basic education needs and, when appropriate, the availability of such equipment as a peak meter, small volume nebulizer, or oxygen. For elective surgical procedures (ie, total hip replacement), the NCM will evaluate the patient preoperatively to determine and arrange posthospital healthcare needs (possibly including extended care facility, home health management, or the travel of family members from other cities to assist the patient in the home). The NCM will follow the patient after surgery (both in the hospital and on return to the home) to ensure proper availability of nursing needs, physical therapy, and any orthopedic appliances. For the "healthy patient," the NCM also can help to coordinate interval wellness programs, both as formal assessments (ie, mammography, childhood immunizations, interval measurement of cholesterol, HDL, LDL, and triglycerides) and as informal education (general "good health habits").

Thirdly, the NCM takes on the new role of patient advocate. While the NCM reports to three "bosses" (the patient, the provider, and the MCE), he or she must never lose sight of the responsibility as the patient's ombudsman. The NCM can help to lighten the red tape to facilitate problem solving, especially in the outpatient setting. Furthermore, the NCM can help to instill within the patient an understanding of his or her expectations of the MCE and also his or her own responsibilities for good health (ie, weight control, appropriate exercise schedule, keeping of appointments, home monitoring of diseases such as diabetes mellitus, asthma, or hypertension).

At times, the NCM may be caught in a seemingly ethical dilemma. With the physician's hands sometimes tied, he or she must be on a constant lookout for the patient's best health interests. In the setting of ongoing changes in healthcare delivery, Ms. Powell's textbook beautifully illustrates the important role of nurse case management. As a pioneer in the field, she draws on her extensive experience at St. Joseph's Hospital and Medical Center, a tertiary care hospital in Phoenix, Arizona.

Part I defines this relatively new field and looks to the qualifications and responsibilities of the NCM. Current goals and duties are discussed; however, in the era of ever-increasing medical technology, even the job description remains in flux. The NCM constantly calls on his or her knowledge of medicine, insurance, health plan rules and regulations, and available outpatient services through the hospital departments and in the community at large. He or she knows "whom to call" to expedite discharge planning and to help to move the patient from the acute care hospital into an appropriate and usually less expensive environment.

In Part II, Ms. Powell clarifies the tools of the trade. She includes the important list of definitions. In earlier years, patient care was often directed toward the concept of "newer is better" (albeit more expensive). The NCM must assess cost-effectiveness of alternative therapies. Some decisions are relatively straightforward (ie, provision of antibiotics for chronic suppression of recurrent urinary tract infections). Others are more complex (ie, assessment of home healthcare versus extended care facility for a patient; choices among varieties of durable medical equipment). Here, he or she is an important advisor to the treating physician, who may not be attuned to cost differentials among therapeutic options. The NCM will interact with multiple insurance plans and managed care organizations and must be familiar with the intricacies of each. Additionally, as managed care guidelines come into further acceptance, familiarity with them and their applications to specific patients is important. A goal of medicine is not just the prolongation of life but rather the extension of quality life. Recent examples of Jacqueline Kennedy Onasis leaving the hospital with pneumonia in order to "die with dignity at home" from her progressive lymphoma and of Richard Nixon's advanced directive (use no heroic measures in the face of a fulminant cerebral edema from a massive cerebrovascular accident) make both the public and the medical profession more aware of ethical dilemmas. The NCM, as the patient's ombudsman, helps to interact with the physician, the patient, and the family in making the most appropriate decisions. The other side of the legal issue is equally important. The elderly patient who is not terminal must not be denied care by the family members whose only interest is the selfish preservation of a potential inheritance.

Part III outlines the case management process. The field is a moving target. Not only must the NCM continually monitor patient progress (always mindful of the quality of medical care, the cost-effectiveness of treatment alternatives, and ethical and legal responsibilities), but she or he must also continually update his or her very job description.

Part IV brings many of the theories presented to actual practice. Much is required of the NCM, and Ms. Powell candidly discusses job stress and opportunities for success in the work. For example, the chapter entitled "A Day in the Life of a Nurse Case Manager" chronicles the simultaneous demands on her time during an often breakneck pace. The reader is left with much better appreciation of the importance of her every interaction with the patients. In order to deliver cost-effective healthcare, hospital discharge must not be delayed by such potential roadblocks as home care agency approval by the insurance company, finding a physician to assume care at an extended care facility, delivery of oxygen or durable medical equipment to the home, or even arrangement of a wheelchair or stretcher van to transport the patient home.

The final chapter presents more than twelve clinical vignettes in order to demonstrate how effective nurse case management can make a very positive difference for both the patient and the physician. No "correct answer" is given, because the task of the clinician is often to choose the best of several alternatives. Rather, the reader is afforded the opportunity to play the game of "NCM by proxy" to determine the most appropriate course of action. She concludes the text with a bibliography of references to further direct the interested reader in specific topics.

With ongoing advances of medical technology, changes in the role of the physician, increasing concern of appropriate expenditures of the ever-shrinking healthcare dollar, and a philosophic move in medical emphasis (from the treatment of acute illness to the prevention of diseases by maintaining good health practices), the evolving field of nursing case management is an important "new player" in the healthcare field. I have enjoyed the privilege of working with Ms. Powell for many years; this text is a wonderful testimony to her experience and talents. It will be well received and frequently referenced by nursing case managers everywhere.

William C. Weese, M.D.
Medical Director, St. Joe's —Preferred Choice Health Plan
St. Joseph's Hospital and Medical Center
Mercy Healthcare Arizona
Phoenix, AZ

Preface

The late Dr. John Miller was an old-fashioned physician in the truest sense. With a medical practice typical of those of the sixties and seventies, he was devoted to his patients and always looked out for their best interests. He was accustomed to making patient decisions and dispensing curatives in a single-handed fashion. Conversely, he was not used to being second-guessed or "policed" by insurance companies.

When the face of healthcare began to change in the eighties, it was difficult for Dr. Miller to come aboard. When "managed care" with its ominous implied restrictions no longer loomed as a threat but became reality, he fought back. In classic Gandhi-like tradition, Dr. Miller carried out his own brand of "civil disobedience," leaving his patients in the hospital longer than what was becoming acceptable by utilization standards. He also penned his disapproval of the "new ways" to several large newspapers and got himself bounced out of favor with a few managed care insurance plans. As a self-professed "medical dinosaur," he did a lot of charity work, made frequent house calls, and taught me a lot about patient advocacy.

Dr. Miller's dilemma is one example of the many different struggles taking place as the beleaguered healthcare system teeters to find its footing. While politicians, doctors, insurance companies, pharmaceutical companies, lawyers, and consumers are pointing fingers of blame at each other, insurance premiums are going up and reimbursements are coming down. Consumers toil to afford their premiums (or agonize over no insurance), healthcare facilities get sicker patients and less money, and physicians grapple with medical practices inundated with new mandates. And still costs continue to rise. The price tag for healthcare in 1993 was a staggering $903 billion—$233 billion *more* than in 1990. It is clear that something had to be done to stem this raging economic tidal wave.

While the debate over "how" rings loud and reaches far, a quiet light has switched on as one avenue to assist. Case management has emerged as a pivot point within the healthcare milieu, a point from which the many facets of medical care can be embraced and directed. The case management function fits well in the role of the nursing professional. In grassroots fashion and on a case-by-case basis, nurse case managers are managing out-of-control resource utilization while helping to ensure quality of care and patient satisfaction.

Case management is becoming an important area of nursing, both for its contribution to humanity and because nurse case managers play a key role in impacting on the healthcare crisis. Yet, a recent article on the subject revealed disillusionment among nurse case managers themselves. They felt ill-prepared for their roles, reporting personal frustration and burnout.

Because case management is relatively new and has not traditionaly been incorporated into nursing school curricula, new nurse case managers often must "fly by the seat of their pants." When situations go awry—sometimes due to poor understanding of basic managed care principles—case managers must dodge verbal bullets from patients, families, physicians, and hospital administrators.

Due to the fluid and changing nature of managed care and, therefore, case management, this book is not intended to be "the last word" but rather a teaching tool and useful reference on pertinent issues. The reader is encouraged to stay current in this field. Even though case management is evolving in the nineties, every attempt has been made to include all applications of this process.

Nurse case management is an exciting challenge for nurses, and NCMs are in a unique position to be recognized for their contribution to managed healthcare. It is my hope that this book, coupled with a solid on-the-job training program, will help develop NCMs who have peak job satisfaction and who will be recognized as shining lights, pulling the fragmented pieces of healthcare together.

Note: All names and nonessential details have been changed for confidentiality. Any resemblence to a real person is coincidential.

Throughout this text, the word "family" refers to any significant person in the client's life. This person may or may not be legally related to the client.

Acknowledgments

With loving thanks to my husband, James, who not only was an inspiration and support but tolerated neglect—and piles of the book all over the house—without a complaint. The best is yet to come.

To Mom and Dad #2 for their constant encouragement and joy in this project.

In special appreciation to Diane Cummings for her guidance, support, and dedication in getting the manuscript onto disk in proper APA format, and for her nonstop enthusiasm for this book.

A special thanks to Patty Wekell for all the expert help and support—and for squeezing this project into her already power-packed schedule.

With gratitude to Dr. William Weese for the helpful suggestions and kind contributions to this book.

To Jennifer Brogan and Lippincott–Raven for making this dream a reality.

To the University of Phoenix and Richard Eisenach. This book is the fulfillment of the essay.

To the wonderful nurses, nurse case managers, social workers, physicians, and staff at St. Joseph's Hospital in Phoenix. Our stories are written here.

To my wonderful friends who have encouraged me to have some fun (through kidnapping when necessary) throughout the duration of this endeavor.

To the patients; may your quality of life be optimized because of nursing case management.

To future nurse case managers.

Contents

NURSING
Case Management

A Practical Guide to
Success in Managed Care

PART I

Introduction to Case Management

"Foolish is the doctor who despises the knowledge acquired by the Ancients."

HIPPOCRATES
c. 460-c. 377 B.C.

PART I
IMPORTANT TERMS AND CONCEPTS

Broker Model

case management across the
continuum

case management/nursing care
management

catastrophic case management

episodic case management

large case management

managed care

Managed Care Model

Service Management Model

CHAPTER 1

What Is a Case Manager?

"What is case management?" "What is a case manager?" I am asked these questions weekly by staff nurses, attending physicians, residents, interns, patients, families, and nursing students, who are especially eager to learn about their future options. Often, what is being asked is, "What does a case manager do?"

The terms case management, nursing case management, and managed care are often used interchangeably, even though they are not exactly synonymous. Add to these terms all the other expressions for this endeavor, such as care management, care coordinator, case coordination, service coordination, and continuity coordination, and much confusion results.

There is not a single, uniform definition for case management or managed care. However, this chapter will attempt to clarify what managed care is all about and then to explore the working definitions of case management. In general:

- *Managed care* is *systems*-oriented.
- *Case management* is *people*-oriented—and negotiates the managed care systems in a way that, ideally, benefits everyone.

Managed Care

Managed care was the natural response to a healthcare system of waste and expanding, expensive technology. In the 1950s and 1960s healthcare was paid for on a fee-for-service basis; essentially, this meant that a bill was rendered and paid for without limitation of any kind. In the 70s and 80s, Medicare reimbursement changed to the DRG/Prospective Payment System, which set a standard: each diagnosis carried with it a set prearranged reimbursement, whether a patient stayed in the hospital 2 days and cost $1000 or stayed 2 weeks and cost the hospital $15,000. This system changed the face of healthcare forever. With new limitations being placed on reimbursement for care, everyone started scrambling to improve the management of that care. Now in the 90s, the ripple effects are still being felt.

Managed care systems sprang up in insurance companies and hospitals, and in virtually all agencies affected by healthcare dollars. HMOs, PPOs, and traditional health plans managed care through various forms of restrictions such as prior authorization, use of networks, preadmission authorization, utilization manage-

Powell: Nursing Case Management. © 1996 Lippincott–Raven Publishers

ment, capitation, DRG reimbursement, per diem payments and gatekeepers (see Chapter 5: Insurance, for a discussion on these issues).

Managed care is a mutating and dynamic force—economically driven—that is constantly trying out new delivery systems. The goal of managed care is to encourage consumers, providers, and payors to all become accountable for the wise use of the limited healthcare resources. The definitions of managed care—perhaps because they are changing at such a velocity—often focus on strategies used in managed care and the restrictions placed on healthcare dollars. This is exemplified in two definitions:

1. "Managed healthcare—A regrettably nebulous term. At the very least, is a system of healthcare delivery that tries to manage the cost of healthcare, the quality of that healthcare, and access to that care. Common denominators include a panel of contracted providers that is less than the entire universe of available providers; some type of limitations on benefits to subscribers who use non-contracted providers (unless authorized to do so); and some type of authorization system. Managed healthcare is actually a spectrum of systems, ranging from so-called managed indemnity, through PPOs, POS, open panel HMOs and closed panel HMOs" (Kongsvedt, 1993, p. 505).

2. "Managed care is defined as a set of techniques used by or on behalf of purchasers of healthcare benefits to manage healthcare costs by influencing patient care decision-making through case-by-case assessments of the appropriateness of care prior to its provision. The implementation of managed care strategies follows a series of other cost control measures including insurance benefit limitations and exclusions, prepaid health plans, prospective payment systems, and fee schedules" (Williams & Torrens, 1993, p. 226).

Managed care conjures up different images to different people. Some see it as an over-bureaucratization, which will lead to rationing of services, limitations on access to care, poor quality of care, and loss of choice and autonomy. Others see managed care as a necessary evil that will allow healthcare coverage to a larger segment of the American population.

The simple days when the physician decided on patient care, ordered it, billed for it, and was paid are over. The new reality of requirements, restraints, restrictions, and rationales have catapulted the healthcare environment into ever-increasing complexity. Issues never before even thought of now must be addressed:

- What will Patient A's insurance company allow?
- What will Patient B's pharmacy benefit cover and which pharmacy must they use?
- What patient is reimbursed under a DRG versus a risk contract or a per diem rate?
- What extended care facility or home health agency can you use?
- What physician is contracted with the plan?
- Is the Medicare coverage of the traditional type or a risk contract type?

- How can the nurse case manager provide a safe discharge plan if the insurance company wants the patient discharged quickly and while the patient is still ill?

Case Management

Nursing was quick to recognize the constraints healthcare was under, and nurses viewed the dilemma as an opportunity to expand their practice and patient advocacy roles. They indeed became the response to managed care. The nature of managed care dictates that healthcare services be limited; it is economics driven. Nursing case management balances this concept by ensuring caring and quality. For this reason, nurses are proving themselves to be the most effective equalizers to managed care.

Definitions of case management found in literature often confuse rather than clarify the issue for several reasons:

- There are a plethora of models of case management. Each model looks at case management from its own perspective and therefore defines its own type of case management rather than supplying a definition that applies universally. Often this definition describes what works for a particular facility or setting.
- The definition often merely restates the nursing case management *process*—what a case manager *does*—rather than contributing a definition.
- Many simply confuse case management with managed care.
- Some definitions make it difficult to differentiate between individual nursing case management *functions*. Like managed care, the nursing case management role is evolving and dynamic. Once a purer role, the nurse case manager is now often a hybrid of the utilization reviewer–quality improvement specialist–nurse case manager.

Future changes in nursing case management may change the definition further. The following is a sampling of some important definitions:

1. "Case management is the process of getting the right service to the right client" (Yee, 1990, p. 31).
2. ". . . a healthcare delivery process whose goals are to provide quality healthcare, decrease fragmentation, enhance the client's quality of life, and contain costs" (ANA, 1991, p. 6).
3. "Case management is a collaborative process which assesses, plans, implements, coordinates, monitors, and evaluates options and services to meet an individual's health needs through communications and available resources to promote quality, cost-effective outcomes" (Anonymous, 1994, p. 60). [This definition was written by the Certification of Insurance Rehabilitation Specialists Commission (CIRSC) Board, the credentialing board which administers the certification exam for Certified Case Managers (CCM). The Case Management Society of America (CMSA) Board of Directors approved this definition (Anonymous, 1994).]

4. "The purpose of care coordination is to work directly with clients and families over time to assist them in arranging and managing the complex set of resources that the client requires to maintain health and independent functioning. Care coordination seeks to achieve the maximum cost-effective use of scarce resources by helping clients get the health, social, and support services most appropriate for their needs at a given time. It guides the client and family through the maze of services, matches service need with funding authorization and coordinates with clinician and provider organizations" (Williams & Torrens, 1993, p. 202).

5. "Case Management—A method of managing the provision of healthcare to members with catastrophic or high-cost medical conditions. The goal is to coordinate the care so as to both improve continuity and quality of care as well as lower costs" (Kongsvedt, 1993, p. 501).

6. "Case management is a coordination of a specific group of services on behalf of a specific group of people. Case management can also be defined by listing its component processes. By widespread agreement, these processes include screening or case finding; comprehensive multidimensional assessment; care planning; implementation of the plan; monitoring; and reassessment . . ." (Kane, 1988, p. 161).

7. "Case management is a process that is concerned with more than simply monitoring or limiting the volume of services. While cost containment is clearly one objective of a case management program, its prime focus is the organization and sequence of services and resources to respond to an individual's healthcare problems" (Merrill, 1985, p. 5).

8. "Case management is a care delivery system that focuses on the improvement of patient goals within a specifically defined time frame, integrating the efforts of all healthcare team members. Case management addresses the entire episode of illness through the use of case management plans or critical pathways. These plans, or critical pathways, define the anticipated length of stay, delineate desired patient outcomes and goals, and provide directions for care for specific patient care types. Case management facilitates primary nursing, which is the general means of patient care delivery, by proactively planning for the patient care, increasing the nurses' time at the bedside, and facilitating communication between members of the collaborative healthcare team" (Latini & Foote, 1992, pp. 51–52).

By combining aspects of these eight definitions the reader can focus on a bigger picture of what case management is all about. Nurse case managers are the pivotal, prime movers of the managed care environment. Their presence adds humanity to an otherwise overwhelming system. More important than the definition of case management or what nurse case managers accomplish is the heart of their role: the holistic and humane care of both the patient and their family.

Who Should Be Case Managers?

Every discipline today seems to have case managers. Depending on the agency, the educational preparation varies from a high school diploma (GED acceptable) to master's level and beyond. In today's healthcare market, the main contenders for the role of case manager are nurses and social workers. Traditionally, social workers held the position of discharge planners in most hospitals until the mid-to-late 1980s. With the advent of prospective payments and managed care (ie, with the goal of getting the patient through the cost-intensive acute care setting as efficiently as possible), the trend is the use of nurses as case managers. But the "nurse versus social worker as case manager" debate still remains a touchy subject. Turf wars have ensued over it, articles have been written about it, and jobs have been lost over it.

So who is more appropriate for the role of case manager? Critical to answering this question is assessing the type of population needing case management. This will help to determine the professional background that will most suitably meet the client's needs. For example, foster children as the target population reflect a predominantly social model, thus needing the expertise of a social worker. Respiratory therapists have been hired as case managers for the pulmonary population, such as for those with cystic fibrosis, chronic obstructive lung disease, or asthma. The cognitively fragile population may also benefit from the use of social workers or from psychiatrically experienced RNs. Rehabilitation facilities may use RNs, social workers, or physical therapists, individually or as teams. Gerontology practitioners may be best suited for the fragile elderly.

Acute hospital care, at first glance, appears to be a purely medical model, so the obvious choice would appear to be professional nurses. Consider some of the responsibilities of a hospital case manager:

- Astute assessment of skills are necessary, recognizing ominous changes in medical status, whereby timely interventions can divert an impending medical crisis; often these changes in the patient status may also necessitate a change in the service plan.
- Direct bedside care may be performed.
- Thorough systems assessment, documentation, and placement into utilization management language are needed for insurance authorization.
- Often descriptions of wounds and surgical interventions must be reported to the insurance company for negotiating hospital authorization.
- Coordination of equipment and other resources for home use will often necessitate a medical perspective. For example, tracheostomies may require a range of supportive equipment from suction catheters and suction machines to home oxygen or aerosol masks.
- Knowledge of medications and of the safe and appropriate time to change from intravenous route to an oral route is important.
- The knowledge of the meaning of various lab and test results must be understood when looking at the total medical picture.
- Teaching may include any aspect of medical care, from teaching the patient the side effects and correct administration of specific medications to how to suction a tracheostomy or to pack and redress a wound in a sterile manner.

For these types of responsibilities, nurses, as specialists in holistic bioassessment and functional health planning, are ideally suited as case managers.

In reality, the acute care setting is often *not* a purely medical model. Trauma units routinely overflow with everything from motor vehicle accidents to gunshot wounds and remnants of gang violence. Intensive care units experience patients who have attempted suicide or drug overdoses. Medical floors treat cellulitis and abscesses from intravenous drug abuse. Obstetric floors routinely witness "babies having babies"—14-year-olds who are already multigravida moms. And all units treat catastrophic conditions and diseases that can bring the strongest families to their knees; all units need social workers, as well—for social assessments and social discharge planning.

A person's professional training elicits its own unique perspective; a nurse case manager and a social worker each have a different point of view about what a patient's needs might be upon discharge. Both contribute important data for a client's successful rehabilitation, illustrating that perhaps the *best* solution is a nurse case manager–social worker team approach. This is ideal in many settings, not only in acute care, but in subacute levels such as hospice or spinal cord rehabilitation.

What Makes the Nurse Case Manager–Social Worker Team Work?

Superimposing nurse case managers on already existing social worker–discharge planners can create turf wars, until both realize their importance and necessity. The nurse case manager–social worker teams may, initially, appear to have some overlapping roles as well as their more obvious distinctly separate responsibilities. However, these overlapping gray areas do not necessarily mean duplication. Good communication within the team and mutual trust regarding follow-through can eliminate the risk of wasted effort from repetition. Some nurse case manager–social worker teams have had difficult times because of attitudes about roles "carved in stone" or an individual need to "do it all." These attitudes make one of the basic tenets of teamwork—pitching in for one another—very difficult.

Perhaps the element that best makes the teams work is the elusive factor known as chemistry. And when all the components of a good nurse case manager–social worker team are met, the client wins, the facility wins, job satisfaction peaks, and managed care becomes quality, cost-efficient care.

NOTE

Those interested in applying for case management certification can write to:

Certification for Case Manager
Certification of Insurance Rehabilitation Specialists Commission
1835 Rohlwing Road–Suite D
Rolling Meadows, IL 60008
(708) 818-0292

References

American Nurses Association. (1991). *CHN Communique* (Council of Community Health Nursing). Washington, D.C.: Author.

Anonymous. (1994). DMSA Standards of Practice. *The Case Manager, 5*(1), 59–71.

Kane, R. A. (1988). Case management: Ethical pitfalls on the road to high quality managed care. *Quality Review Bulletin*, pp. 161–166.

Kongstvedt, P. R. (1993). *The Managed Health Care Handbook.* Gaithersburg: Aspen Publishers.

Latini, E. E., & Foote, W. (1992). Obtaining consistent quality patient care for the trauma patient by using a critical pathway. *Critical Care Nursing Quarterly, 15*(3), 51–55.

Merrill, J. (1985). Defining case management. *Business and Health,* July/August, pp. 5–9.

Williams, S. J., & Torrens, P. R. (1993). *Introduction to Health Services.* New York: Delmar.

Yee, D. L. (1990, July). Developing a quality assurance program in case management service settings. *Caring Magazine,* pp. 30–35.

CHAPTER 2

Goals of Case Management

Optimal Versus Inadequate Outcomes

The target goals of managed care and nursing case management are quality care and cost efficiency. Many smaller goals contribute to those ultimate aims and, when achieved, culminate in "good case management." When these goals are not met, the consequences are poor quality of care or poor utilization of healthcare resources.

Unmet managed care–nursing case management goals may occur for many reasons. The following are examples:

- No formal nursing case management in the facility or agency
- Poorly trained nurse case managers
- Inadequate social service staffing to support the psychosocial aspect of the case
- Case loads that are too heavy for all details to be adequately attended to
- Patient–family resistance
- Patients who are incorrigibly noncompliant
- Unrelenting patient–family dissatisfaction
- Lack of cooperation from the payor source
- Lack of payor source
- Lack of understanding among staff regarding nursing case management–managed care principles
- Substandard care in the facility/agency

The following tables display outcomes of the case management process. On the left are optimal outcomes, characteristics resulting from proper case management. The right side exhibits consequences that occur when those objectives are lacking or inadequately met.

As the issues and game rules of the healthcare environment change during the 1990s, the goals must also transform to match new priorities. It is certain, however, that quality and efficiency will never go out of style.

Quality of Care Issues

Outcomes From Optimal Case Management	Outcomes From Inadequate Case Management
• Increased patient/family satisfaction	• Patient/family dissatisfied with care; possible increase in lawsuits
• Ensures optimal clinical outcomes through monitoring and adherence to quality standards of care	• Increased quality of care issues; possible risk management scenarios, complaints, and grievances
• Comprehensive and accurate assessment of clients' deficits, health status, resources, formal and informal support systems, and outcomes	• Increased complications/ineffective care
• Matching assessed needs to valuable services	• Duplication or gaps in services and client's needs unmet
• Continuity of care emphasized, thus reducing or eliminating fragmentation, duplication or gaps in treatment plan and/or services	• Fragmented, inefficient care
• Careful monitoring of safety issues	• Misses risk factors that lead to risk management issues (eg, falls)
• Reduced adverse patient outcomes	• Increased adverse outcomes
• Proactive: prevents adverse occurrences when possible and intervenes quickly if prevention is not possible, thereby minimizing poor outcomes	• Adverse occurrences maximized before anyone recognizes them
• Maximum recovery; minimum complications	•Minimal recovery; maximum complications

Collaboration

Outcomes From Optimal Case Management	Outcomes From Inadequate Case Management
• Physician satisfaction with the case management process and the quality of patient care	• Alienation and frustration of physicians
• Effective collaboration and coordination strengthened among all members of the healthcare team	• Treatment delays; fragmented care; frustrates and obstructs efforts to improve health status of the patient
• Communication enhanced among the multidisciplinary team	• Each discipline singing in different key, resulting in discordant care for the patient; miscommunications and misunderstandings among the team alienates team members

Fiscal Responsibilities

Outcomes From Optimal Case Management	Outcomes From Inadequate Case Management
• Provider–payor satisfaction	• Uncooperative providers
• Balancing fiscal responsibility for the client, the facility/agency, and the reimbursement source	• Conflict of interests; mixed or inequitable loyalties; poor or unethical allocation of resources
• Appropriate and efficient use of benefits and resources	• Suboptimal use of healthcare resources; unnecessary waste; over- or underutilization
• Cost-efficient care through timely use of appropriate level of care for the client's needs	• Expensive and inappropriate level of care; may not be reimbursed by payor source; may leave facility or client fiscally responsible for excess payment
• Appropriately reduced length of hospital stays	• Increased length of hospital stays
• Reduced number of intensive care days	• Increased number of ICU days
• Reduced visits to emergency department	• Increased number of emergency department or clinic visits
• Prevents unnecessary admissions; reduces acuity upon admission; reduces number of admissions	• Preventable admissions; higher acuity upon admission; frequent readmissions
• Careful identification and matching of clients' needs with resources available (both public and private resources)	• Suboptimal use of healthcare system and public or private resources
• Maximizing reimbursed services at all levels of care by meeting established criteria, performing precise utilization reviews, accurate and thorough documentation, and timely discharges	• Agencies/facilities at increased financial risk because of lost revenue for the facility from uncompensated patient care; increased charges to clients; clients unable to pay or leaving them financially destitute
• Successful negotiation of cases for appropriate continuation of length of stays or extension of services	• Same as above
• Accurate interpretation of benefits for the client and the facility	• Same as above

Patient Advocacy

Outcomes From Optimal Case Management	Outcomes From Inadequate Case Management
• Personal attention in a large, complex, and impersonal healthcare system	• The client is alone and afraid
• Nurse case manager to advocate for client/family	• No one to advocate for client/family
• Optimizes patient's quality of life, autonomy and, if possible, independence through thoughtful, appropriate placement at discharge	• Warehouses patients in inappropriate environments; poor quality of life
• Fosters educated, independent choices in all aspects of care and services	• Uninformed decisions
• Education on disease processes, allotted services, rehabilitation techniques, self-care; education matched to individual needs	• Poor education resulting in noncompliance of treatment plan, "out-of-control" feelings, decreased self-care capabilities, and inability to avoid or allay the disease process
• Patient and family empowerment through participation in decision-making	• Paternalism; decreased freedom of choice; decreased autonomy of client
• Promotes optimal function of family unit	• Frightened, exhausted, stressed-out families
• Optimizing self-care capabilities by assisting patient to become fully functional as quickly as possible; if return to independence not possible, assists family unit and client in obtaining supportive care	• Minimal time for patient to become independent and optimally healthy; family may become exhausted or dysfunctional and utilize excessive healthcare services
• Patient/family understand the direction of the plan of care and knowledge of the disease process through education, clinical pathways, and so on	• Confusion, anxiety, and out-of-control feelings of patient and family
• Monitors and advocates for a clinically appropriate treatment plan	• Duplication of services; gaps in treatment plan; wasteful services, inappropriate levels of care; excess costs being billed to client
• Assist client/family in accessing the complex healthcare system, thus utilizing available and necessary resources	• Underutilization of resources, leaving some needs unmet; services ordered that are not covered by the health plan, thus creating wasted effort and possibly extensions of hospital stays because of delays in accessing needed services for a safe discharge
• Finds solutions to noncovered services	• Families' funds exhausted through noncoverage of services necessitating private pay

Outpatient Management

Outcomes From Optimal Case Management	Outcomes From Inadequate Case Management
• Thorough identification of discharge needs including medical, educational, durable medical equipment, and social support	• Frustrated and exhausted families who are suboptimally caring for patient
• Facilitates timely, coordinated, safe, and appropriate discharges	• Unsafe, incomplete dispositions
• Links the client with appropriate level of care and services: acute, subacute, supervisory, homebound, or community-based services	• Service gaps; higher readmission rate
• Comprehensive and consistent posthospital or post–extended care facility followup	• Complications during convalescent phase with setbacks and possibly readmissions to acute hospital care
• Optimal outpatient management that reduces or avoids acute hospital readmissions through early identification of health status changes or changes in self-care capabilities	• Poor outpatient management leading to increased complications and increased utilization of acute facilities
• Chosen level of care for client matches client's need and financial capability	• Client/family's financial resources are exhausted through nonreimbursed placement of client into expensive care facility

Professional Nursing Practice

Outcomes From Optimal Case Management	Outcomes From Inadequate Case Management
• Promotes nursing professionalism by creatively and proactively finding solutions to the problems facing the healthcare system in the 90s	• Results in nursing being in a subordinate and supportive role, rather than a collaborative partnership
• Acknowledges research opportunities about efficient, effective care for the chronically and acutely ill	• Diminished credibility due to lack of serious research
• Promotes job satisfaction	• Promotes job stress and burnout

CHAPTER 3

Essential Characteristics and Job Responsibilities

Not long ago, the task of case managing belonged to the family physician. Choices were simple; insurance companies usually paid for the services that the doctors deemed necessary. Enter the age of convoluted insurance plans (or no insurance plan): multiple specialists for a single client; multidisciplinary teams that include dozens of members; the rush to get clients through the system and into less cost-intensive settings; increasing chronicity of health problems; ethical dilemmas; increased patient and family expectations—the list goes on.

Much of the management of clients has been transferred to the nursing arena. But staff nurses, already overloaded with daily nursing tasks, barely have time to read a patient's chart, let alone try to fill in the gaps between the patient's needs and his or her reality, assess the availability of resources and support systems, and figure out insurance benefits.

As Figure 3–1 shows, the nursing case management role is a pivotal one. This chapter discusses essential *characteristics* that affect how well the nurse case manager (NCM) performs the role. The *job responsibilities* section explores what a NCM does. Although the list is extensive, it should be noted that the role of the NCM is evolving and, therefore, the list may still be incomplete. Because nursing case management responsibilities are extensive, on some days case managers may feel that they are "dancing as fast as they can!"

Nursing case management roles vary according to the population being served and the case management perspective. The job priorities of each case management position must also be weighed; a hospital case manager may have a perspective different from one who is employed by an insurance company; a NCM for a private insurance company may encounter different issues than one who works for Medicaid or Long Term Care; an entrepreneurial NCM may have a different point of view and priority set from one who works for a privately owned or state-run company; a case manager who is responsible for clients across a continuum of health-care settings may have a different perspective from one who is responsible for episodic (ie, one episode of illness) case management. Roles and responsibilities also differ because of the case mix of clients whom the NCM works with; geriatric

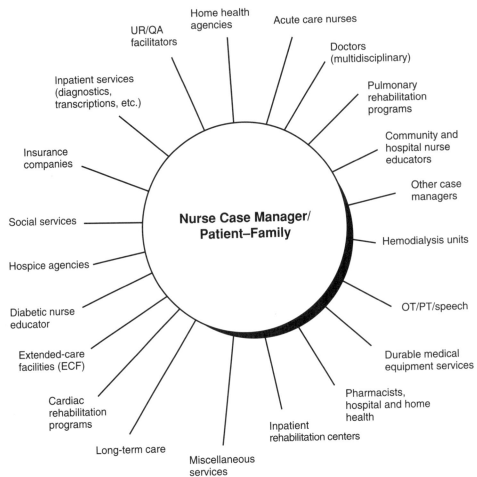

Figure 3-1. Case management wheel.

clients have different needs than high risk obstetric, or people with AIDS, or cancer patients, or cystic fibrosis—virtually each clinical category has its own needs.

At times, the NCM may find the various roles conflicting. As a patient advocate, the case manager wants the best of everything for the client; as the procurer of healthcare resources, the NCM may not be able to obtain all that the client wants or needs. Perhaps it is "not a covered service," or the client has already used up that particular benefit, or the insurance company does not feel the patient is entirely "homebound" and denies home nursing services (see Chapter 8, Ethical Issues and Dilemmas). Fortunately, there are other characteristics that can come to the rescue. A knowledge of alternative and community resources—and the nurse's own creativity—can often ease the dilemma.

Essential Characteristics

The following characteristics are important strengths to develop and will greatly aid all nursing case management daily activities. Not everyone is organized or is a "detail person" or a top-notch negotiator, and not every nursing case manager needs all these characteristics. Many excellent case managers are weak in some areas and compensate very adequately with other talents. But if any shortcoming is causing problems, the nurse should look for ways to grow; all the characteristics can be enhanced if desired.

Commitment and Desire to Be a Nurse Case Manager. Each professional will have his or her own personal reasons for wanting to become a NCM. Perhaps it is to help level some inequities observed as managed care regulations become tighter; or, perhaps it is the unique nature of the NCM–client relationship that is appealing. A clear view of your commitment may get you through challenging cases and stressful days.

Ability to Prioritize. This is simply doing the most important task first. In general, good nurses excel at prioritizing. Each hour and each day has its own priorities. Meetings have been missed because of a "Code Blue," and interfacility transfers have been delayed in order to meet the safety needs of a suicidal patient. Distinguishing between urgency and importance is vital. Urgent tasks must be attended to immediately—no matter what. Important tasks come next. The ability to decide what is important and what is more or less routine is often a matter of common sense. Having a "feel" for the pacing and sequencing of a case is important; sometimes nurse's intuition plays a role and pushes a case "up the list," which averts an urgent scenario later on. For example, getting a code status or calling a family meeting may ward off a crisis situation. Often delegation of tasks helps to get several tough jobs done.

Clinical Expertise and Critical Thinking. Keeping up to date on new treatments and technologies in your area of case management is a necessary edge, and it is important to update clinical knowledge regularly through seminars and texts. It is impossible to completely case manage in a medical environment without clinical expertise. Many extra days have been authorized by insurance companies because important clinical data were provided by the NCM. Accurate assessment of discharge needs depends on knowledge of the disease process. Practice standards also change as safer and improved methods are discovered. A clinically sharp NCM offers an important advantage, and it is important to apply the most up-to-date knowledge and standards to your clients.

Understanding of Insurance Idiosyncrasies. I often describe one of my roles as a "game keeper." Each insurance company has its own rules, covered services, interpretation of Intensity of Service/Severity of Illness (see InterQual, Chapter 6), and type of reimbursement. To obtain the full hospital stay authorization, to maximize the chance of a successful discharge plan, and to minimize last-minute surprises, know the game rules for your client's insurance plan (see Chapter 5: Insurance, and Chapter 6: Utilization Management.)

Ability to Read Poor Penmanship (or Tracking Down the Perpetrator!). One day I was squinting myself nearly blind trying to read an important note on a client's chart, when Dr. "Finehand" walked in. He gave the chart a bemused look and threw up his hands; even he couldn't read his script. Fortunately, he remembered what he had written. If all else fails offer the doctor a typewriter!

Good Follow-Through. Gaining physician trust is not always easy, but perhaps the most important activity as an inroad to trust is follow-through once a plan has been agreed on. If something impedes the plan, a phone call to the physician to discuss the problem and to offer a potential solution or new course of action keeps the trust level high.

Respect and Trust by Peers. This does not come with the job title. It is earned!

Team Player. This is a multidisciplinary world; all players are important.

Self-Esteem and Confidence. Nursing case management isn't a job for the meek. Sometimes it involves risk taking. At times, being a patient advocate requires going toe-to-toe with everyone from physicians to insurance companies. Self-confidence often comes from a good knowledge base and a history of solid, successful case plans. Novice NCMs should be gentle with themselves and realize that it takes time to learn how to fit together all the pieces of the managed care jigsaw puzzle.

Ability to Work With People. Many employers list this ability among their top three priorities. In case management, it is essential. Each client may have several agencies on board and many individuals involved in their case plan. Not only must the case manager be able to work with all of these agency members, he or she must be able to coordinate them and the services they represent. This is not always easy when there are conflicting ideas about what is right and best for the client.

Diplomacy. This is a skill and an art. When several of the team players are singing in different keys, the NCM must possess the tact and finesse to bring the group through negotiation and help them to decide which "key" is best for the client.

Adaptability, Flexibility, and Creativity. NCMs must adapt to different units, facilities, doctors, client cultures, other case managers, changing medical conditions and changing transitional plans. Sometimes a case plan must "turn on a dime"; this requires flexibility and creativity, so that no hospital day or resource is wasted. Rigidity can lead to poor case management and stress or burnout.

Strong Interpersonal Communication Skills. The case manager, as the hub of the wheel (see Fig. 3–1), must channel information to all other parties. Almost every nursing case management task requires some form of communication. This can be verbal, nonverbal, or written. The four primary purposes of communication are (1) to inquire, (2) to inform, (3) to persuade, and (4) to entertain (Leddy & Pepper, 1989). Three of the four are essential in the nursing case management process. Inquiring can be done through written communication or verbally, either in person or by telephone. Written communications must be succinct and unambiguous; verbal communication often involves tact and diplomacy.

Informational communication is a large part of nursing case management transactions. Insurance companies must be informed and updated about their members' progress; thoroughness and creative persuasion are often important here. Physicians and other team members need frequent information about how the client is faring according to the other modalities (coordinating information). Clients need information about their disease process and treatments. An important case management communication skill is the ability not only to understand complex and technical information but to be able to translate this information into layman's terms, so that it is understandable to a client. This is not always easy, since other factors may block the exchange of information. The client may have suboptimal receptive and retention abilities because of several factors such as shock, illness, high anxiety level, fear, depression, developmental age, language or cultural barriers, and being already on "information overload," or because the client is harboring an "I don't care" attitude.

Perhaps the most important communication act is that of listening. A wise person once directed, "Listen twice as much as you speak. That is why you have two ears and one mouth." The ability to listen sends a message that the case manager places the needs of the client before his or her own needs.

Excellent Assessment Skills. With the multitudinous levels and facets of assessment needed, missed details at this critical juncture can delay or imbalance the whole case plan (see Chapter 13: Stage II: Assessment).

Attention to Detail. If you are not a detail person, bone up. Each case has so many variables—multiply these by the number of cases you have—and your total is perhaps thousands of details. Again, missed details can destabilize the whole case.

Organizational Skills. With all the details that must be attended to, organization skills are a must. Also, time is prime; time constraints are frequent and often everything must be accomplished precisely and quickly (see Chapter 18: Job Stress Versus Success Factors for Case Management).

Management Skills. As the title implies, nursing case management requires a wide array of management skills: delegation, conflict resolution, crisis intervention, collaboration, consultation, coordination, identification, and documentation.

Knowledge of Community Resources. To have a good, knowledgeable social worker aboard is probably the closest thing to nursing case management "heaven." The social problems of many clients are overwhelming, and many would benefit from their expertise. However, social service support is sometimes unavailable, and therefore knowledge of community resources is needed.

Resourcefulness. The NCM may be called on to provide everything from a translator for an obscure European dialect to a macrobiotic diet. Creativity is often the first step in solving unusual problems. Tenacity and persistence are the other keys.

Knowledge of Legal and Quality Issues and Standards of Practice. Quality outcomes are a main goal of case management. Astute case managers routinely avert potential disasters by recognizing potential problems and resolving them before they get too far out of line (see Chapter 7: Legal Issues for Case Managers, and Chapter 9: Quality Improvement and Risk Management).

Competency and Accountability. This translates into doing things well and taking responsibility for the outcomes. In her book, *From Novice to Expert*, Patricia Benner discusses competency using the Dreyfus Model of Skill Acquisition. This model theorizes that a student must pass through five levels of proficiency when acquiring and developing a skill. Stages I and II, Novice and Advanced Beginner, describe those who have little or no experiences from which to draw when performing their new responsibilities. This stage may describe a staff nurse who enters the role of nursing case management with little understanding of insurance principles, utilization review modalities, quality issues, or discharge planning.

The final three stages, *Competent, Proficient,* and *Expert,* describe a progression of advanced skills and perceptions. This holistic understanding goes beyond a merely analytical response of a situation to an intuitive grasp of the events taking place. According to Benner, an intuitive grasp is not wild guessing; it is a *direct* comprehension of a situation that is only available when a broad base of knowledge, experience, and a deep understanding have been encountered. Therefore, advanced competency is often more visible in its absence and thus may go unnoticed and unrewarded. Experienced nurses (NCMs) learn to organize, plan, and coordinate multiple patient needs and requests and to reshuffle their priorities in the midst of constant patient changes (Benner, p. 149).

Self-Directedness. Nursing case management is not a position for someone who needs constant direction. NCMs must make many independent decisions each day and must prioritize their caseload according to their own judgment. For those who love autonomous nursing, nursing case management is a real fit.

Caring Attitude and Behavior. Caring involves being concerned about another's welfare; it is the root of the role of patient advocacy and the heart of nursing. Caring between the nurse and patient requires reciprocal communication, trust, respect, and commitment (Hein & Nicholson, 1994). Almost every task a NCM performs is done out of involvement with and caring for the quality of patient care. Specific caring actions cited include being present in a reassuring manner; providing information; assisting with pain; spending time with the patient; promoting autonomy (1994); nurturing hope and faith; cultivating sensitivity in order to promote comfort, recovery, and wellness in others; extending altruistic behaviors such as empathy and kindness; acceptance of others; using creative problem-solving processes for the client's best outcome; provision of a supportive or protective environment; assistance with gratification of basic human needs; and allowance for each person to express him- or herself spiritually as he or she chooses (Wadas, 1993). Negotiations to achieve the optimal resources for a client and the scrutiny of the case for quality of care issues are expressions of caring.

Negotiation Skills. In the 90s environment of scarce resource availability and declining benefits, the art of negotiation is extremely important. Few people are natural-born negotiators, and it may require some practice. The effort is well worth it, because advocating for a client's needs frequently requires this skill. Understand that rarely will things just "happen" for your client unless you make them happen and that usually takes negotiation.

Before negotiation begins, it is wise to do some research; understand the other side before negotiation. For example, know what services are covered, know the approximate readmit rates if a client does not receive a particular service, be prepared to ask for a supervisor—by name, if possible—if you feel strongly about a particular service need. Negotiation starts by stating the problem(s) and the goal and stating what is needed to solve the problem. Explain the reasons why the services are imperative and the benefits of the service to all concerned (ie, less costly readmissions to the acute care setting). State the request in a positive and thorough way. Use active listening and acknowledge the other side's concerns; ask how some of the problems may be overcome. Be realistic; attempting to negotiate for a service that absolutely will not be covered wastes everyone's time and energy.

Common mistakes can create a defensive environment not conducive to negotiation. Some behaviors that may be problematic include poor listening skills, poor use of questions, improper disclosure of ideas, mismanagement of issues, inappropriate stress reactions, rejecting alternatives too quickly, misusing a negotiating team member, not disclosing true feelings, improper timing, and being aggressive rather than assertive (Hein & Nicholson, 1994). (See Assertiveness skills in the following text.)

If negotiations start sounding like something from a professional wrestling match, use the following techniques to overcome the deadlock. Try resummarizing ideas, discussing the remaining alternatives, asking hypothetical questions, evaluating the differing points of view, and analyzing past and future needs of all concerned (Hein & Nicholson, 1994). Always remember that the most important focus is the patient.

Assertiveness Skills. Assertiveness skills are an important part of the NCM's communication repertoire. Not infrequently, case managers are placed in tense situations; any NCM who has *never* been told off by a physician is either an expert at assertiveness or is topping the scale of wishy-washy passivity. Historically, nurses have always tried to please everyone. "We hate to offend anyone. We pride ourselves on being fair, flexible and open minded. Someone quipped that we try to be so open-minded our brains fall out" (Chenevert, 1988, p. 69). Flexibility is necessary in some situations, backbone is necessary in others. Passive behavior (ie, giving up your seat when a doctor enters the room) is no longer applauded or condoned.

Substituting self-doubt with self-assurance is the first step in assertiveness and takes patience and practice; after changing your *outlook*, you can change your *behavior* (Hein & Nicholson, 1994). First, an understanding of the differences between passive behavior, aggressive behavior, and assertive behavior is helpful. In passive behavior, you may violate your own rights by ignoring them and allowing others to infringe on you (Bradley & Edinberg, 1986); doing as you are told can lead to feelings of anxiety, helplessness, and depression. With aggressive behavior others may be violated, dominated, humiliated, or put down (1986); aggressive behavior may lead to feelings of guilt, bitterness, and loneliness. Assertive behavior is direct, honest, and lacking in excuses; you must be able to trust your feelings, to like yourself, to respect your own hunches and feelings, and to be willing to accept the consequences of your assertive behavior. Assertiveness is a tool, not a weapon (Chenevert, 1988).

Fundamental to assertiveness practice is the substitution of "I" messages for "you" messages (Hein & Nicholson, 1994). "You" messages often put the recipients on the defensive. Simple questions such as "Why did you...," "When do you plan to...," "What did you intend by..." immediately cause people to put on their armor. "I" messages such as "I feel...," "I understand that...," "I want...," "I expect...," "I choose...," "I plan...," or "I am..." provide a clear, honest, and direct expression of one's feelings, thoughts, opinions, and beliefs. Other verbal techniques include choosing words carefully, speaking clearly, using a full well-modulated voice, and projecting the message boldly, confidently, positively, frankly, and concisely (Chenevert, 1988). Nonverbal techniques include good posture, head held up, good eye contact, and hands quiet and relaxed (1988).

Assertiveness allows you to act instead of react in a given situation. It is the perfect tool to get not only your own needs met, but those of your clients; it is the perfect tool for the patient advocate to use. "Focus on the patient and you will be amazed at how the petty, peripheral things will float away, and your work will seem less complicated and cluttered" (Chenevert, 1988, p. 156).

Sense of Humor. Used with taste and in discriminating proportions, laughter and humor add an important dimension to your work and increase job satisfaction (see section on humor in Chapter 18: Job Stress versus Success Factors for Case Management).

Job Responsibilities

As stated earlier, the job responsibilities of each case manager may be different, depending on the employment focus (independent nurse case management versus hospital case management versus insurance company case management, and so on) and the case mix diagnosis you are working with. Not all of the roles and responsibilities that follow may apply to your clinical area of expertise and your type of case management; yet, many are essential in every form of case management.

Coordination of Plan of Care and Services. This is the umbrella role under which all other roles fall; it is "where the rubber meets the road" in case management. If done well, case management provides a seamless and smooth-running system in which everyone benefits. If done poorly, case management is a rough ride with team members colliding into one another. Collaboration and coordination of the many caretakers, of their perspectives, orders, and suggestions—and matching those with the patient and payor's permission—constitute not a small task. The "what" and "how" of the coordination of services make up an individual sequence that depends on the nature of each patient's illness, the psychosocial support, the insurance coverage, and many other factors.

Patient Advocate. Think for a moment about a time when you felt especially vulnerable, when few elements of your life were within your control. Perhaps you were told you had a large tumor, or the dreaded test came back positive, or a loved one was seriously ill. Times such as these leave people feeling overwhelmed. Those who can ask pertinent questions are already on their way to healing, but many are too overcome with the enormity of their situations to even articulate their needs.

The role of patient advocate is one of the most important of all the NCM's charges; it is also one of the greatest challenges. Historically, nurses have always acted as client advocates to some extent. "Advocacy for the client was given highest priority unless it conflicted with advocacy for the physician or advocacy for the employing institution" (Leddy & Pepper, 1989, p. 378). And in today's healthcare environment, advocacy for the payor source (which may also be the employer) further muddies the issue. It is the NCM's responsibility—an obligation, if you will—to remember that the most relevant unit is the *patient*, not the payor, not the utilization review modality, not the service offered or not offered, and not the institution.

How does a NCM act as a patient advocate? In a sense this whole book readies the NCM for that role; by understanding the principles of case management and managed care, the NCM can best position the client to maximize his or her chances for optimal services.

One tenet of advocacy is to assist clients to achieve autonomy and self-determination, to assist them to become empowered. This is done by helping clients to articulate their views and choices or those of an incapacitated family member. The NCM is obligated to act in the client's interest, but the client will determine what the definition of "best interest" will be, according to personal beliefs (Prins, 1992).

Autonomy in decision making and self-determination also requires informational support. The quality and relevancy of the information are important, and the quantity of data must be delicately balanced. Giving information that the patient did not seek, is not ready to hear, and is too much—causing information overload—violates the basic principles of patient advocacy. Giving too little information may be considered paternalistic and prevents self-determination and informed consent.

One of the biggest challenges the NCM often has to face is the ethical dilemma of the conflicting roles of patient advocate versus that of the gatekeeper (see Chapter 8: Ethical Issues and Dilemmas). It is difficult to balance the demands of these two strict taskmasters—one that necessitates optimal care and services for your client and the other that demands cost containment and stringent allocation of resources. Wise allocation of resources fulfills the requirement for the role of gatekeeper, but may violate the concepts of advocacy; on the other hand, if NCMs can successfully perform the role of patient advocate, they can often "become the levelers" for inequities in the system (Dubler, 1992, p. 85).

Advocacy at its most basic essence is caring for another human being. If we lived "in a perfect world with equal access to healthcare and patients who are powerful players in the healthcare system, advocacy would not be necessary..." (Hein & Nicholson, 1994, p. 166). But the reality is that inequities in our healthcare environment *do* exist, and most of the population does not have the knowledge or the savvy to access this convoluted system. Through the NCM's caring, attention, and support, perhaps one more client will be prevented from slipping through the cracks, will receive the help needed for one more try at independent living, or will have a last wish acknowledged and carried out. Supporting a client's own choices with available means and services is the gift of advocacy.

Protector of Privacy and Confidentiality. In today's age of telephonics, computers, and FAX machines, maintaining privacy and confidentiality is no easy task. It seems as if everyone has access to the medical record, including many types of medical caretakers, quality improvement specialists, insurance companies, auditors, billers, case managers, and others. "Indeed, much of modern medicine, with the computerized passing of data, is designed to preclude privacy, not to protect it. Healthcare providers regularly set aside the patient's needs for secrecy in pursuit of the kind of communication that permits all to strive together toward a shared goal of care" (Dubler, 1992, p. 84). See Chapter 7: Legal Issues for Case Managers, for recommendations on the preservation of privacy and confidentiality. But these are not sure measures. "The lawyer/client relationship is more protected, more fully confidential, than the physician/patient relationship. Unlike a hospital chart, records of the attorney/client dialogue cannot be subpoenaed. They are guarded and protected" (Dubler, 1992, p. 84). And new problems are arising because of computer charting; fail-safe ways must be provided to keep patients' medical records from computer sport hackers, employers, and others without a right to know or a need to know. Still, the NCM has an obligation—as a patient advocate—to protect the clients' privacy as much as possible. By doing so, the NCM is protecting that person's dignity and is practicing within the standard of nursing.

Direct Patient Care. NCMs may or may not be involved with hands-on care of the patient; some may provide direct patient care for a limited number of hours in the work week (see further discussion later in this chapter).

Conducting Multidisciplinary Patient Care Rounds. Various types of multidisciplinary rounds may take place; these include daily rounding with physician groups, weekly rounds discussing all cases on the NCM's caseload, and patient care conferences that focus on one particular client with extensive needs. The NCM is usually responsible for facilitation and coordination of the latter two types of rounds. A few tips for well-coordinated rounds are included in Display 3–1.

Case Screening. It would be overwhelming, unrealistic, and unnecessary to case manage all the patients in any facility or diagnostic group. It is often the NCM who identifies those patients who would most benefit from case management. A more thorough discussion on case screening can be found in Chapter 12: Stage I: Case Screening and Selection.

DISPLAY 3–1
Tips for Patient Care Rounds

1. Know the case histories of the patients being discussed in as much detail as possible. Be able to give a good overview of the patient's present status, and state the problems that need discussion clearly and completely.

2. Involve everyone on the patient's healthcare team. Each member knows the patient from a different perspective, and the sum total of all the perspectives allows a more complete picture. As the patient advocate, do not forget the patient's perspective.

3. Try not to allow interruptions during conferences with the healthcare team. If possible, hold calls and pagers until completion of rounds.

4. Anticipate problems that might arise with all of the solutions discussed and have a second possible course ready in case the first one falls through.

5. Bring each case to closure with a plan that everyone can work with, if possible. Be in the habit of making rounds an effective use of time.

6. Set time limits to help make rounds an efficient use of time.

Assessing and Reassessing. The needs of patients can change daily, even hourly. Constant reassessing of clients' physical status, psychosocial support, mentation, and spiritual needs is important. The case must also be monitored for financial resources. Attention to the patient's and family's goals will keep the case on track; be alert for changing goals, too. Good case managers keep a flexible attitude about each case, allowing creativity to flow when tough situations and sudden changes occur.

Informational Guide. There are times when patients and families do not know what they need, what is available to them, or even what they want, because the situation they have found themselves in is simply too overwhelming. Eliciting preferences and priorities from patients or their families is a great relief to them; it also steers the NCM in the right direction. In turn, the case manager keeps the family/patient unit updated and informed on how plans are progressing. Changes and detours can be discussed when the need arises.

Crisis Intervention/Grief Counseling. Most hospice NCMs are well trained and prepared for this role, but some nurses may need to seek out training. Not everyone is comfortable with this assignment; yet in the healthcare field, it is inevitable that NCMs will be involved when loved ones deteriorate or when death occurs. Some situations may be more difficult for a particular NCM to feel comfortable with than others. I personally find it easier to comfort children of an aged parent than parents who have lost their "child"—no matter what the age. On some level, parents feel that for a child to die first is not the natural order of things. Yet pediatric patients, young trauma victims, and young AIDS patients are disrespectful of that order. Inherent in the populations that require case management are those who are dying. This skill is very important; if needed, attend seminars or peruse the literature to become more proficient.

Conflict Resolution Expert and Referee. Fear and anger are emotions commonly expressed by patients and families. Often attentive listening is all that is needed to defuse the anger. Some simply need validation or some control over their seemingly uncontrollable situation. Honest and thorough answers are often what are required. The skills used for crisis intervention and conflict resolution may be similar. However, crisis intervention often revolves around pure grief, whereas conflict resolution requires detective work to get to the core problem, which is often hidden behind various acting-out behaviors. Also, be prepared to play referee when conflict enters the multidisciplinary team; patients and families are not the only dispensers of acting-out behaviors. Stay objective and bring the focus back to the patient.

Integrator. Murphy's law of medicine says that the more medical specialists on a case, the less they speak to one another. The NCM is often the integrator and collaborator of the fragmentation of care caused by this.

On Call. Some programs—hospice, for example—must have persons on call at all times for their clients' safety and support. Problem resolution can often be done by telephone rather than on site or at the home, but the situation, the agency, and the type of case management determine what is most expedient.

Staff Development. The NCM is a resource person to all levels of staff. In teaching hospitals, this extends to medical students, interns and residents, as well as attending physicians, who will look to you to help them develop the best transitional plans for their patients. Nurses, too, appreciate the nursing case management perspective in such foreign areas as insurance idiosyncrasies and utilization review. Time spent in developing staff and helping doctors and nurses understand the concepts of managed care will be repaid in cooperation, timely changes in levels of care, reduction time spent trying to make excuses to the payors as to why that patient is still here, and improved patient care and patient satisfaction.

Case Presentation. A case manager may be asked to present a particularly difficult case to the interns and residents during teaching rounds for educational purposes. It is a wonderful opportunity to explain the concepts of utilization review, go over the case's budget (and losses, if necessary), and explain potential ways improvements in the case plan might have been initiated. Case presentations can be used equally effectively among seasoned case managers to elicit new insights and further hone case management skills.

Educator. The opportunities for NCMs to teach are unlimited. Topics for education of patients, families, or significant others are wide-ranging and varied, including medication administration and side effects, disease processes and treatment, information so that informed decisions can be made, insurance coverage and noncoverage, tube care, and any other needs that have been individually assessed. Staff nurses often help with medical topics, but patients also ask insurance questions, such as what pharmacies they are allowed to use, how much is their deductible and copay, how can they change Medicaid plans, or can they change doctors. And the case manager is the expert in these areas.

Careful assessment of teaching needs and education of knowledge deficits is cost-effective and leads to greater patient satisfaction. Readmissions due to noncompliance are reduced when the client understands the disease process and the treatment needed. If a patient has a newly diagnosed condition, it is critical to thoroughly educate the client; insufficient understanding can lead to a deteriorated medical condition, more emergency room visits, complications, and hospital readmission.

Often case managers see patients who, after a long discussion with their physician, are more confused than ever. The ability to clearly explain difficult concepts in simple, easy-to-understand terminology is an asset to the NCM–patient relationship. It helps to build trust, and the patient doesn't feel "stupid" or condescended to. A ready-made file of handouts and information is a timesaver; bilingual handouts are also needed in many populations.

The teaching process may require repetition. It is unrealistic to teach a new tracheostomy patient all the care needed on the day of discharge (see Chapter 20: A Case Study With and Without Case Management). Other factors can hinder learning: too much information in too short a time, fear, anger, shock, depression, medications, any number of things patients in hospitals routinely go through. When preadmission or preoperative teaching can be carried out, this is an excellent choice. Also, note that some insurance plans may attempt to deny readmission payments if they feel the hospitalization was caused by poor discharge preparation (ie, education).

Liaison Between Hospital and Payor. The first step here is often the identification of the primary and secondary payment sources. In this "PR" position, the ability to speak the insurance company's language is very useful when requesting extended hospital days (see Chapter 6: Utilization Management). A good NCM–utilization reviewer can save financial stress for both the patient and the facility. Sloppy reviews can lead to "grievance trials" which would be unnecessary if the insurance company had all the facts in the first place. Attention to detail and a thorough knowledge of utilization modalities are important for the role of liaison.

Discharge Planning. Many NCMs enter the world of case management through the role of discharge planner. This task requires an assessment of the total medical, psychosocial, and financial elements of each case. Although some cases may be similar, no two cases are exactly alike. Start discharge planning on admission or, if possible, during preadmission screening (see Part III: The Case Management Process).

Facilitates Changes in Levels of Care. Discharge planning requiring changes in levels of care from a hospital to an extended care facility or to home or from a subacute facility to home are two types of transitional changes in levels of care. NCMs must also be alert for a client's readiness to change levels within a facility. This may include transfers from the intensive care unit to a step-down or floor level. Often the NCM must alert and gently prompt the physicians that the patient may be ready for this change.

Postdischarge Follow-up. Some NCMs perform episodic case management, which involves following up the client through the episode of acute illness. Other NCMs follow up their clients at wherever stage the clients are, whether acutely ill or chronically stable. Still others perform intermittent postdischarge follow-up on a "need-to" basis. How often a case manager needs to follow up after discharge depends on the acuteness or chronicity of the client and assessment of the following:

- Is the care optimum? Is your client receiving quality care?
- Does the client still match the level of care he or she is residing in?
- Is the client/family still satisfied with the arrangement and care, or is modification needed?
- Are the treatment goals being met, or are new goals needed? (More on postdischarge is discussed in Chapter 17: Final Evaluation: Postdischarge Follow-Up and Case Closure.)

Negotiating and Procuring Resources and Services. Some call this brokering of services. The first place to look to meet client needs is the client's own support system. If skilled services are required, most insurance companies cover them. Community resources may be what are needed to fill in gaps that family and insurance can't cover. But many people don't have a family, friend, or church support; some don't have health insurance, since universal coverage is not yet a reality. Sometimes the only options are charity care. Many hospitals and social service departments have some funds in reserve for these very tough cases. Usually, persistence and creativity eventually yield enough services for a safe discharge or transition. Here, the NCM acts as a general problem solver.

Benefit Analyst. Some types of case management require intensive analyzing of benefits. This is especially true for freelance or entrepreneurial case managers. At one time or another, most case managers will be asked to do a cost comparison of some aspect of a case. Occasionally, family members need comparative financial information, and insurance companies, inclined to refuse payment for a requested plan if they feel that a less cost-intensive solution is available, may request prices. Some case managers are required to make a formal documentation of savings per case for accounting and research purposes.

Documenter of Plans. As with any aspect of the nursing profession, NCMs are accountable for their actions. Documentation is important for obvious legal reasons. Thorough documentation is necessary when, for example, the case manager is not present and a situation arises in which contacts must be made immediately; therefore, all important contact phone numbers and plans should be visible on the chart for quick reference. The documentation theme is important and recurs often throughout this text.

Physician Support. Some NCMs accompany physicians on rounds, informing them of the patient's status and progress. This informational role may repeat throughout the day when any change in patient's condition or critical values (labs, vital signs) present. If a NCM feels a consultant may help in the case, that is suggested. For example, a case manager may hear a disturbing report or comment from a patient and suggest a psychiatric consultation, thereby averting a full-blown crisis.

Monitors Quality of Care Issues. Quality improvement monitoring is required for all aspects of patient care. One of the main tenets of case management is quality care, and identifying deviations from standards of practice is an important obligation. Case managers, being on the front lines, often pick up potential or actual variances from standards of care; this is another potential way in which case managers can avert a full-blown crisis.

Concurrent Coding, DRG Assignments, ICD-9-CM Coding Issues. Occasionally, a hospital-based NCM has as one job responsibility, concurrent coding using ICD-9-CM coding or DRG assignments. Although this usually is done somewhere in the medical records department after discharge, *concurrent* coding is advantageous. Coding is done in a timely manner, allowing hospital reimbursement to take advantage of "quick pay" discounts. Because the NCM knows the medical details of a case, few potential charges will be missed. It also encourages physicians to thoroughly document the disease process, which decreases the risk of insurance companies or Medicare denying hospital reimbursement.

Selection and Monitoring Clinical Pathways. Many institutions have been using clinical pathways over the past several years. Clients with a "pure" diagnosis (pneumonia, total hip replacement, asthma, myocardial infarction, for example) have a clear and definite pathway to choose from. This isn't always the case. Multimedical mix patients or those who develop severe complications may require more careful choices; sometimes the NCM may choose to change pathways if a new complication overpowers the original diagnosis. Clinical pathways have many advantages in the managed-care arena and are discussed in more detail in Chapter 6: Utilization Management.

Utilization Review. This is the process of monitoring Intensity of Service and Severity of Illness (ISSI) (see InterQual, Chapter 6), medical necessity, and appropriateness of level of care the patient is presently in. Monitoring ISSI also reveals the patient's changing condition. This provides a cue to the case manager to speed up a discharge plan if the patient is doing exceptionally well or change a discharge plan if the patient deteriorates and remains debilitated. Utilization review is the language that an insurance company can understand; authorization for extensions of hospital days is often based on utilization modalities (see Chapter 6: Utilization Management).

Utilization review functions in another capacity, too: reviewing for appropriate utilization of hospital services and resources during the patient admission. Overutilization of tests and services can have many causes:

- The facility is a teaching hospital in which medical students, interns, and residents are trying to find the balance between good and complete care.
- Patients insist on expensive, high-tech procedures.
- Physicians are cautious if a litigious event arises (eg, a patient falls).
- Physicians practicing defensive medicine overcautiously order multiple tests to prevent lawsuits.
- A test has a duplicate order and no one caught it.
- The monitoring frequency (eg, of hemoglobin/hematocrit or prothrombin/partial thromboplastin time) could be changed due to patient's stability, but no one has done so.
- An intravenous medication can be changed safely to oral.

The list is endless.

The utilization review role can be touchy. Conflicts can arise if the physician feels the NCM is telling him or her what to do or is "policing" the patient and patient care. Utilization tools such as clinical pathways are helpful. When a care plan goes off the path, that clinical pathway—and the patient—can be the focus of the discussion, which directs the conversation away from any personal physician practice.

Devil's Advocate. It takes a healthy dose of objectivity and chutzpah to play this part, but often, like brainstorming, the devil's advocate breaks apart any stagnant thinking and helps to provide a fresh new review.

Have Fun. It's an attitude!

References

Benner, P. (1984). *From novice to expert. Excellence and power in clinical nursing practice.* Menlo Park: Addison-Wesley.

Bradley, J. C., & Edinberg, M. A. (1986). *Communication in the nursing context.* Norwalk, CT: Appleton-Century-Crofts.

Chenevert, M. (1988). *STAT—Special techniques in assertiveness training for women in the health professions,* 3rd ed. St. Louis: C. V. Mosby.

Dubler, N. N. (1992). Individual advocacy as a governing principle. *Journal of Case Management, 1*(3), 82–86.

Hein, E. C., & Nicholson, M. J. (1994). *Contemporary leadership behavior.* Philadelphia: J. B. Lippincott.

Leddy, S., & Pepper, M. (1989). *Conceptual bases of professional nursing.* Philadelphia: J. B. Lippincott.

Prins, M. M. (1992). Patient advocacy: The role of nursing leadership. *Nursing Management, 23*(7), 78—80.

Wadas, T. (1993). Case management and caring behavior. *Nursing Management, 25*(9), 40–46.

CHAPTER 4

Opportunities in Nursing Case Management

As the managed care environment tightens, more positions for nurse case managers (NCM) are opening up, both in the public and private domains. Also, managed care strategies are changing, so it is reasonable to speculate that some of the current nursing case management job responsibilities may become more diverse and new ones may be emphasized. At any rate, the basic functions of case management—ensuring quality care in a cost-efficient manner—will not become less relevant.

The Future of Managed Care

The managed care crystal ball reveals various probabilities. One trend is that purely episodic case management (case managing one episode of a client's illness) will lose some favor. Although necessary, the scope of the role will expand to include case managing a client across a continuum of care. This may include acute and subacute levels of care, including the client's home. In this vertically integrated system, there is more continuity for the patient with a single NCM overseeing all levels of care. Some nursing case management delivery systems already include this multicontinuum style of case management, although these models appear to be in an evolutionary stage. The team approach mentioned previously will expand to include all the key players in the client's individual case, which may include extended care facility staff, hospice personnel, or different physicians from those attending the client in the hospital.

In some ways, this book focuses on acute hospital case management, as it is the most cost-intensive level of care. But some medical soothsayers predict that in the near future hospital care will consist mainly of intensive care unit (ICU) treatments. As care moves out of the costly hospital setting and into the community, new models of nursing case management will generate. The vision of keeping clients out of the hospital may become reality through, so far, unexplored nursing case management strategies. Case management across all levels of care has several potential advantages including the following:

- Its primary focus is on wellness and optimizing quality of life, autonomy, independence, and optimal family functioning
- Detour of potential problems can be accomplished through preventive practices
- Foreseeably fewer readmissions to the acute level of care
- Less acuity when the client is readmitted through early identification of medical changes, resulting in less costly hospitalizations and reduced lengths of stay
- Prevention of unnecessary admissions. This may include low acuity admissions or those known as "social admissions," primarily for disposition problems.
- Provision of a contact person for clients to help them access the complex healthcare system
- Decreased complications due to careful medical monitoring
- Fewer visits to emergency rooms; fewer "911" calls

Just as hospice nurses presently stave off many unnecessary 911 calls, so will NCMs in this expanded responsibility of managing clients across all levels of healthcare. A study done in 1992 by the US Department of Health and Human Services revealed that of the 90 million emergency room visits that year, only 45% were deemed urgent or emergent (Anonymous, 1994). Almost as many people went to emergency rooms for coughs and sore throats as for chest pain and level I traumas. Rather than an emergency room, upon assessment the NCM may send the client to his PCP or an ambulatory care site, or will call in an extra home health nurse visit, a respiratory professional, a social worker, or a psychiatric RN to visit the client. Or perhaps the far-sighted payor source is contracted with one of the new, futuristic, entrepreneurial physician groups who specialize in the age-old activity of house calls. Surely, even a physician-assisted house call is less expensive than a 911 ambulance charge plus the emergency room treatment charges.

Matching Personal Goals and Beliefs With the Appropriate Case Management Model

This chapter discusses several types of nursing case management in the contemporary healthcare environment. Those interested in nursing case management as an employment opportunity would be advised to evaluate the job description and responsibilities carefully to see whether the model of case management offered is compatible with personal beliefs and goals. Some might prefer the episodic version of case management, whereas others would find long-term relationships with clients very satisfying. If home-based case management services are included in your job description, would you be at ease going into others' homes and assessing their medical and psychosocial needs? Are you comfortable and effective with issues such as self-neglect, noncompliance, or abuse (child or elder)? Are you clinically astute enough to safely triage a client at home and make appropriate care decisions?

Another issue for your discernment is whether you feel that direct care is part of the nursing case management role. In varying degrees, some nursing case management delivery systems combine the nursing case management role with bedside nursing. In this combined role, the NCM–bedside RN may assess acute care needs and discharge planning for the patient. A plan of care would be developed by the RN and sent to the multidisciplinary team for additional recommendations. It is then sent back to the RN for evaluation. The team then assists the RN in the implementation of the plan (Bair, Griswold, & Head, 1989).

Variations on this type of NCM–staff RN model exist, but universal acceptance of this style of case management is lacking. In one survey, 52% of the experts questioned felt strongly that NCMs should not perform direct bedside nursing care (Taban, 1993). Another magazine article implied that combining these roles was a main cause of frustration, burnout, and the eventual demise of an initial attempt at case management in one facility. This article unequivocally stated that "the staff nurse should not be used in a dual staff nurse/case manager role" (Biller, 1992, p. 145).

When assessing job openings in case management, note that many employment opportunities are available for various aspects of the total NCM role; these are not the whole picture, but can provide valuable experience in the management aspects of healthcare. Some of these areas are preadmission case management, utilization management, quality improvement, risk management, telephone triage, and discharge planning. When interviewing or in a pre-interview phone call, it is wise to ask about the expected job responsibilities because some job ads may be misleading. For example, an ad for utilization reviewers may actually be more akin to an NCM position, or vice versa. It is wise to ask about the expected job responsibilities when interviewing or in a pre-interview phone call.

Experience in the above roles is important, since considerable skill and an extensive knowledge base are useful to perform nursing case management functions well. In the evolving definitions of what a NCM *is* and *does*, more of these roles are being included in the hybrid interpretation of an NCM. Many NCMs who come into the profession with utilization management or quality improvement backgrounds have made the transition with more ease than even the most clinically competent staff RN. All experience is valuable and will add to your expertise as a NCM.

Three basic models of case management further delineate your choices. These models revolve around the different ways resources can be allocated.

Brokerage Case Management Model

In the Brokerage Case Management Model, the NCM identifies needed services and makes referrals to various sources, both private and community, but does not provide the direct provision of services (Williams & Torrens, 1993). The NCM may broker services to various home health agencies, infusion companies, durable medical equipment companies, or community agencies. Payments are usually agreed upon in advance and range from health insurance paying for home nursing or equipment to sliding-scale fees for community-based services. Here the NCM has no authority over service delivery.

Service Management Model

In the Service Management Model, the NCM manages both the client's service budget and the services provided, and there is usually a predetermined limit on how much can be allocated (Westhoff, 1992). For example, many full-service home health agencies furnish durable medical equipment, intravenous infusion care, pharmacy services, skilled nursing, home aides, social work, psychiatric assistance, and caretaker services; some even have branches across the United States.

Although both the broker model and the service management model offer services to complement the needs of the client, the full-service agency has the advantage of "one-stop shopping." Care must be taken when the agency's services do not best meet the client's needs. A potential ethical dilemma for the NCM may result from this scenario.

Managed Care Model

In the Managed Care Model, the provider has been paid for services prospectively. Although the NCM has no predetermined cap on spending, the provider is at a greater risk, which is a clear fiscal incentive to use resources efficiently and wisely (Williams & Torrens, 1993; Westhoff, 1992).

Case Management Career Opportunities

The following reflect some of the nursing case management opportunities that are available in our contemporary healthcare environment.

Acute Care Case Management

Acute care case management is usually short, episodic nursing case management at the hospital level. This type of case management may be managed in four different ways. First, it may be unit-based, in which NCMs manage patients while on a particular unit such as ICU, orthopedic, medicine, or telemetry.

In a second scenario, acute care case management may mean that NCMs follow clients from admission to discharge. These NCMs often do prehospital teaching if the admission patient is nonemergent and planned. The same NCM will follow up a client in whichever level of care/unit is required, thus ensuring continuity of care.

In addition, acute care case management may be service-based, following up clients according to their primary illness. Each setting requires unique components, skills, and knowledge for effective care. Some nursing case management specialties are included in Display 4-1.

Finally, acute care case management may be represented through primary nursing case management. NCMs also practice hands-on care of the patient. They identify acute care needs, discharge needs, and help to develop the treatment plan with the multidisciplinary team.

DISPLAY 4–1
Nursing Case Management Specialties

- Pediatrics
- Surgical
- Medicine
- Cardiac
- Oncology
- Pulmonary–ventilator
- HIV
- Burn injury
- Spinal cord injury
- Head truama
- Cerebral vascular accident

- High-risk neonatal
- High-risk pregnancy–gynecology
- Transplant specialist
- Miscellaneous catastrophic cases
- Trauma
- Orthopedics
- Rehabilitation (head, trauma, spinal cord, neurorehabilitation)
- Substance abuse rehabilitation
- Psychiatric care

Large Case Management

In another type of service-based nursing case management, also known as "catastrophic case management," the case selection includes those who are at risk for extremely high healthcare costs, eg, patients with AIDS, premature infants in neonatal intensive care units, and patients with possible kidney/liver/heart/bone marrow transplant, high spinal cord injury, and end-stage renal disease clients on hemodialysis.

Insurance (Third Party Payor) Case Management

NCMs must balance quality care/patient advocacy with the responsibility for carefully shepherding that plan's dollars. If there is a conflict between the expectations of the insurance company and the member or the facility to which the member is currently admitted, the NCM must depend on communication and negotiation skills. The NCM is the company's liaison. Third party payor case managers often have the power to authorize services and levels of care. NCMs may perform their job responsibilities in either of two ways:

Telephonics

Some case managers for large insurance companies have clients all over the United States and must rely on telephone review. Since their assessment and planning are only as good as the information they can extract from the facility/member, they must be skilled in asking tough, pertinent questions. If they do not get the right answer, a hospital admission (or specified days) may be denied coverage.

On Site

On-site case management is preferable to telephonics. The chart can be reviewed, staff members can be interviewed, if necessary, and the patient can be seen. Proximity to the patient is an advantage. It allows the NCM to develop a therapeutic relationship, see a patient's wounds first-hand, and make personal observations when assessing the patient's interaction with family members for discharge assessment purposes. Sometimes a picture is worth a thousand words.

Hospice Case Management

NCMs in hospice case management coordinate the care and comfort of the dying and their families. The nurse becomes the primary manager of the case; the physician becomes a consultant.

Home Health Case Management

In home health case management, NCMs service the needs of the chronically ill in the home setting. Coordination of several therapeutic modalities may be necessary in an individual case. These may include wound care, infusion therapy services, physical therapy, speech therapy, occupational therapy, coordination of durable medical equipment, tube feeding, medication monitoring, assessments, tube/tracheostomy care—almost anything done in hospitals. If the patient is stable, home care can also include such intensive services as ventilator assistance. These NCMs monitor for early warning signs, contact the client's primary physician for treatment, and can thereby prevent or lessen the severity of exacerbation of the illness and reduce the frequency of readmissions to the hospital. The therapeutic home health NCM's relationship usually begins and ends with insurance authorization. But acting as a client advocate, the NCM can help to extend authorization from the insurance company if tangible reasons can be cited and the NCM is adept at negotiation skills.

Extended Care Facility (ECF) Case Management

When a patient's self-care needs exceed their self-care capabilities after an episode of acute illness, an ECF placement may be necessary. NCMs act as liaisons between the acute care and subacute care levels. They also assist the convalescent period by determining appropriate needs and services and obtaining required payor funds for the ECF care. Many other responsibilities that resemble an acute care NCM may be required during the client's ECF admission.

Public Health/Community-Based Case Management

This model helps families and clients access appropriate services needed for independent functioning. A wide range of target populations may receive services, depending on the focus of the agency. Community health nursing, such as that on Indian Reservations or with high-risk/low-income maternal/child health has long been taking care of families' health on a case-by-case basis. Other areas or populations needing case managers include mental health, geriatric, catastrophic diseases such as AIDS, homeless families, or substance abuse clients. Some populations can be well served with a social service professional; others require medical knowledge, especially in the HIV and geriatric populations. Like home health nursing, community-based case management also works to prevent exacerbations of illnesses by early assessment of changes in client's conditions and early interventions.

Rehabilitation Specialists

Many rehabilitation units (both freestanding and those in acute care facilities) have discovered the efficacy of the NCM–social worker team concept. Clients enter rehabilitation units for many reasons, such as cerebral vascular accidents, motor vehicle accidents, traumas, gunshot wounds, head injuries, spinal cord injuries. Most clients are not even allowed in rehab unless they are functioning at a low enough level to require intensive rehab services. Inherent in the criteria for acceptance into this unit is a precipitating illness or event that requires a full-scale biopsychosocial assessment, planning, and intervention. The goal is to bring that person back to a functional level that matches his or her baseline level as much as possible. Depending on the precipitating event, this type of case management requires the utmost in creativity, pulling in both private and community resources.

Vocational Case Management

Vocational case management may be a component of rehabilitation case management, a part of workers' compensation case management or a separate form of employment. Vocational case managers assist clients in returning to meaningful employment, given their new limitations. A thorough knowledge of disability laws and excellent assessment skills (both of functional ability and employability) are necessary.

Case Management Firms

NCMs working in private case management agencies will need a national network of resources. Often clients are willing to travel in order to receive the best care for their particular illness. NCMs may need to identify the most up-to-date treatment for a specific disease and locate the facility where that treatment is offered. Clients may be admitted to hospitals anywhere in the United States or even world-wide, if traveling. This type of case management holds the same limitations as telephonics review (ie, reliance on asking the right questions and receiving accurate information from a nurse on the other line, who may have little time to spare for telephone consultation).

Entrepreneurial Case Management

Several brave nurses have been willing to risk starting their own NCM businesses. Also known as case management consultants, these independent NCMs may be contracted by clients, family members, physicians, or insurance companies. Entrepreneurial NCMs need good business skills and the ability to work autonomously. There are some perils involved in this type of case management; if a client sustains a poor outcome from a referred physician or treatment, the company may be sued for liability. On the positive side, independent NCMs often have increased freedom to fulfill the client's desires and needs, especially if the client has funds to supplement private insurance. Without financial constraints and insurance policy restrictions, patient choices can be implemented to the benefit and satisfaction of the client, family, and physician. As in other forms of case management, independent NCMs coordinate all aspects of care, in the home and in any level of care needed. Specialties such as geriatrics or rehabilitation may dominate a professional group practice, depending on the skill and experience of the NCMs. Clients may reside in various parts of the country, and travel may be part of the job description.

Before considering entrepreneurial case management, self-assess whether you have both the background skills required for the job and the personality makeup. Successful NCMs benefit from some of the entrepreneurial characteristics listed in Display 4–2 (Tassel, 1994, p. 143).

In 1990, some entrepreneurial nurses employed by St. Mary's Hospital in Tucson, Arizona, seized an opportunity to contract NCMs and community nursing services to a medical health maintenance organization (HMO), forming a nursing HMO group. Their vision included a better way to manage clients, enter the managed care arena, strengthen business opportunities for NCMs, and advance the

DISPLAY 4–2
Entrepreneurial Characteristics

- *Opportunist*—Sees opportunities but also the risk involved
- *Risker*—Accepts risk and attempts to manage it
- *Visionary*—Sees a better way and takes advantage of the situation
- *Actor*—Is action-oriented with little patience for frequent committee meetings
- *Strategist*—Focuses on the best solutions
- *Innovator*—Unafraid to try a new way of doing something
- *Learner*—Is open-minded and asks questions to develop new strategies
- *Confident*—Assesses opportunities confidently and produces favorable changes
- *Flexibility*—Adapts to fast-paced changes

(From Tassel, M. V. [1994, August]. Case managers use entrepreneurial skills. *Hospital Case Management*, 143).

nursing profession (Michaels, 1992). With the fast-changing healthcare climate, opportunities for entrepreneurship abound. An unselfish vision in the proper hands can benefit the client, the nursing profession, and all those touched by the dilemmas inherent in the managed care arena of the 90s.

References

Anonymous. (1994). Emergency departments visits mostly non-urgent. *Arizona Hospital Association Weekly Newsletter, 8*(33), 1.

Bair, N., Griswold, J., & Head, J. (1989). Clinical R. N. involvement in bedside-centered case management. *Nursing Economics, 7*(3), 150–154.

Biller, A. M. (1992). Implementing nursing case management. *Rehabilitation Nursing, 17*(3), 144–146.

Michaels, C. (1992). Carondelet St. Mary's nursing enterprise. *Nursing Clinics of North America, 27*(1), 77–85.

Taban, H. (1993). The nurse case manager in acute care settings. *JONA, 23*(10), 53–61.

Tassel, M. V. (1994). Case managers use entrepreneurial skills. *Hospital Case Management,* August, 143.

Westhoff, L. J. (1992). Care management: Quelling the confusion. *Health Progress, 73*(5), 43–58.

Williams, S. J., & Torrens, P. R. (1993). *Introduction to health services.* New York: Delmar.

PART I
Study Questions

1. How do case management and managed care differ? In what ways are they similar?

2. Explore various target populations. Who should case manage these populations?

3. Who would be in your "ideal" case management team? Why?

4. Cite an example in which case management was done poorly. Explore reasons and illustrate ways in which improvements could be made next time.

5. Do the characteristics necessary for a NCM differ from those needed for a direct care nurse? If so, how?

6. How do the job responsibilities of nursing case management differ from traditional direct care nursing?

7. Cite an example in which you demonstrated the role of the patient advocate. What might have resulted if you were not there to advocate for the patient?

8. Evaluate your own strengths and weaknesses in terms of essential characteristics of a NCM. How would you turn weaknesses into strengths?

9. What would motivate you to pursue a position in case management? What type of case management appeals to you? Why?

PART II

Basic Concepts in Case Management

"Quality is never an accident; it is always the result of high intention, sincere effort, intelligent direction and skillful execution; it represents the wise choice of many alternatives."

WILLA A. FOSTER

CHAPTER 5

Insurance

IMPORTANT TERMS AND CONCEPTS

ABCs—adjusted billed charges
AFDC—Aid to Families with Dependent Children
CAP
capitation
catastrophic claims
catastrophic reinsurance
categorically eligible
CHAMPUS—Civilian Health & Medical Program of the Uniformed Services
CMPs—Competitive Medical plans
COBRA—Consolidated Omnibus Reconciliation Act
coinsurance
copayment
Corporate Alliances
CPT-4—Current Procedural Terminology Fourth Edition
days per thousand
deductible
deferred liability
PHO—Physician Hospital Organization
Direct Contract Model
disenrollment
DRGs—Diagnostic-Related Groups
eligibility worker
employer mandate
EPO—Exclusive Provider Organization
fee-for-service
gatekeeper
grievance
Group Model
Guaranteed Health Benefit Package

HCFA—Health Care Financing Administration
Health Alliances
HMO—Health Maintenance Organization
ICD-10—International Classification of Diseases-10th Revision
indemnity plans
IPA—Independent Practice Association
JCAHO—Joint Commission for the Accreditation of Health Care Organizations
Lifetime Reserve Days
LOS—length of stay
LTC—long-term care
Managed Competition
MAO—Medical Assistance only
MCO—Managed Care Organization
Medicaid
Medicare
Medicare benefits periods
Medicare Part A—Hospital Insurance
Medicare Part B—Medical Insurance
Medicare Risk Contracts
Medicare Select
Medigap Plans
MIP—managed indemnity plans
MIS-Management Information System
MN/MI—medically needy/medically indigent
National Health Board
National Health Security card
Network Model

open enrollment period
OPHS—Office of Prepaid Health Care
outliers
OWA—Other Weird Arrangement
PAS—Professional Activity Study: Norms
  Handbook
PCP—primary care physician
POS—Point of Service
PPA—Preferred Provider Arrangements
PPO—Preferred Provider Organization
PPS—Prospective Payment System
premiums
Regional Health Alliances
reinsurance

S.O.B.R.A.—Sixth Omnibus Budget
  Reconciliation Act
spend down
SSD—Social Security Disability
SSI—Social Security Income
Staff Model
stoploss
third party payor
Title XIX of the Social Security Act
TPL—third party liability
Universal Health Care Coverage
Wickline v State of California
Workers' Compensation

Insurance provides the financial motor through which the medical system runs. Although it may be the most confusing part of case management, it is perhaps the most important aspect to understand. Each insurance company has its own rules and by-laws. Some companies carve these rules in stone, whereas others modify them slightly on a patient-by-patient basis, especially if they foresee a favorable chance at lessening the prospect of a future expensive hospital admission. If at times you feel like the "master of ceremonies" in the insurance game, you'll be in good company. However, without a solid knowledge of covered services, a case manager's best intentions, plans, time, and energy will be wasted if he or she hears the words "insurance refused to pay" for this plan. It is better to know up front what the limitations are and try to negotiate from there than to have to throw away the entire plan.

Working closely with a knowledgeable social worker provides valuable information and may also prevent a true disaster for some patients. More than one HIV patient has been lured into accepting Medicare's Social Security Disability (SSD) category instead of the SSI category, the latter of which pays out less money. In these instances, when the financial statement was checked by Medicaid, it was found that those who were paid the SSD rate no longer qualified for medical insurance under the Medicaid plan. They had too much monthly income (by about $35 to $85 per month). Therefore, these ill members had no money to buy expensive medications, and if they need hospitalization, it would have to be through hospital charity until they could "spend down" (see Spend Down, discussed in the following text) into a Medicaid plan.

This type of scenario can be more than just confusing and financially troublesome. For some, it means life or death. Consider the case of a single mother in her late 20s from Arizona. The woman worked full-time as a clerk and went to school part-time to improve her future prospects for a better-paying job. When she was diagnosed with leukemia in 1992, she eventually qualified for AHCCCS (Arizona's form of Medicaid). She was on AFDC (Aid to Families with Dependent Children), which allowed her the right to the state's Medicaid coverage and a chance at a bone marrow transplantation. But when she became too ill to work and was persuaded to apply for Social Security Disability (SSD) at $456.80 per month, this put her and her son $86.00 over the limit for AFDC. She fell off the AFDC rolls—and with it the AHCCCS roles. Her chance for a bone marrow transplantation was gone, and she died of leukemia a short time later.

The information in this chapter does not cover all that a nurse case manager (NCM) must know about insurance, because each plan has its own standards for coverage or interpretation of coverage. In addition, the rules change yearly or sometimes more frequently. When describing different types of plans such as an HMO or a PPO, it must be understood that even their basic structure is changing. As the insurance company's vision of the healthcare crisis becomes clearer, the definitions of these plans become more blurred; this is in an effort to become more efficient.

Insurance Systems

From mathematics to physics, every classification of knowledge has its own terminology. NCMs learned to be fluent in "medicalese" in nursing school. Now we must also be fluent in "insurance-ese"; therefore, some of this chapter is in glossary form. As patient advocates, NCMs must understand the convoluted system that insurance is and be wary so that our plans do not saddle patients and their families with unexpected bills or, worse, place them in "catch-22" scenarios like those previously mentioned.

Spend Down

Spend down is the process by which a patient or family can financially qualify for welfare medicine, most commonly known as Medicaid. In essence, the patient must impoverish him- or herself with medical bills. These medical expenses are subtracted from the patient's annual income until the income eligibility limits are met. This yearly financial income allotted depends on such factors as family size and personal property ownership. Following is a simplified example of a spend down in a patient with no extra variables: Mrs. Barrett receives $12,000 per year income. To qualify for Medicaid, it had been assessed that Mrs. Barrett must not earn over $5000 per year. Therefore, she must incur $7000 in medical expenses or, in other words, spend down $7000 to qualify for Medicaid. Mrs. Barrett was in the hospital in February and was billed $4500. She spent $1000 in medications and outpatient doctor bills. It is May and she is presently in the hospital as an inpatient. Her hospital bill has exceeded the remaining $1500 charge, so she has "met her spend down." Mrs. Barrett can now qualify for Medicaid.

PCP

PCP is an acronym for Primary Care Physician, the main doctor assigned to a member of a healthcare plan. Often insurance companies use PCPs in a gatekeeper role (see below).

Gatekeeper

The gatekeeper concept is an important one in the world of managed care. It is an informal term used to define the role of the primary care physician. Essentially, the PCP stands at the gate of available medical services and decides which services each member requires. The gatekeeper is responsible for the basic medical care of the patient and also determines when that member needs lab tests, an x-ray, a specialist, or virtually anything medicine has to offer. True emergencies are excluded when members may be serviced in emergency rooms. The gatekeeper concept is a predominant characteristic of Health Maintenance Organizations (HMOs) (Kongstvedt, 1993).

Although the gatekeeper concept can be an excellent method to manage healthcare, it can also become a barrier to access of specialty services. Depending on a physician's practice patterns and financial incentives, the PCP may under-refer or over-refer to various specialists or services (Williams & Torrens, 1993).

Reimbursement and Protective Strategies

The following terms and concepts refer to reimbursement and protective strategies for physicians or facilities. New ways to control costs and to reimburse for care are continually being evaluated, and the NCM should stay current on this issue.

Capitation

Capitation is a fixed monthly payment to a provider, paid in advance of services; a full range of medical services may be expected for each member capitated (Kongstvedt, 1993). Capitation started out as a popular method for reimbursing PCP-gatekeepers. Now many hospital risk contracts use capitation as a cost management tool as well.

Here is a simplified fictitious example of how capitation works for a PCP: Dr. Jones has 100 members from Insurance Company A. The capitated rate is $15.00 per month per member, so Dr. Jones will receive $1500 per month from Insurance Company A to manage its 100 members.

Capitation rates vary widely across the country and even among counties in one state. Also variable is what the PCP includes in the capitation rate. For example, a capitation for office visits would be less costly than a capitation that includes office visits and all laboratory tests. The capitation rate will be still higher if the PCP agrees to see these members in the event that they are hospitalized.

Capitation provides a powerful incentive to contain costs, but balances in this system are delicate. Some feel that the capitation system is unfair to those PCPs with sicker patients who require more office visits per month. From the HMO standpoint, capitation allows the plan to budget for medical costs. For years, capitation was used essentially as a budget tool for outpatient services such as physician office visits. With capitation moving into the acute hospital setting, more NCMs will be needed to manage the use of cost-intensive hospital services and resources.

CAP

Not to be confused with capitation, a CAP is the maximum dollar amount allowed in an insurance policy. Some policies are capped at $25,000, whereas others are capped at $1 million or more for a lifetime. Yearly caps are occasionally specified. Some insurance sources have no maximum cap, such as most Medicaid plans.

Fee-For-Service

Fee-for-service is the old method of reimbursement, in which a healthcare provider sends a bill to the insurance company and then the insurance company pays it. With this form of reimbursement, healthcare costs go up as more services are provided. Some feel that fee-for-service was a major reason for the healthcare crisis, and at this time most insurance companies are agreeing to pay only "reasonable" charges.

Preferred Provider Organizations (PPOs) use a variation of fee-for-service: the physician gets paid each time the member requires services (in contrast to capitated physicians), but at contract rates agreed upon in advance.

High-level specialists may be paid fee-for-service by some insurance plans.

Prospective Payment System (PPS)

In 1983, Social Security amendments initiated the Medicare Prospective Payment System. Under this system, hospitals are no longer reimbursed for inpatient services on the basis of what services were performed, how long the patient stayed in the hospital, or the costs of care. Rather, hospitals are reimbursed for certain types of insurance, most notably Medicare, according to Diagnostic-Related Groups (DRGs, discussed below). DRGs set predetermined rates of reimbursement; the hospital is permitted to keep excess dollars if the patient does not incur that limit of cost. Conversely, the hospital is required to absorb losses for patients who are more resource-intensive than given in the DRG allotment (Williams & Torrens, 1993).

Diagnostic-Related Groups (DRGs)

DRGs, developed in the 1970s by Yale researchers, were originally designed as a patient classification system, not as a reimbursement method (InterQual &

Tennant, 1993). Four-hundred-and-ninety-four diagnoses are listed and divided into 25 major diagnostic categories. Several variables account for the choice of DRG for a patient including the primary diagnosis, comorbidities (preexisting conditions), treatment procedures, age, sex, complications, secondary diagnosis, length of stay (LOS) and discharge status. Each DRG is scored according to its potential consumption of resources.

A dollar amount is placed on each DRG, and hospitals are most often reimbursed a flat rate for all patients who fall within each DRG category. If a particular case has been extremely cost-intensive or had a very long LOS when compared with other cases in the chosen DRG, extra reimbursement is possible for these *outlier* cases. For example, a simple appendectomy would not be considered an outlier case until the patient stayed for 15 days. Then the case must cost the hospital more than two times the DRG rate of payment, or $44,000, whichever is greater (Williams & Torrens, 1993). As a comparison, Milliman & Robertson (see Chapter 6: Utilization Management) has a goal LOS for a simple appendectomy of 1 day; with abscess or peritonitis, the goal LOS is 4 days.

Perhaps more than any other factor, DRGs provided the impetus for hospitals to utilize NCMs. With the exception of the above outlier cases, the hospital will receive the same basic DRG reimbursement whether the case is managed well or poorly and regardless of the costs incurred.

Compare the two following cases:

- Patient A with Medicare coverage came into the emergency room with abdominal pain. Gallstones were found on the emergency room ultrasound. An open cholecystectomy was performed on the evening of the patient's first hospital day. She was tolerating clear liquids on the evening of postop day (POD) #1. On POD #2, she tolerated full liquids and was ambulating short distances. Her diet was advanced as tolerated. On POD #3, she tolerated a soft diet, her bowels were functioning, and she was on oral pain medications. She was discharged in the evening of POD #3, her fourth day in the hospital.
- Patient B with Medicare coverage came into a different emergency room with abdominal pain. Gallstones were found on the emergency room ultrasound. The next afternoon an open cholecystectomy was performed. This patient received nothing by mouth for 2 days postoperatively. On POD #3, the doctor wrote orders for a clear liquid diet. On POD #4, the patient was allowed to advance diet as tolerated. He tolerated a full liquid diet at lunch and a soft diet for dinner. His bowels were functioning, he was ambulating in the hallway, and he was on oral pain medications. The following day, POD #5, the physician came in and discharged the patient—on hospital day #7.

These two disparities are not uncommon. Both hospitals received the same DRG reimbursement. Studies have shown that case management has made a difference in cases such as these. Hospitals can no longer afford not to manage their resources wisely, and NCMs are proving to be one of the best resources for this. A list of DRGs can be found in the Appendix: Medicare DRGs. The 10 most common DRGs are detailed in Display 5-1.

DISPLAY 5–1
The Ten Most Common DRGs

DRG Name	DRG Number
1. Heart failure and pleurisy	127
2. Simple pneumonia and pleurisy with complications, age > 17	89
3. Specific cerebrovascular disorders except transient ischemic attack	14
4. Angina pectoris	140
5. Psychoses	430
6. Major joint and limb reattachment procedures	209
7. Esophagitis, gastroenteritis, and misc. digestive disorders with complications, age > 17	182
8. Nutritional and misc. metabolic disorders with complications, age > 17	296
9. Cardiac arrhythmia and conduction disorders with complications	138
10. Bronchitis and asthma with complications, age > 17	96

(From HCFA [Baltimore, MD] in Managed Healthcare, December 1993. Ranked by all Medicare inpatient discharges—FY 1991)

Length of Stay (LOS)

Some insurance companies allow the hospital a standard number of hospital days for a patient's condition. A laparoscopic cholecystectomy may be given a 1-day length of stay. An uncomplicated appendectomy may be given a 2-day LOS. The Professional Activity Study (PAS) *Norms Handbook* has LOS broken down by regions in the country and diagnosis. They are further delineated by age and other factors. The estimated LOS for each category is given in percentiles—10%, 25%, 50%, 75%, 90%, 95%, and 99% (Health Care Knowledge Resources, 1991). For example, a patient 65 years of age or older with paroxysmal supraventricular tachycardia may be given an LOS of 1 day (10th percentile) to 7 days (99th percentile). Most insurance companies use the 10% to 50% range for assignment of LOS. (*LOS: Length of Stay by Diagnosis and Operation* is published by Health Care Knowledge Resources, Ann Arbor, MI.)

A landmark legal case developed around an assignment of an LOS in *Wickline v State of California* in the late 1980s (Saue, 1988). This case involved a Medi-Cal (California's Medicaid plan) patient, Mrs. Wickline, with peripheral vascular disease and occlusion of the abdominal aorta. Mrs. Wickline was admitted to a California hospital where an artery was removed and replaced with a synthetic graft. The postop course was described as "stormy" with several complications, so the attending physician asked the state agency for 8 additional days after the LOS was established. The LOS was extended for only 4 more days, at which time the patient was discharged in stable condition. Home health nursing was provided, but within days after discharge, the patient's leg became more painful and started to change color. At about 9 days after discharge, the leg pain became unbearable. It was determined that at some point Mrs. Wickline developed a clot in her leg and a graft infection. Antibiotics, anticoagulants, and bed rest failed to save the leg and a below-knee amputation was deemed necessary and performed. Nine days later, the patient needed an additional above-knee amputation.

Subsequently, Mrs. Wickline filed a multimillion dollar lawsuit against the state of California, stating that Medi-Cal forced her out of the hospital prematurely and that the physician was intimidated by the Medi-Cal program and complied with their LOS. This case went to the California Supreme Court, which ruled in favor of the State. In its judgment, the Court stated that the attending physician—not Medi-Cal—was ultimately responsible for treatment decisions concerning the care of patients and that the physician cannot abdicate that responsibility for any reason. It is important then for NCMs to know that physicians are legally responsible for the treatment plan. As the court warned in the Wickline Case, "...a physician could not shift legal responsibility for his patients welfare to a third party payor by complying with a cost containment program." (Saue, 1988, p. 83).

At the time of this case, Medi-Cal did not have an appeals process, but now hospitals have a grievance procedure whereby additional funds or LOS days can be argued. Physicians, NCMs, and the treatment team *must* put the patient before the payment. Know that appeals are frequently won on the side of the hospital.

Insurance companies frequently give short LOS—24 to 48 hours—for admission diagnoses that are more symptomatic than diagnostic (eg, chest pain, abdominal pain). As the case develops, additional LOS days can usually be negotiated. If a patient is stable after several days and care can be given at a less cost-intensive setting, the company may not extend the LOS further, but may agree to pay for an alternative plan. (More on length of stay can be found in Chapter 6: Utilization Management, under Utilization Management Modalities.)

Per Diem Reimbursement

Per diem reimbursement is based on a set dollar amount per day, rather than on charges (Kongstvedt, 1993). Many insurance companies favor this method of payment. They often pay for the day of admission, but not the day of discharge. Occasionally certain expensive items can be billed separately. Per diem reimbursement may be a different dollar amount for different service lines. Intensive care services have a higher per diem rate than surgical service lines; a medicine patient may be reimbursed more per diem than a mental health patient in a per diem system.

Adjusted Billed Charges (ABCs)

Some health plans reimburse hospitals using formulas outlined in state revised statutes. Popular in the 80s, ABCs may be falling out of favor as managed care concepts strengthen.

Bundling and Unbundling

Bundling case rates indicate that the facility charges and the physician charges are all "bundled" together. For example, a plan may negotiate a rate of $20,000 for a cardiac bypass. This would include everything from the surgeon and anesthesiologist to postoperative hospital care (Kongstvedt, 1993).

Unbundling is a term that explains the practice of billing separately for items that were once bundled together in a single bill (Kongstvedt, 1993). For example, a minor surgical procedure was once a single charge. When unbundled, it may include a procedure fee, physician services, a fee for instruments, and one for dressings.

Current Procedural Terminology

Current Procedural Terminology, 4th edition (CPT-4) codes list procedures and services and differentiate them with a 5-digit number. These codes function as a record of physician utilization practices by HMOs and are useful for billing purposes. The American Medical Association revises and publishes CPT-4 annually (InterQual & Tennant, 1993).

International Classification of Diseases

International Classification of Diseases, 9th revision—*Clinical Modifications ICD-10*, (formerly called ICD-9-CM) ICD-9 and ICD-10 are the most widely used classification of diseases in the world. These alphanumeric codes are used by hospitals and other providers when reporting diagnostic information about members of federally funded programs such as Medicare, Medicaid, and Maternal and Child Health. All third party payors are required to submit ICD codes for billing purposes (InterQual & Tennant, 1993).

Reinsurance

Reinsurance is purchased by an insurance company to protect it against extremely expensive cases (Kongstvedt, 1993). Just as an individual may purchase an insurance plan with a $500 deductible for protection from high medical bills, health plans also purchase reinsurance with deductibles. A *stoploss* is a form of reinsurance that protects a health plan when a medical case exceeds (for example) $100,000 (Kongstvedt, 1993); any charges over $100,000 are paid out at 80% from the reinsurance company. Stoploss amounts differ, just as an individual may purchase higher or lower deductibles on their insurance plan. These high dollar claims are known as *catastrophic claims.* Since certain diagnoses carry proven statistics of being expensive cases, *catastrophe reinsurance* may be tied to diagnoses such as acquired immunodeficiency syndrome (AIDS) and human organ transplants.

Deferred Liability

Deferred liability offers Medicaid plans protection in specific circumstances. Suppose a patient is admitted through the emergency room without medical insurance and spends down to where he or she is eligible for membership in a Medicaid plan. Under deferred liability, a portion of the medical expenses are deferred by payments from federally funded coffers. This helps the plan to maintain some financial control, especially if the new member is very ill. In many states, sick newborns are an automatic deferred liability category.

Cost-Sharing Strategies

The following three terms relate to cost-sharing strategies used by most insurance companies. The beneficiary is usually responsible for copayments, coinsurance, and deductibles.

Copayment

Copayment is a set amount of money specified by each health plan that the member must pay at the time services are rendered (Kongstvedt, 1993). This payment may range from $1 (for Medicaid recipients) to $15 or more. Pharmacy copayments are common. Some patients are unable to pay even small copayments, so many physicians and emergency rooms waive them.

Coinsurance

Coinsurance is another type of out-of-pocket expense for the member. This type of cost sharing limits the amount of coverage by a health plan to a certain percentage—commonly 80% (Kongstvedt, 1993). The member is responsible for the remaining 20%, but normally there is a ceiling dollar amount (usually $5000). Private/indemnity plans often use coinsurance strategies.

Deductible

A third type of out-of-pocket expense for a member, medical deductibles, must be paid out typically every year before the health insurance becomes active. In the 1980s, the deductibles amount was frequently $100 to $300. With the rising cost of healthcare, high deductibles of $1000 to $1500 are now offered to keep the monthly premiums lower. Deductibles are common in private plans and PPOs; HMOs rarely use deductibles.

Premiums

Premiums are the monthly fees that most insurance companies charge the member for insurance coverage.

Enrollment

Enrollment in a health plan may require specific qualifications. Medicaid, for example, requires the patient to be financially impoverished; Medicare Part A requires a specified amount of work hours into which social security is paid and may have age restrictions or a disabled health condition. Private insurance plans may refuse enrollment for persons with preexisting medical conditions, or they may accept a chronically ill member for a high monthly premium. The following three definitions explain aspects of a member's enrollment.

Open Enrollment Period

Open enrollment is a time period, usually during a specified month of the year, when a member may change health plans (Kongstvedt, 1993). As a rule, most managed care plans (specifically HMOs) have their open enrollment period in the fall, which becomes effective January 1. In Arizona, open enrollment for the state's Medicaid plan is in August and goes into effect October 1. For members unhappy with their health plan, it is important to know when open enrollment periods come around, since it is the one time of year that a plan change can be made without financial penalty to the member, regardless of health status. This feature will probably survive regardless of any legislative changes in healthcare in the 90s.

Disenrollment

Disenrollment is the process of terminating insurance coverage (Kongstvedt, 1993). Voluntary termination involves a member quitting simply out of personal desire. Involuntary termination can include reasons such as losing or changing jobs (see COBRA). A serious form of involuntary disenrollment can be for reasons such as fraud, abuse, nonpayment of agreed-upon copayments or premiums, or a demonstrated inability to comply with recommended treatment plans. Disenrollment for some of these reasons may be very difficult to prove and is therefore rare.

Consolidated Omnibus Budget Reconciliation Act (COBRA)

Under COBRA, employers with 20 or more employees are required to offer terminated employees an opportunity to continue health coverage under the present medical plan in exchange for a monthly premium. This premium may cost up to 102% of the actual cost of the premium, with 2% being administrative expenses (Williams & Torrens, 1993). The former employee has 60 days to decide if he or she desires to purchase insurance under COBRA (1993). If a COBRA policy is desired, the employee can keep it for up to 18 months, after which time another type of insurance needs to be obtained (1993).

Insurance Types

The following section discusses various types of insurance strategies. Matching needed services for patients with available resources is a primary nurse case management responsibility. Few people can afford medical services without the benefit of some form of insurance.

A basic understanding of insurance types is essential for the NCM. What is covered; how are the services reimbursed; what is the patient's fiscal responsibility; with whom is the patient allowed to follow up; where must the patient fill prescriptions—these and many other questions must be assessed with the insurance company for effective care planning.

Medicare

Perhaps the most well-known of all insurance plans in the United States, Medicare is a federally funded program under Title XIX of the Social Security Act. Medical services are provided to US citizens over the age of 65 who have worked at least 10 years (40 quarters, considered work credits), to those who qualify for Social Security Disability for at least 24 months, and to persons with permanent kidney failure who are on dialysis (Williams & Torrens, 1993). This federal health insurance program is overseen by the *Health Care Financing Administration (HCFA)* of the US Department of Health and Human Services.

Not all citizens automatically receive Medicare on their 65th birthday month. Often, they need to file an application. For a client who is 65 years old or older with a reliable work history and who does not show coverage under Medicare, social services may be able to help get the person on Medicare. Persons with renal failure must also apply (HCFA, 1994). Renal patients are eligible for Medicare after 3 months on hemodialysis. No age limits are imposed. Benefits will continue until 1 year after hemodialysis stops or a kidney transplantation is performed (InterQual & Tennant, 1993).

The care of Medicare patients is monitored by Peer Review Organizations (PROs) in each state. These are groups of physicians or other healthcare professionals hired by the federal government to assess whether the care meets standards of quality, is reasonable and necessary, and is provided in the most appropriate level of care. They also review any complaints from Medicare members; these range from poor care to premature discharge (HCFA, 1994).

Medicare Part A

Medicare is divided into two distinct and separately financed parts. Part A is known as the *Hospital Insurance* and includes coverage for hospital care, inpatient stays at a skilled nursing facility, home healthcare, and hospice care. Part A is premium-free and is earned based on a person's, or spouse's, employment credits (HCFA, 1994). It is financed through part of the Social Security (FICA) tax that all employees and employers pay out. Part A may be purchased under certain circumstances.

Medicare benefit periods are also known as "spells of illness." They measure the beneficiary's use of Part A or inpatient care. The information below is taken from the *Medicare 1994 Handbook* with 1995 price updates from the *Federal Register*; be aware that the dollar amounts change almost yearly.

- A benefit period *begins* upon admission to an inpatient facility.
- A benefit period *ends* when the member has been out of a hospital, skilled nursing facility, or rehabilitation facility for 60 consecutive days (including the day of discharge).
- There is no limit to the number of benefit periods the member can have for hospital and other skilled nursing facility care.
- Each time a benefit period is begun, a $716 hospital deductible charge is incurred.
- Medicare will pay for 100% of the beneficiary's hospitalization (minus the above deductible) for the first 60 days of any benefit period.
- From the 61st day until the 90th day in the hospital, the member is responsible for $179 per day. This $179 charge is called the coinsurance.
- If greater than 90 inpatient days are needed in a benefit period, Lifetime Reserve Days help offset medical expenses.
- Only 60 lifetime reserve days are given per beneficiary. These may be used up in one, two, or any number of benefit periods. If 10 reserve days are used up in 1 year, the member has 50 left to use any time that a benefit period exceeds 90 days. They are not renewable.
- Lifetime reserve days pay all hospital expenses but $358 per day. This $358/day is the responsibility of the member.
- Members can opt out of using the reserve days by telling the hospital in writing of their wishes.

Long or frequent inpatient admissions can cause eventual loss of Part A benefits. To lose these benefits, this patient would have to be in the hospital or an extended care facility (ECF) for 150 days (using up 90 days plus the 60 lifetime reserve days), without a reprieve of 60 consecutive days *out* of the hospital or ECF. Although this rarely happens, NCMs need to be aware of its possibility. Medigap plans cover an additional 365 hospital days after the lifetime reserve is used up. If the patient does not have a Medigap plan, that patient will most likely have to spend down to become eligible for a Medicaid plan.

Medicare Part A also pays for some posthospital skilled nursing facility (SNF) care. The patient must have been in the hospital under an acute admit (*not* observation status) for 3 days at the minimum. The patient may be discharged directly into a Medicare certified SNF or can go home and, if a skilled SNF need is discovered, can be admitted to a SNF within 30 days of the hospital discharge date (HCFA, 1994).

Medicare Part A helps pay for a maximum of 100 days *in each benefit period* for skilled care in an extended care facility (Table 5-1). The member pays nothing for the first 20 days; Medicare pays 100%. If the patient still needs additional skilled care at a SNF level, 80 additional days will be paid for, but the coinsurance to the member is $89.50 per day (1995). After 100 days in each benefit period, Medicare will not be financially responsible.

Medicare Part A also pays for home healthcare provided in lieu of hospitalization if certain criteria are met. Essentially, the member must be homebound, have a physician-ordered home healthcare treatment plan, and must require intermittent (rather than intensive) skilled nursing or skilled rehab services. As long as the above criteria are met, the Catastrophic Coverage Act of 1988 ensures that home health services can be covered for a maximum of 38 consecutive days (Corkery, 1989). If the services are deemed appropriate, they will be reimbursed at 100%.

Durable medical equipment (DME) has a coinsurance payment of 20%; Medicare will pay for 80% of covered DME (HCFA, 1994). Hospice care is also covered under certain conditions. Inpatient psychiatric care is reimbursed for up to 190 days, if needed (HCFA, 1994). Detailed requirements for skilled nursing facilities, home health services, rehabilitation care, and hospice coverage are discussed in Chapter 10: Discharge Planning: Understanding Levels of Care and Transfers.

Medicare Part B

Part B is also known as the *Medical Insurance*, and it includes coverage for physician services, outpatient hospital services, durable medical equipment, and other miscellaneous services. Monthly premiums for Part B in 1995 are $46.10 for most beneficiaries.

Medicare Part B can be purchased even if Part A requirements have not been met. Some Medicaid plans purchase Part B for their ineligible (for Part A) members as a cost-saving method. Part B has an annual deductible of $100, and any Part B

Table 5-1. Payment According to Level of Care in Each Benefit Period (1995)

	Hospital	
	Member Pays	Medicare Pays
Day 1–60	Deductible $716	All other qualified expenses
Day 61–90	$179/day coinsurance	All other qualified expenses
Day 91–150 Lifetime Reserve Days*	$358/day	All other qualified expenses
	Extended Care Facility	
Day 1–20	0	All other qualified expenses
Day 21–100	$89.50/day	All other qualified expenses

* Unlike other benefit periods, Lifetime Reserve Days are not renewable and can be used only once in a member's lifetime.

service can be used to fulfill that deductible. A 20% coinsurance is also owed by the member for many Part B services.

In general, Part B helps cover physician services, outpatient hospital care, diagnostic tests, radiology and pathology services (inpatient or outpatient), durable medical equipment, home health services, physical/occupational/speech therapies, and *limited* chiropractic, podiatry, dentistry, and optometry services (HCFA, 1994).

Like Medicare Part A, Part B will pay for 100% of approved home health services and 80% of durable medical equipment (HCFA, 1994), but not until after the $100 annual deductible is met. Kidney dialysis and kidney, liver, and heart transplantations may be partially covered under Part B when strict criteria are met (HCFA, 1994).

Both Part A and Part B cover blood components such as red blood cells, platelets, fresh frozen plasma. Both sections of Medicare require the recipient to pay for any replacement costs on the first three units. This replacement fee is the amount charged for blood that is not replaced. The replacement fee criteria can be satisfied with use on either the Part A or Part B side. Part A pays all costs from the fourth pint each calendar year. Part B pays for 80% starting with the fourth pint. The annual Part B deductible must also be met (HCFA, 1994).

Under certain circumstances, Medicare Part B pays for antigens, epoetin alfa when self-administered by dialysis patients, hemophilia clotting factors, hepatitis B vaccine, immunosuppressive drugs within 1 year of organ transplantations, flu and pneumococcal pneumonia vaccines (no deductible or coinsurance needed—100% reimbursed), and certain oral chemotherapy for cancer (HCFA, 1994).

In late 1993, traditional Medicare approved a limited number of IV medications to be administered in the home setting. Previously no IV medications were covered in the home. Because the cost of the medications is so high, many otherwise independent patients had to be transferred to nursing homes where IV medications are covered for long-term IV antibiotic regimens.

According to the Medicare DMERC Guide (1993–1994), the criteria for home IV medications include use of an infusion pump and a prolonged infusion of at least 8 hours or infusion of the drug at a controlled rate in order to avoid toxicity. Another means of accomplishing the infusion is not acceptable.

Some approved medications (with the above criteria) include acyclovir, foscarnet, amphotericin B, vancomycin, ganciclovir, selected narcotic analgesics such as morphine sulfate, and some chemotherapeutic agents when administered by continuous infusion over at least 24 hours. The home health agency called in to care for the patient can help the NCM in assessing which home intravenous medications are covered under Medicare.

Most prescription medications are not covered under either part of Medicare. This is a real hardship for chronically ill persons on a fixed income. Frequent readmissions should be assessed for "noncompliant patients" who are not taking their prescribed medications. Assess reasons for noncompliance:

- Can they afford them?
- Are they carefully doling them out, cutting the dose so the bottle will last longer?

- Some patients hoard old prescriptions for "emergency" use; they may be expired or the dosage may be too low or too high. People with no pharmacologic insurance coverage should be assessed and possibly helped to acquisition needed medicines.

Tables 5-2 and 5-3 help summarize the detailed list of hospital insurance covered services in both Part A and Part B. These tables are based on 1994 figures.

The Medicare system is not only complicated, but subject to changes in any year. Case managers may benefit from a recent copy of *The Medicare Handbook*, which is available from any Social Security Administration office.

NOTE

or write to the following address:
Health Care Financing Administration
6325 Security Blvd
Baltimore, Maryland 21207-5187
(Publication No. HCFA 10050)

Combined Medicare/Managed Care Plans

The combined plans are also known as Medicare Risk Contracts and offer prepaid, comprehensive health coverage. Instead of paying hospitals the traditional DRG payment, these risk contracts are actually health maintenance organizations (HMOs) or competitive medical plans (CMPs) and contract with members and hospitals like HMOs and CMPs. These HMO and CMPs contract with HCFA to provide services to Medicare patients for a fixed monthly payment. The plan is "at risk" if the services needed are more costly than the fixed payment.

From a member perspective, the out-of-pocket costs may be less than traditional Medicare, and added services such as preventive care, dental care, hearing aids, and eyeglasses may be included. All services must be approved and HMO/CMP authorized facilities must be used, unless urgent care is required, outside the plan's service area. Gatekeeper-style PCPs are generally required.

The NCM may now have to coordinate care with this Medicare's utilization review (UR) coordinator for necessary services and discharge planning. These plans offer less freedom of choice in that the NCM must match the Home Health Agency or ECF (for example) to the Medicare HMO-contracted facilities. Some advantages include more home intravenous medication coverage and added pharmacy coverage for the client.

Medigap Plans

In July 1992, the federal government approved a list of 10 standardized insurance policies designed to supplement, or fill in the gaps, of Medicare coverage. Before these plans were standardized, Medicare beneficiaries had to choose among so

Table 5-2. Medicare (Part A): Hospital Insurance-Covered Services for 1994

Services	Benefit	Medicare Pays	You Pay
Hospitalization			
Semiprivate room and board, general nursing, and other hospital services and supplies	First 60 dys	All but $716§ per benefit period	$716§
	Day 61 to 90	All but $179/day§	$179/day§
	Day 91 to 150*	All but $358/day§	$358/day§
	Beyond 150 days	Nothing	All costs
Skilled Nursing Facility Care			
Semiprivate room and board, general nursing, skilled nursing and rehabilitative services and other services and supplies†	First 20 days	100% of approved amount	Nothing
	21–100 days	All but $89.50/day§	Up to $89.50/day§
	Beyond 100 days	Nothing	All costs
Home Healthcare			
Part-time or intermittent skilled care, home health aide services, durable medical equipment, and supplies and other services	Unlimited as long as Medicare conditions are met	100% of approved amount; 80% of approved amount for durable medical equipment	Nothing for services; 20% of approved amount for durable medical equipment
Hospice Care			
Pain relief, symptom management, and support services for the terminally ill	For as long as doctor certifies need	All but limited costs for outpatient drugs and inpatient respite care	Limited costs for outpatient drugs and inpatient respite care
Blood			
	Unlimited if medically necessary	All but first 3 pints per calendar year	First 3 pints‡

Note: 1994 Part A monthly premium: None for most beneficiaries
Either $245 or $184 if you must buy Part A (either amount may be higher if you enroll late)
* This 60-reserve-days benefit may be used only once in a lifetime.
† Neither Medicare nor private Medigap insurance will pay for most custodial care.
‡ Blood paid for or replaced under Part B of Medicare during the calendar year does not have to be paid for or replaced under Part A.
§ Denotes 1995 costs.
(From Health Care Financing Administration [HCFA]. *The Medicare 1994 Handbook*, p. 39)

Table 5-3. Medicare (Part B): Hospital Insurance-Covered Services for 1994

Services	Benefit	Medicare Pays	You Pay
Medical Expenses			
Doctors' services, inpatient and out-patient medical and surgical services and supplies, physical and speech therapy, diagnostic tests, durable medical equipment, and other services	Unlimited if medically necessary	80% of approved amount (after $100 deductible) 50% of approved charges for most outpatient mental health services	$100 deductible,* plus 20% of approved amount and limited charges above approved amount
Clinical Laboratory Services			
Blood tests, urinalyses, and more	Unlimited if medically necessary	Generally 100% of approved amount	Nothing for services
Home Healthcare			
Part-time or intermittent skilled care, home health aide services, durable medical equipment, and supplies and other services	Unlimited as long as you meet Medicare conditions.	100% of approved amount; 80% of approved amount for durable medical equipment	Nothing for services; 20% of approved amount for durable medical equipment
Outpatient Hospital Treatment			
Services for the diagnosis or treatment of illness or injury	Unlimited if medically necessary	Medicare payment to hospital based on hospital cost	20% of billed amount (after $100 deductible)*
Blood			
	Unlimited if medically necessary	80% of approved amount (after $100 deductible and starting with 4th pint)	First 3 pints plus 20% of approved amount for additional pints (after $100 deductible)†

Note: 1995 Part B monthly premium: $46.10 (premium may be higher if you enroll late).

* Once you have had $100 of expenses for covered services in 1994, the Part B deductible does not apply to any further covered services you receive for the rest of the year.

† Blood paid for or replaced under Part A of Medicare during the calendar year does not have to be paid for or replaced under Part B.

(From Health Care Financing Administration [HCFA]. *The Medicare 1994 Handbook*, p. 40) many vague Medicare supplemental policies that often the NCM would find that their clients had supplements that were both inadequate and duplicative.

Although the federal government does not offer these policies, since they are private insurance policies, the government requires strict adherence to guidelines. Both federal and state laws govern the sales of Medigap insurance. They may not sell a policy that duplicates the member's present health plan or sell a policy that is not one of the approved standard policies (HCFA, 1994).

The 10 plans are identified by the letters A through J (Table 5-4). Each plan must include a core package of benefits. And all 10 plans cover an additional 365 days of approved inpatient hospitalization after the long-term reserve days (see section under Medicare) have been used up (HCFA, 1994).

The core benefits include (Grimaldi, 1992):

- Part A hospital coinsurance—equaling $179 per day (1995), starting from day 61
- Part B coinsurance, which is 20% of Medicare approved charges
- First 3 pints of blood each year

Note that the core benefits do not include such basics as the Part A inpatient deducible ($716 per benefit period in 1995) or the Part B deductible ($100 annually in 1994).

Medigap's Plan A covers only the core benefits. Plans B through J include the core benefits plus a menu of variable coverage. Of course, the more coverage, the higher the premium rate. Plan J includes all nine benefits, which are as follows:

- Basic (core) benefits

Table 5-4. Ten Standard Medigap Policies (Plan A-Plan J)

Benefits	Plans									
	A	B	C	D	E	F	G	H	I	J
Core benefit	X	X	X	X	X	X	X	X	X	X
Skilled nursing coinsurance			X	X	X	X	X	X	X	X
Part A Deductible		X	X	X	X	X	X	X	X	X
Part B Excess 100%						X	X		X	X
Foreign travel emergency			X	X	X	X	X	X	X	X
At-home recovery				X			X		X	X
Basic drugs $1250 limit								X	X	
Basic drugs $3000 limit										X
Preventive care					X					X

(Adapted from *Federal Register* (1992, August 21) *57*, 37999; and Grimaldi, P. (1992). Medigap insurance policies standardized. *Nursing Management*)

- Skilled nursing coinsurance—$89.50 (1995) per day while in an ECF from day 21 to day 100.
- Part A deductible—$716 per benefit period in 1995
- Part B deductible—$100 annually in 1994
- Part B excess (100%)
- Foreign travel emergencies
- At-home recovery—provides short-term assistance with various activities of daily living (ADLs) for members who are recovering from an episode of illness, injury or surgery. Services may include a homemaker or personal care aid. The maximum payment allowed is $40 per visit up to $1600 per year (Grimaldi, 1992).
- Prescriptions—Plans H and I have a limit of $1250 annually. Plan J has a limit of $3000 annually. The prescription benefit has a $250 deducible per calendar year and pays for 50% of the outpatient drug charges until the maximum is reached (Grimaldi, 1994).
- Preventive care—includes such services as vaccines, hearing tests, urinalysis, occult stool testing, serum cholesterol, thyroid function testing, and mammogram. A $120 annual limit is enforced (Grimaldi, 1992).

Medicare Select

Medicare Select is a Preferred Provider Organization (PPO) arrangement in which Medicare beneficiaries agree to use the network of preferred providers in return for lower premiums. It is a Medigap type insurance approved in 15 states: Alabama, Arizona, California, Florida, Indiana, Kentucky, Michigan, Minnesota, Missouri, North Dakota, Ohio, Oregon, Texas, Washington, and Wisconsin. The member may lose coverage if an outside (not network) provider is used, except in an emergency (HCFA, 1994).

Medicaid

Medicaid, like Medicare, is a federally funded healthcare program under Title XIX of the Social Security Act. Medicaid was enacted into law on July 20, 1964 (Williams & Torrens, 1993) and is part of the federal and state welfare system. Prior to 1965, physicians and hospitals often gave out charity care or billed on a sliding-scale basis. Eligibility for Medicaid is based on income and/or various welfare categories such as Aid to Families with Dependent Children (AFDC) (1993).

Many Medicare recipients financially also qualify for Medicaid. If a client has both Medicare and Medicaid, a supplemental policy may be redundant. The Medicaid portion will cover all Medicare deductibles, coinsurance, medically necessary care, and prescription medications. Home IV medications may also be covered under this insurance arrangement.

The member with only Medicaid generally has no premiums, deductibles, or coinsurance costs. Prescription drugs are paid for, although some states have a "negative formulary list," which excludes some medications and substitutes others. Some states may also require a small out-of-pocket charge for doctor visits or prescriptions; this is rarely enforced.

Medicaid programs are subject to state regulatory agencies; therefore, wide variations in coverage and eligibility exist among the different states. Title XIX of the Social Security Act does mandate certain basic health services. Each state, however, may determine the scope of services offered or may offer optional services such as clinic services and dental or optometry services (Williams & Torrens, 1993).

Some core Medicaid benefits include (Williams & Torrens, 1993):

- hospital inpatient care
- hospital outpatient services
- prenatal care
- laboratory and x-ray services
- skilled nursing facility care for ages 21 and older
- home health services
- physician services
- family planning services and supplies
- rural health clinic services
- EPSDT—early and periodic screening, diagnosis, and treatment for children under 21 years of age
- nurse-midwife services
- certain federally qualified ambulatory and health center services

Because of the vagueness of some covered Medicaid services, the NCM may be able to negotiate resources for the client. If services requested are in lieu of hospitalization or an ECF placement or are necessary for patient safety, the Medicaid plan *may* choose to accommodate the request. Because of budget cuts, however, fewer nonemergent services are being provided. This makes the patient advocacy role even more critical when it comes to planning safe and adequate discharges.

Most Medicaid plans do not cover services such as inpatient drug or alcohol programs. The NCM and social worker may be limited to community programs, which might be free or on a sliding fee scale. A baseline knowledge of what your state's Medicaid coverage services includes can save the NCM from assessment of time-consuming plans that will not be fulfilled.

Medicaid began as a fee-for-service program in the 1960s. Now many states have changed to capitated payments or per diem rates as a primary method of reimbursement. In Arizona, the state's Medicaid Plan is known as AHCCCS (Arizona Health Care Cost Containment System) and pays hospitals on a per diem basis. As an example, the Medical patient receives approximately $750 per day for care in the hospital. An MRI (magnetic resonance imaging) uses up most of that, but also included in the per diem rate is all care from labs to radiology to nurses. Since hospital patients are so ill (or they are not admitted—see Chapter 6: Utilization Management), it is easy to see that for many multisystem failure patients who are resource intensive, this rate will be inadequate. Tight utilization of resources is important. The challenge is providing medically necessary care to ill patients while striving for a fiscally healthy institution—all within the confines of a Medicaid per diem rate. Reimbursement styles may change again this decade, and awareness of this will help the NCM to plan appropriate care.

Medicaid Eligibility

The following are some of the categories that allow Medicaid eligibility. To be *categorically eligible*, individuals must fit into a category that makes them eligible according to Title XIX (Medicaid) of the Social Security Act. Recipients of Supplemental Security Income (SSI) and those who qualify for Aid to Families with Dependent Children (AFDC) are automatically eligible for Medicaid (Williams & Torrens, 1993).

Medical Assistance Only (MAO). A special category of Medicaid recipients under AFDC or SSI who receive only Medicaid benefits and not financial assistance.

Medically Needy/Medically Indigent (MN/MI). A category of Medicaid recipients in which Medicaid receives funds only from county and state treasuries. Other categories may also receive matched federal funds.

Sixth Omnibus Budget Reconciliation Act (S.O.B.R.A.). One of Medicaid's maternal and child health reforms that was passed by Congress and became effective in 1987. Pregnant women and children with family incomes at or below the poverty level become eligible for Medicaid.

Blind and disabled persons who also receive SSI, and certain other specifically defined categories, are also eligible for Medicaid (Williams & Torrens, 1993). If an NCM has a patient who may qualify for Medicaid, most large hospitals and DES (Department of Economic Security) or Social Security Administration offices have eligibility workers. These are employees of a county, DES, or Social Security, whose job is to determine eligibility for Medicaid through interviews and assessing medical and financial data.

CHAMPUS

CHAMPUS is an acronym for Civilian Health and Medical Program of the Uniformed Services. It is a program of medical benefits for covered military personnel and eligible family members. By strict definition, CHAMPUS is not an insurance program. It doesn't involve a contract guaranteeing medical coverage in exchange for a premium, and it is not subject to the state regulatory agencies that cover most insurance plans. CHAMPUS is provided for by US governmental funds, which are appropriated through Congress. Medically necessary and certain psychologically necessary services are covered and are detailed in the Department of Defense (DOD) directive (Kongstvedt, 1993). Benefits under CHAMPUS are equivalent to high-option plans of the public sector. Because of CHAMPUS's historical generosity to its members, expenditures and claims have doubled since 1985. Reform initiatives are changing the face of CHAMPUS, and now some CHAMPUS programs strongly resemble HMOs and PPOs; like Medicare, they reimburse hospitals at a DRG rate (1993).

Workers' Compensation

The Workers' Compensation laws began in 1908 by federal statute. The first state to enact the law was New York in 1914, in response to a factory fire in which 146 women lost their lives. Mississippi was the last state to enact the law in 1950 (Williams & Torrens, 1993). Workers' Compensation is compulsory in most states and is designed to provide compensation and medical benefits if an employee is hurt or disabled while on the job (1993).

Three types of benefits are provided, although the scope is mandated by individual states.

1. Indemnity cash benefits in lieu of lost wages (Williams & Torrens, 1993)
2. Reimbursement for necessary medical expenses (1993)
3. Survivors' death benefits (1993)

Workers' compensation, like all facets of the healthcare industry, is a victim of a system out of control. In 1992, Workers' Compensation claims reached an estimated $70 billion. That is triple the benefit figure of 1980 (InterQual & Tennant, 1993). To offset the spiraling costs, recent changes are being implemented, including adaptations of PPOs, HMOs, and hospital utilization review. These types of managed care modalities are expected to grow rapidly and have already proven effective in reducing LOS and even avoiding medically unnecessary admissions.

Workers' Compensation claims frequently involve trauma, repetitive motion, or neuromuscular impairment. There is a growing trend toward alleged soft tissue claims with nonspecific diagnosis. These claims pose a challenge from the UR perspective, since they often lack objective physical findings. From a patient advocate perspective, an admitting diagnosis of severe back pain (especially without positive test results) often opens up these patients to denials of insurance-covered hospitalizations and even judgmental attitudes among hospital staff. Yet, as nurses (who are especially prone to back injuries) know, the most painful sprains, muscle spasms, and pinched nerves don't show up on scans, but can lead to inability to work and frequent reinjuries. Often the patient needs reassurance that care is necessary and that it can be provided for at a different level of care (ie, it doesn't always need to be done in the hospital). The primary goal of Workers' Compensation is for the client to return to work.

Indemnity Plans

Indemnity Plans are the traditional plans before the days of managed care. Although they now use some managed care concepts such as prehospital certification and catastrophic case management, indemnity plans still offer the most flexibility (Kongstvedt, 1993); virtually any hospital or doctor can be chosen by the member. Monthly premiums are generally higher for this freedom, and other out-of-pocket expenses may include deductibles and a percentage of the bills (usually 20%) up to a ceiling of $500 to $5000 per year. As with all insurance companies, the case manager needs to know the specific types of allowable coverage and possible patient costs to formulate a workable discharge plan. Indemnity plans often cover mental health and alcohol and drug detoxification treatment, both inpatient and outpatient, within certain limited time frames and dollar amounts.

Managed Indemnity Plans (MIP)

The evolution of the old indemnity plans, MIPs use utilization management (UM) strategies such as hospital preadmission screening, concurrent review, second surgical opinions, outpatient procedure services review, and case management. They keep the traditional indemnity approach of members' freedom of choice of physicians/providers and fee-for-service payment to these providers (Coleman, 1994).

Managed Care Organization (MCO)

MCO is a generic term that applies to managed care plans. These plans have programs that include utilization management (UM) modalities: preadmission, concurrent and retrospective review programs, case management, referral management, utilization reporting and evaluation programs, and provider incentive programs. MCOs also focus on quality assurance activities, such as credentialing, quality assessment studies, and peer review. The evolution of healthcare is toward some variation of managed care organization, such as HMOs, PPOs, and POS plans (Kongstvedt, 1993).

Health Maintenance Organization (HMO)

In its purest form, an HMO is nearly synonymous with managed care; a member must go through the chosen PCP (primary care physician) who acts as a gatekeeper for any needed services (Kongstvedt, 1993). Only HMO-contracted facilities and physicians are allowed. Members who use unauthorized doctors or facilities are usually required to pay for services rendered. Limited psychiatric and dental care and limited coverage when traveling are other disadvantages.

HMOs have potentially the least expensive premiums, often with no deductibles, coinsurance, or claim forms to fill out. Some copayments at the time of service may be expected. Physicians and other healthcare professionals are paid for through capitation, thereby sharing the risk of financing the healthcare for the enrolled population. If the provider incurs expenses exceeding budgeted cost, they would be required to absorb those excesses, not the member.

HMO Models

There are five models of HMOs: Staff Model, Group Model, Individual Practice Association (IPA), Network Model, and the Direct Contract Model. The relationship between the HMO and the physicians distinguishes the various models.

Staff Model. In this model, the HMO employs the physicians who work in HMO clinic–type settings (exclusively) for salaries. This model is considered the most cost-effective, but also the most restrictive (InterQual & Tennant, 1993).

Group Model. Here, the HMO contracts with multispecialty physician groups. These groups provide all services to its members. The members' choice of providers is wider in this model (1993).

Independent Practice Association (IPA). IPA model HMOs recruit physicians from all specialties to care for their HMO members. These physicians are also free to service non-HMO patients, if desired. The IPA is paid on a capitation basis by the HMO, and the physicians are in turn paid in either a fee-for-service or capitated manner (Kongstvedt, 1993).

Network Model. This model combines elements of the staff, group, and IPA styles. The HMO contracts with more than one group practice (Williams & Torrens, 1993).

Direct Contract Model. In this model, the HMO contracts directly with the physician, rather than through an intermediary such as an IPA (Kongstvedt, 1993). The gatekeeper approach is common in this model. Fee-for-service or capitation is the reimbursement method, although capitation is the preferred method because it limits financial risk for the HMO.

Preferred Provider Organization (PPO) (also called Preferred Provider Arrangements [PPA])

This model falls somewhere between an HMO and an indemnity plan. PPOs use a "preferred" panel of physicians who have been selected because of their cost-efficient and quality care (Kongstvedt, 1993). The member has a monthly premium, a deductible and often a 10% to 20% coinsurance up to a specific ceiling of about $500 to $2000 per year. A major advantage for some members is the ability to use doctors who are not on the plan, but reimbursement is at a lower rate (ie, more out-of-pocket for the member). This is important to some people who hesitate to choose an HMO because HMOs don't pay at all if outside facilities or physicians are used. Members are encouraged, but not obligated, to use the gatekeeper PCP concept in many PPOs (InterQual & Tennant, 1993).

Exclusive Provider Organization (EPO)

An EPO is very much like a PPO in the choice of physicians and their organization. The major difference between a PPO and an EPO is that EPO members do not get any reimbursement if they use physicians outside the EPO network. EPOs may also use the gatekeeper approach (Williams & Torrens, 1993).

Point of Service (POS)

POS plans combine elements of an HMO model and an indemnity plan. The member does not have to choose how to receive services up front; when a service is needed, the member may choose to stay in the plan or use outside providers (Kongstvedt, 1993). Significant differences in out-of-pocket expenses for the member may apply (eg, 100% compared with 60%). The physicians may be reimbursed through capitation or performance-based methods and may act as a gatekeeper. POS plans were hybrids of HMOs mainly in response to a market that clearly wanted freedom of choice to pick a well-known specialist if the need should arise.

Physician Hospital Organizations (PHO)

The PHO model bonds a hospital with the attending staff for the purpose of linking with a managed care plan (Kongstvedt, 1993). Like IPAs, PHOs have their own internal political structure and therefore can define on their own terms what is high quality or cost-effective. Some PHOs use outside utilization review firms, which allows some degree of objectivity.

Long-Term Care (LTC)

In some ways, LTC becomes one of the biggest challenges for the case manager. Although an increasing number of people are buying LTC insurance policies and many states have coverage for poor, chronically ill patients, there are often waiting periods of up to 3 months for all the paperwork to be approved and placement to commence. Sometimes families can manage for the interim. Often, this is a time of frequent readmissions into the acute care setting. Medicare, Medicaid, and most private insurance will pay for short stays in a nursing home for *skilled* care. A case manager can assess clients for a possible need of greater than 3 weeks of nursing home care or a probable deterioration of the patient's condition with little chance of recovery. It is vital to start LTC paperwork quickly; early, careful assessment of postdischarge needs (sometimes with a Plan B in mind) is also essential. Custodial care needs, as well as skilled needs, are assessed. Many LTC programs have home-based and ECF-based support. Family support and available respite can be assessed for possible home-based LTC placement. A case manager who is familiar with the eligibility requirements and enrollment process of their state's LTC program will be better prepared to meet these challenging situations.

Other Weird Arrangement (OWA)

OWA is an acronym that applies to any new, nonconforming managed care plan that provides a new twist (Kongstvedt, 1993).

Third Party Payor

In this arrangement, the two primary parties are the patient and the vendor (ie, physician or hospital). The third party is the payor of the medical care that is provider to the patient, usually a private insurance carrier, prepayment plan, employer, or government agency (InterQual & Tennant, 1993).

Third Party Liability (TPL)

TPL can best be understood by an example. Suppose an automobile accident victim is admitted to the hospital. Mr. Victim was sitting at a red light when Mr. Careless hit him from behind. Mr. Victim had lacerations and facial swelling caused by his hitting the steering wheel. He had to be monitored for a possible cardiac contusion. Mr. Victim and Mr. Careless both had medical and automobile insurance. Most likely, Mr. Careless's auto insurance would be the third party who is liable for Mr. Victim's hospital bill.

Insurance companies keep a close eye on certain red-flag indicators that may signal third party liability. Some target diagnoses may include motor vehicle accidents, multiple trauma, near-drowning, unnatural events such as explosions, burns, assaults, fractures, and lacerations. Insurance sources that may be liable include automobile, homeowner's, workers' compensation, malpractice, and product liability insurance.

Important Miscellaneous Organizations and Terms

JCAHO

JCAHO, also known as Joint Commission, also known as Joint Commission for the Accreditation of Health Care Organizations, is a private organization founded in 1951. It establishes quality standards and surveys hospitals, nursing homes, and other outpatient facilities to accredit the facilities. Accredited facilities are deemed to meet DHHS's (Department of Health and Human Services) certification requirements. It is hoped that the accreditation process encourages the facility to maintain the highest quality and performance levels (Williams & Torrens, 1993). JCAHO accreditation is necessary for hospitals and other facilities to be eligible to receive reimbursement from Medicare and other health plans.

Days per Thousand

Days per thousand is a measurement commonly used by insurance companies, which states the number of hospital days used per year for each 1000 members (Kongstvedt, 1993).

Grievance

Grievance is a term that refers to the complaint process that can occur when an adverse action, outcome, decision, or policy is challenged (Kongstvedt, 1993). A member can file a grievance for any number of reasons, such as a physician complaint, denial of a medical claim, denial of a piece of equipment, or a poor hospital outcome. A hospital or other facility may file a grievance for a denial of a claim they felt was medically justified.

MIS-Management Information System

MIS-management information system is the computer term for hardware and software that provides support for managing health plans, including case management (Kongstvedt, 1993).

Office of Prepaid Health Care Operations and Oversight (OPCOO)

OPCOO is the federal agency that is part of HCFA; it oversees eligibility and compliance of HMOs and CMPs.

Clinical Data Abstraction Centers (CDACs)

CDACs are utilization review firms contracted by HCFA. These centers are expected to collect clinical data from 3.5 million records by 1999. The data are then analyzed by the Medicare PROs to identify areas of care for quality improvement projects (Anonymous, 1994).

Contemporary Issues in Healthcare

The following are terms used in various healthcare reform proposals. Some were components of the failed efforts by the government to reform the nation's health system. The bill for this effort reached approximately $9.6 million, according to the US General Accounting Office (GAO), but final audits are expected to be as high as $15 million (Arizona Hospital Association Weekly Newsletter, April 7, 1995). If efforts resurface in the future, some of the following terminology will be meaningful.

Notch Group. The term *notch group* refers to the portion of the American population whose annual income is too low to afford medical insurance premiums but too high to be eligible for Medicaid programs. This concept seems innocuous enough, but a staggering statistic is attached to it: over 38.9 million Americans were uninsured in 1992!

Universal Healthcare Coverage. It was the notch group that prompted Congress to attempt to provide universal healthcare coverage, that is coverage for all Americans. The target date for this was January 1, 1998 (Connell, 1994). Several plans were examined, each addressing how this could be accomplished: The American Health Security Act (the plan proposed to Congress by President Clinton), the Affordable Health Care Now Act, the Managed Competition Act, the Consumer Choice Health Security Act, the Health Equity and Access Reform Today Act, and the Comprehensive Family Health Access and Savings Act (Cannella, 1994).

All the plans approached the problem of spending $900 billion annually on healthcare from a different perspective (Cannella, 1994). Most agree on several fundamentals: that preexisting conditions as a reason for denial of coverage must be eliminated; that the red tape must be reduced; that the policies should be portable (taken from job to job with the member); that malpractice liability must be reformed; and that the government provide subsidies for low-income persons so that insurance is affordable (Cannella, 1994).

Guaranteed Health Benefit Package. The package of benefits that all Americans would be guaranteed is called the Guaranteed Health Benefit Package.

The proposal resembled a basic managed care policy. Out-of-pocket expenses include deductibles and copayments (usually 20%), with annual maximum expenditures of $1,500 per person or $3,000 per family (Cannella, 1993). Basic benefits include inpatient hospitalization, approved outpatient and emergency services, home healthcare, preventive care focusing on prenatal and well-baby, outpatient physical and speech therapies, prescription medications, and limited dental and vision services (Cannella, 1993).

Health Alliances. Health alliances are healthcare "brokers" who purchase healthcare services for large groups of consumers. Regional health alliances were proposed to be created by each state and corporate alliances by large corporations that exceed perhaps 5,000 employees. Under the American Health Security Act Plan, a state would be permitted to fold beneficiaries into their alliance when they become eligible for Medicare, thus creating another option to Medicare (Cannella, 1993).

National Health Board. A National Health Board was proposed to oversee the states' creation of regional health alliances. This federal panel would interpret the healthcare packages, enforce the healthcare budget, monitor the quality of care, and investigate pharmaceutical pricing.

Employer Mandate. The proposed employer mandate consisted of the mandated contributions to healthcare coverage that an employer must make for its employees. Mandating businesses to buy health insurance for workers and their families was the topic of much debate and contention. Opponents felt that the employer mandate could drive up costs and put some companies out of business. Others simply didn't want to be forced (mandated) into this decision. It was proposed that larger businesses may be required to pick up 80% of the premiums, with the employee paying 20%. Low-income workers would receive subsidies. Smaller businesses would be required to pay a 1% or 2% payroll tax rather than 80% of the premium (Connell, 1994).

Managed Competition. Managed competition is an interesting marriage, uniting the concepts of free-market enterprise and government regulation. For example, large groups of consumers would be able to buy healthcare from networks of providers who are under government regulations. The goal would be to create business competition among the networks, which in free-enterprise fashion should encourage cost restraints and quality of care (Cannella, 1993). If managed competition did not prove to keep prices down, two backup mechanisms were discussed: (1) insurance premiums can be capped based on regional targets, and (2) a national health board can review the benefit package and recommend changes that would keep the benefits within a target budget. These would have been in the form of revisions to Congress but with the stipulation that if Congress didn't act quickly to reject them, the recommended revisions would become law (Connell, 1994).

National Health Security Card. This card would identify the member's eligibility for government guaranteed benefits (Cannella, 1993). Some suggested adding the beneficiary's medical history and physical , leaving new ethical and privacy issues open for debate.

The future change of the face of healthcare leaves the possibility of wide revisions on many types of medical insurance. Even Medicare—almost a part of the American tradition—is dramatically changing in an effort to lower the budget by several million dollars. Many visions of future healthcare have been proposed. Although the first major attempt at national health reform was unsuccessful, one thing is certain: the cost of healthcare is high and rising rapidly, and change is still sorely needed to cover the needs of millions of uninsured Americans. The crystal ball has not revealed the final answer, but one probability looms large: that NCMs, in grassroots fashion and on a case-by-case basis, can make an impact on the high cost of health services and help ensure quality care in the bargain.

CASE STUDY

Mr. Anderson, age 72, presents with fevers, malaise, and shortness of breath. He has had these symptoms for more than 3 weeks. At an office visit, his primary care physician appreciated a cardiac murmur; his temperature was 38.8° C. Mr. Anderson was admitted for further workup.

An echocardiogram was performed showing some vegetations. Blood cultures were positive. Mr. Anderson was diagnosed with endocarditis and was started on intravenous penicillin every 4 hours and gentamicin every 8 hours. The expected length of treatment was 4 to 6 weeks of intravenous therapy.

Mr. Anderson has been a healthy, active man who has loved golfing, boating, and traveling with his wife. Mrs. Anderson retired 2 years ago as a registered nurse supervisor at a large teaching hospital and was capable of taking care of her husband's medical needs at home.

Mr. Anderson's insurance coverage includes traditional Medicare A and B and a standard supplemental policy. Like most Medicare policies, this one would pay for intravenous antibiotics in a hospital or an extended care setting. These medications would not be paid for in a home setting.

After assessing the weekly cost of the doses of penicillin and gentamicin, Mr. and Mrs. Anderson felt they could not afford to pay without the aid of insurance for 4 to 6 weeks. After Mr. Anderson spent 3 days in the hospital, he and his wife reluctantly agreed that he would be transferred to an extended care facility for 4 to 6 weeks for his treatment.

CASE STUDY QUESTIONS

1. Was there a way to discharge this patient home and get insurance to pay for his IV antibiotics? Consider his social support. Consider the frequency of his antibiotic doses.
2. If this patient had Medicare and Medicaid (as a supplement), would discharge options have been expanded? What if the patient had a newer "risk" type of Medicare?
3. If the patient had private insurance, would discharge options be different?
4. Discuss admitting symptoms. Do they meet intensity screens for acute hospitalization?
5. Did the patient need to wait 3 days before being admitted to the extended care facility? Why?

References

Anonymous. (1994). HCFA awards $66 million to UR firm, PRO to abstract records for PROS. *Medical Utilization Management, 22*(17).

Anonymous. (1995). Federal efforts to cure healthcare were costly. *Arizona Hospital Association Weekly Newsletter, 9*(14).

Cannella, D. (1993, September 19). Proposal could turn family doctor into medical dinosaur. *Arizona Republic*, A9.

Cannella, D. (1994, January 30). Shaping the debate on health: Clinton faces competing plans. *Arizona Republic*, A1, A6, A7.

Coleman, J. (1994). The managed care organization evolution. *The Case Manager, 5*(1), 75–82.

Connell, C. (1994, June 10). Health care plan gets initial approval. *The Phoenix Gazette*, A1, A14.

Corkery, E. (1989). Discharge planning and home health care: What every staff nurse should know. *Orthopaedic Nursing, 8*(6), 18–26.

Grimaldi, P. (1992). Medigap insurance policies standardized. *Nursing Management, 23*(11), 20, 22, 24.

Health Care Financing Administration. (1994). *The Medicare 1994 Handbook*. DHHS Publication No. HCFA 10050. Baltimore, MD.

Health care Knowledge Resources. (1991). *Length of stay by diagnosis and operation*. Ann Arbor: Author.

InterQual & Tennant, T. (Eds.) (1993). *Utilization review and management training manual*. North Hampton: Author.

Kongstvedt, P. R. (1993). *The managed health care handbook*. Gaithersburg: Aspen Publishers.

Saue, J. M. (1988, August). Legal issues related to case management. *Quality Review Bulletin*, JCAHO, Chicago, IL, pp. 80–85.

Williams, S. J., & Torrens, P. R. (1993). *Introduction to health services*. New York: Delmar.

CHAPTER 6

Utilization Management

IMPORTANT TERMS AND CONCEPTS

admission review
appropriate level of care
concurrent authorization
concurrent review
continued stay review
Clinical Pathways/critical pathways
denial
discharge reviews
discharge screens
Healthcare Management Guidelines
   (HMG)
Intensity of Service (IS)
InterQual
ISD-A criteria
lag days
Length of Stay (LOS)
medical necessity

Milliman & Robertson
Optimal Recovery Guidelines (ORG)
patient advocacy
pending review
preadmission review
precertification
prospective authorization
prospective review
retrospective authorization
retrospective review
Severity of Illness (SI)
subauthorization
subsequent reviews
telephonics
utilization management (UM)
utilization review (UR)
variances

Nurse case managers (NCMs) who came from the ranks of the utilization review (UR) nurses of the 80s feel at home in the UR role. But many NCMs who came straight in through the clinical doorway (ICU nurses, staff nurses) find UR overwhelming and frustrating. The purpose of this chapter is to break down the concepts into clear and usable pieces. It is not difficult; so relax. Sometimes it is frustrating, however; not all patients fit neatly into the allotted categories, and the criteria are getting stricter and more demanding each year.

Good UR includes the use of medical instincts or "nursing intuition." Often a patient does not meet official criteria to be hospitalized, but the NCM senses something unstable about the patient. Within 24 hours, the patient crashes and is admitted to the intensive care unit. Perhaps the NCM spoke to the insurance UR department earlier and received a "denial" notice; a second phone call would rescind the denial and substantiate why the NCM was hesitant to "push" for a discharge or transfer to a lesser level of care. Occasionally, an insurance reviewer is very set on using the company's chosen utilization modality as though it were law. "Cookbook" UR is very frustrating and probably accounts for the number one reason why many NCMs prefer root canals to UR responsibilities.

Utilization review is the process by which the utilization of hospital resources and days are monitored. UR modalities use established criteria to evaluate medical services for necessity, level of care for appropriateness, and the timeliness of discharge (Sederer, 1987). The goal is to use the healthcare resources to provide the highest quality of patient care in the most cost-efficient setting. Perhaps a more appropriate term is *utilization management* (UM), since NCMs are managing the utilization of healthcare resources and not merely reviewing them.

Utilization management is primarily a cost-containment activity; therefore, it is essential for the NCM to focus on the patient advocacy role. The NCM assesses the whole clinical picture. If an insurance company comes in with inappropriate threats of "denied stays," the NCM may let the company know that it will be challenged for reasons of patient safety or medical necessity. This requires thorough knowledge of UR modalities and criteria—and a thorough assessment of the patient. Bear in mind that UR nurses are constantly asking themselves, "What is it about this case that makes it impossible for the patient to be safely cared for at a lesser level of care?" The NCM must be prepared to answer this question and to back up the answer with clinical facts.

Utilization management is important. It allows services to be authorized by insurance companies; simply put, hospitals must get paid for services in order to stay open. Utilization modalities also encourage fiscally responsible length of stays and offer the NCM an efficient aid for determining medical necessity as the patient moves through the healthcare maze.

Although utilization management is within the scope of the NCM's responsibilities, case management goes beyond UM, enhancing *all* aspects of patient care—psychosocial as well as medical. In a sense, UR is *reactive* to medical criteria, whereas nursing case management is *proactive*. Cookbook UR (ie, poor UR) has the goal of removing the patient from cost-intensive settings as quickly as possible. Good nursing case management may have the same end point, but it uses patient advocacy and a multidisciplinary team approach to planning and implementation of care to achieve that end point. Sometimes merging the roles of utilization management and patient advocacy seems to cause conflict (see Chapter 8: Ethical Issues and Dilemmas) This conflict may signal the need for discussion between a physician and an NCM, or even a full conference with the multidisciplinary team on the case.

Utilization Review Services

The following reflect the main types of UR services. Each one also provides a career opportunity for those who would like to focus on utilization management.

Preadmission Review

Also called precertification or prospective review, preadmission review is a certification that takes place before ("pre") services are rendered (CMRI, 1990). Here the reviewer determines whether admission to the facility (ie, hospital, rehab unit, surgicenter, extended care facility [ECF]) is reasonable and medically necessary. Since the attending physician has the ultimate responsibility for the patient, this physician will determine admitting status, regardless of authorization. A compromise may be a 24-hour authorization to see whether the patient needs that particular level of care or a "pending review" status.

Concurrent Review

A concurrent review is performed while the patient is in the facility. The reviewer often visits the facility for this role, but with more UR firms cropping up, telephone review is equally as common. Here, the utilization management nurse would be assessing the appropriateness of the level of care such as intensive care unit, step-down, telemetry, floor care, extended care, rehabilitation care, or home with home health. Medical appropriateness is gauged by monitoring and evaluating the medical condition of the patient against the services performed. Concurrent review has two parameters:

1. *Admission review*—performed within 24 to 48 hours.
2. *Continued stay review*—performed at specific points during the patient's stay. If the patient is critical, a review every 2 to 3 days may be an acceptable time frame. If the patient is nearing a change in level of care, daily reviews are necessary.

Retrospective Review

A retrospective review is performed after discharge (CMRI, 1990). Medicare charts are often reviewed retrospectively. Reviewers come to the facility, request patient charts from medical records, and perform their review. They may authorize the whole hospital admission or deny payment in whole or in part. Although concurrent review feels more honest and up front, retrospective review is a reality that NCMs need to be aware of.

Retrospective review is a useful tool for looking at quality control. Monday morning quarterbacking can often prevent similar quality issues from repeating themselves if a preventive plan is assessed and implemented.

Telephonics

Telephonics is UR done by telephone, usually concurrently. This is a less expensive way for insurance companies to perform UR, but the reviews are only as good as the information elicited. Poor or inadequate information can result from the reviewer's not knowing medically important questions to ask for a particular admitting diagnosis. If the hospital does not have a case management or UR department, the information must be elicited systematically from the staff nurse taking care of the patient. The reviewer must ask the questions that will efficiently demonstrate whether the patient needs continued stay at the present level of care. The staff nurses should know what IVs the patient is on, some lab results, and the patient's response to treatment. But their time is limited, and many staff nurses resent speaking to insurance companies or feel they cannot give out information over the phone because of confidentiality issues.

Telephonics without a good UR nurse or NCM on the patient end is the least effective means of UR. Yet a good NCM or utilization management nurse combined with insurance telephonics may be good for everyone. It keeps hundreds of UR nurses out of your facility and still maintains that the institution is "user-friendly." For insurance companies, use of telephonics is the least expensive method of acquiring the information they require.

Insurance Authorizations

Types of insurance authorization follow logically from the types of UR:

Prospective or Precertification Authorization. This is authorization given prior to services rendered. Prospective payment usually refers to a diagnosis-related group (DRG) payment, in which one amount is given for all services needed based on a specific diagnosis (Kongstvedt, 1993; see Chapter 5: Insurance).

Concurrent Authorization. This authorization is generated at the time the service is rendered (1993).

Retrospective Authorization. This authorization is approved after the services have been performed (1993).

Pended (for Review). Here the hospital keeps their fingers crossed in hopes of a real authorization (1993). *Pending review* has been described as a state of "authorization purgatory," since the institution is unsure *if* an authorization will be given. This state may lead to retrospective review and authorization or a denial of services in whole or in part.

Denial. No authorization was given for services (1993). Grievance procedures may commence and are often won, especially with good physician NCM and UR documentation.

Subauthorization. One authorization number allows other services to piggyback on it. For example, a single authorization number is given for a cholecystectomy. This number can be used by the surgeon, radiologist, pathologist, or anesthesiologist, and for labs or x-rays (1993).

Utilization Management Nursing Skill

The most important skills that a utilization management nurse—or NCM with utilization management responsibilities—needs are a first-rate clinical databank and excellent communication techniques. Many physicians feel that UR nurses are "nurses telling doctors how to practice medicine." They resist reviewers, feeling that their toes are being stepped on. Yet UR nurses should not necessarily be looked on as adversarial during this questioning process; their documentation can often prevent the insurance denial process. Some doctors inadequately document assessment or plans in the medical record; this often leads to insurance denials. Poor physician documenters often have acceptable plans, but it takes time and communication skills to elicit them.

The following are some practical ideas to help in utilization management responsibilities:

- Focus on the patient. The patient-centered approach diffuses suspicion and allows the reviewer and the physician to focus on the same goal.
- Be colloquial and not adversarial in your approach to physicians. Gain a reputation for solving problems, not becoming one.
- Be succinct and to the point about your needs and concerns. Physicians are busy and often have a low tolerance for rambling conversation from reviewers.
- Make sure you have an accurate and thorough clinical assessment of the situation prior to a conversation with the physician.
- When discussing discharge plans, make sure you have the patient's/family's cooperation in a plan before you discuss it with the physician; this saves wasted steps. On the other hand, some physicians have known their clients and families for many years and can provide preliminary information that will be very helpful when assessing a discharge plan.
- Be assertive, not aggressive.
- Keep lines of communication open and follow through on what is discussed. More trust has been gained because of good follow-through than any other approach I have used.

Utilization Review Documentation

As in all aspects of medical care, documentation for utilization management activity is vitally important. If, for example, you are working with a poor physician documenter, your documented conversations with the physician(s) and insurance reviewer may make the difference between an insurance authorization or a denial of hospital days or services. Note that some insurance companies demand physician documentation in the charts, so the NCM responsibility will be to attempt to obtain that documentation.

UR documentation does not have to be lengthy, but proper documentation of facts is necessary to validate the diagnosis and support the necessity of the treatment plan. Most insurance plans will not pay for services if a doctor's order is missing or if they could not find documentation that the service was in fact performed.

Documentation from a utilization management perspective should include the following:

- Record all clinically pertinent data. Objective data should be exact. For example, record a patient's temperature as 39.2° C, rather than "high temp." Other clinical data may include results of lab work, x-rays, scans, vital signs, biopsies, cultures, and so on. Subjective data may support the facts. All data should validate the diagnosis and necessity of the treatment plan.
- Record the patient's response or lack of response to the treatments and services.
- As stated earlier, accurately document conversations with physicians, insurance reviewers, and all other people pertinent to the services needed and treatment plans. I remember one novice UR nurse who denied a patient with a persistent high fever because all intravenous antibiotics had been discontinued (this patient had been on three antibiotics). What was lacking in the chart was the plan to discontinue the antibiotics and pan-culture the patient in the hopes of "catching" the offending bug. The reviewer missed the order to pan-culture, and the documentation lacked a clear picture and a black-and-white plan. After explaining to the reviewer that this was an approved standard of treatment for a fever of unknown origin, she rescinded the denial, but required physician documentation of the medical plan.
- Include times and dates of conversations. Many insurance companies (not all) give the facility 24 hours to supply requested data before the denial goes into effect. Other companies simply end the length of stay. If the NCM or physician can give them pertinent data, the insurance companies will also approve the day of the conversation (usually until midnight).
- In documentation, demonstrate the patient's status at any given point in time. If another reviewer picks up the case, no backtracking should be needed.
- Make careful documentation of discharge planning. If a discharge plan needs to be changed, include reasons for the changes in the report. Also include the level of care that is planned, home health nursing services, durable medical equipment needed, transportation and all other arrangements made, and the reasons for medical necessity. It is also important to reveal the person's name and title in the insurance company who approved payment of these discharge services.

Utilization Management Modalities

The out-of-control economics of healthcare were apparent in the 1980s. Various ways and modalities of managing the utilization of healthcare resources have come and gone; more will likely emerge in the 90s. The staggering dollar amounts being spent for healthcare are forcing this search for better management. Some utilization management tools have changed and become more efficient. Still others are in their adolescence—raw, but with good potential. The four modalities discussed here are the most commonly used utilization management tools at this time: Length of Stay, InterQual, Clinical Pathways, and Milliman & Robertson. Lag days will also be discussed as they affect all forms of utilization modalities.

Length of stay (LOS) as a utilization management modality assigns a number of days allowance to a particular episode of illness. InterQual is a criteria-based system that includes objective and measurable symptoms and services. These criteria should guide the utilization management reviewer in assessing medical necessity and appropriateness of the level of care (InterQual & Tennant, 1993a). Clinical pathways gives a daily plan of care for a particular illness and sequences all aspects of that care for optimal quality and efficiency. Milliman & Robertson is a combination of clinical pathways and length-of-stay modalities.

When using utilization management tools, keep in mind that they are just that—tools. They are not mandatory law. More important, they are only a part of total case management. They do, however, speak a language that insurance companies understand, and insurance companies pay the hospital bills, which ensures that ill people will have a hospital to go to in the future.

There have been times when I have felt sandwiched between an insurance company's threat to deny payment unless the doctor moves the patient to a lesser level of care and a physician angry over the insurance company's decision. At these times it helps to get everyone's focus back on the patient and what that patient needs to be safely cared for. At other times, the physician is grateful for the added "support" of an insurance denial if the patient or family is adept at manipulating or malingering. In either case, knowledge of utilization modalities will aid the NCM; impending insurance denials will not be a surprise because the NCM already predicted the possibility and therefore the discharge plan was already in place well into the case management process.

Lag Days and Variances

Inappropriate hospital days, also known as lag days, may occur at the beginning of a hospital stay (on admission), during, or at the end of a hospitalization in which a patient could have been discharged or transferred sooner than was actually done. These days are considered nonacute by insurance companies; here *over-utilization* of resources becomes apparent. It is not uncommon for insurance companies to deny portions of a hospitalization (on admission, during, or at the end of a stay) if they feel it is due to avoidable delays. Good case management can minimize these lag days, and hospitals are seeing an encouraging impact in this area. At times, unavoidable lag days still occur; when this happens, the NCM should help to get the case back on track as quickly as possible.

Given all the people involved and factors that make up each case, it is not surprising that lag days occur with monotonous consistency. The reasons for lag days are varied, and closely related to these nonacute days is the issue of *variances.* Variances are deviations from normal, quality care. Unexpected or worrisome occurrences that affect the course of illness can be identified through analysis of variance data (Anonymous, 1989). These data, in turn, can identify possible opportunities for improvement. Sources for variance identification used by NCMs include nurses and physician documentation and verbal communication with the multidisciplinary healthcare team (Bueno & Hwang, 1993). Clinical pathways are also an excellent tool to trend variances (see Clinical Pathways). The patient or family members are another source (and sometimes a cause) of variances.

The causes of variances, which may lead to lag days, are generally assigned to three categories: (1) patient/family reasons, (2) practitioner reasons, or (3) institution/systems reasons. Variances can be caused by social factors, environmental factors, patient or family responses or lack of responses, physician-induced reasons, or hospital (institution) responsibilities. The following are some examples of variances that may lead to lag days. The list is by no means complete, as very creative and interesting circumstances can and do pop up unexpectedly!

Patient/Family Variances

- The patient and/or family is indecisive about a test, procedure or surgery.
- The patient or family insists that the patient is too ill to be discharged.
- The family does not show up to pick up the patient after arrangements were made.
- The patient is ready for discharge on Friday, but the family member responsible for at-home care cannot arrive from out of state until Saturday or Sunday.
- The patient is uncooperative with the medical program, causing delayed diagnosis and treatment.
- The patient suffered an intraoperative myocardial infarction or other medical complication (eg, hemorrhage, shock, ileus, postop infection, or pneumonia).
- Educational needs were attended to early in the admission, but the patient or family still had a significant knowledge deficit and needed additional teaching.
- The transfer or discharge is delayed because of inadequate discharge planning details.
- Family members change their minds about the discharge plan at the last minute (eg, the NCM's suggestion that an extended care facility may be appropriate suddenly sounds good!).
- A chronically ill patient has inadequate (or lacks) insurance support and poor social support. This causes a difficult discharge dilemma (if available, "charity" care may be needed).

Practitioner Variances

- This variance can be attributed to patient/family or physician, depending on how one looks at it. That is, all ECFs where the patient's physician will follow are full; the physician will not go to other suggested ECFs; or the patient refuses care by a "strange" physician.
- The doctor writes the discharge order at 10:00 PM, when visiting hours are over and patients and their families alike are usually asleep!
- The patient was admitted for a problem outside the expertise of the attending physician. Delays occurred getting specialist consultations.
- The physician's practice pattern is such that only one test is ordered at a time, and the results must be back before any other diagnostic action is taken.

- The physician comes in early—before the day's lab tests are back and before patient's progress for the day can be assessed—and will "discharge tomorrow" if the patient is rock stable today.
- Tests are ordered in poor sequence, causing delays because of extensive prepping.
- Poor practitioner's techniques causing complications.
- Delays in ordering needed services (ie, social service, physical therapy, rehab consultation).

Institution/Systems Variances

- Scheduling delay for tests, procedures, or surgery may be the result of full operating room or tests that run only on specific days of the week.
- Test or biopsy results are delayed, which postpones further procedures or discharge.
- A lower level of care would have adequately met the needs of the patient, but traditional Medicare requires 72 hours in acute care prior to transfer to an ECF level.
- The institution does not have the necessary equipment, so that transfer to another hospital is necessary for a test or procedure.
- Equipment malfunctions or breaks down.

The causes of variances are seemingly endless. The more complicated the discharge, the more opportunities for variances and lag days to occur and the more a detailed social evaluation is needed. I heard of one case in which the NCM worked very hard putting together a complicated discharge with various pieces of durable medical equipment. On the day of discharge, someone in the family happened to mention that there was no electricity at home! Assessment had missed this crucial fact. This, of course, delayed discharge. Be alert for possible changes, and be prepared with a Plan B.

Length of Stay

Length of stay (LOS) is perhaps the most basic attempt at controlling costs of healthcare (see also Chapter 5: Insurance). A LOS is essentially a number of days that a patient should stay in the hospital for a specific diagnosis or operation. The statistics were calculated from over 4 million hospital discharge records from hospitals that participated in the Professional Activity Study (PAS) of the Commission of Professional and Hospital Activities (Health Care Knowledge Resources, 1991).

These statistics were broken down by region in the United States, by specific year, by cause of hospitalization (ie, primarily diagnostic or surgical), by age, and by percentile. The LOSs were calculated by counting the admission day as Day 1; the day of discharge was not included (Health Care Knowledge Resources, 1991). Percentiles include 10th, 25th, 50th, 75th, 90th, 95th, and 99th. Patients over the 99th percentile were excluded from the study (1991).

Those who compiled these statistics feel they assisted in the following aspects of managed care:

- Projecting extended stay reviews
- Identifying candidates for utilization review
- Establishing baselines
- Developing forecasts
- Service planning (Health Care Knowledge Resources, 1991)

A goal LOS is used within the Milliman & Robertson Guidelines, although Milliman & Robertson probably use stricter guidelines than even the 10th percentile of the PAS lengths of stay. However, Milliman & Robertson, Inc, also includes this cautionary note. "Length of stay assignment has an over assignment problem because it is usually based on retrospective data, assigns number of days without explicit references to expected clinical care, and is often viewed by physicians as an uninformed negotiating stance" (Milliman & Robertson, 1992).

This modality does leave little room for individualization and is rarely used by insurance companies as the sole consideration for authorization of hospital stays. It is, however, a useful tool for case managers to grasp *average* length of time a patient should stay in the hospital. If a patient is admitted to your NCM service with a less familiar illness or procedure, knowing the usual LOS may be a comforting place to start. Making a "cheat sheet" of 10%, 25%, and 50% for common problems encountered on your service may be worth the time.

Figure 6–1 illustrates changes in hospital LOS over the past 10 years. Figure 6–2 discusses a variety of trends that explain the decrease in LOS. Examples of lengths of stay by diagnosis and by operation are included in the chapter Appendix 6–A. These numbers change (usually getting smaller for tighter LOS), so use of the most up-to-date PAS book is recommended.

NOTE

For more information on the Length of Stay manuals contact:
HCIA, Inc.
300 E. Lombard Street
Baltimore, MD 21202
1 (800) 521-6210

InterQual

InterQual was first introduced in 1978 with many subsequent revisions and additions (InterQual & Tennant, 1993b). It is perhaps the most well-known and commonly used of all the utilization parameters; therefore, it is important for the NCM to understand. It is also somewhat complicated and has intimidated its share of case managers.

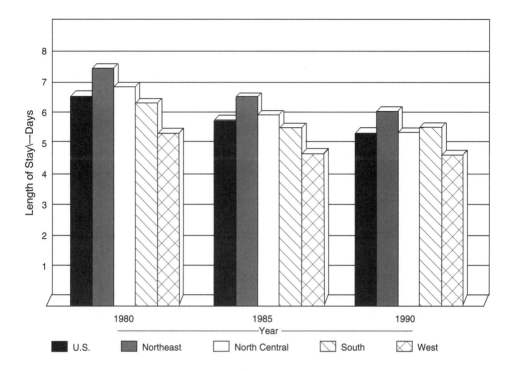

Figure 6-1. Average length of stay—United States and regions* (All patients—1980, 1985, 1990; short-term, general nonfederal hospitals.) Ten-year length of stay comparison. (Length-of-stay data included in this publication are provided with permission from HCIA, Inc, Baltimore, MD.)

The Length of Stay publications present statistical data that describe hospital stay in the United States. Companion volumes display data for census regions and the pediatric and geriatric populations. The 1990 LOS series, published by Healthcare Knowledge Resources, is derived from the database developed and maintained by the Commission on Professional and Hospital Activities (CPHA) and is drawn from over 4 million hospital discharge records.

Hospital stay data provide a valuable perspective for healthcare professionals who make decisions based on hospital utilization. Length of Stay has been published since 1963 and can be used to track trends, examine patterns of care, and conduct comparisons between years.

The above graphs illustrate changes in hospital stay over a 10-year period.

It is the intent of this section to breakdown the *ISD-A Criteria* into user-friendly pieces and to dispel some of the anxiety associated with use of this modality. Presented here is a brief and basic overview of InterQual's main points. Attendance at one of their informative seminars is suggested, as is access to their criteria sets. Three ISSI criteria sets have been included in chapter Appendix 6–B, so that the reader can be more familiar with the ISSI format.

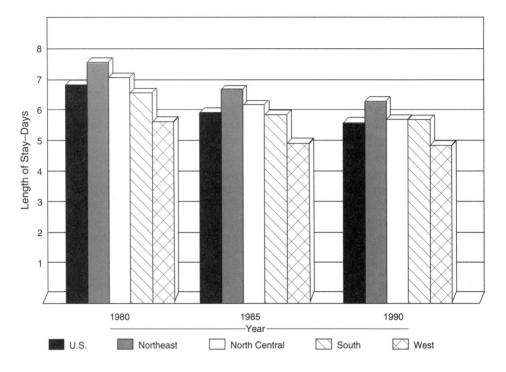

There is a steady decline in length of stay over the time period studied, with a 12% drop observed from 1980 to 1985 for all patients in the United States. From 1985 to 1990, the decline continued, but slowed to a 5% decrease.

Traditionally, hospital stays are highest in the Northeast and North Central, and lowest in the South and West. This regional pattern remains consistent until 1990, when the North Central and Southern regions display an almost equivalent length of stay.

A variety of factors can be looked at to explain the decline in hospital stay. Studies show that the prospective payment system implemented by the federal government had an impact on reducing hospital stays by reimbursing at a fixed rate for inpatient care. The introduction of utilization review to monitor costs and resource consumption helped to shorten hospital stays by ensuring medical necessity of admissions.

Other factors that affect hospital stay include introducing new medical technology and techniques that require shorter hospitalization and recovery time, discharging patients as soon as medically feasible to less acute care settings, providing more home-based services as an alternative to impatient care, and managing catastrophic cases.

The growth of HMOs and PPOs provides yet another explanation for the decrease in hospital stays. Because services are prepaid, all medical care is closely monitored to control costs and utilization.

Figure 6-2. Average length of stay—United States and regions (Short-term, general non-federal hospitals). All patients excepts newborns—1980, 1985, 1990. (Length-of-stay data included in this publication are provided with permission from HCIA, Inc, Baltimore, MD.)

Interqual's Criteria

InterQual's criteria are named ISD-A, which stands for:

I—intensity (of service)

S—severity (of illness)

D—discharge (how stable is patient for discharge)

A—appropriateness of level of care; used for specialty units such as telemetry, intensive care, rehab, coronary care, observation (InterQual & Tennant, 1993b)

In general, the criteria are broken down into 15 categories. One category is generic and is a catch-all division. Although still being used at this time, the generic category is expected to be incorporated into the remaining divisions in future revisions of the ISSI criteria. The other 14 classifications are anatomically divided as follows (InterQual & Tennant, 1993):

- Blood and lymphatics
- Cardiovascular
- Central nervous system/head
- Endocrine/metabolic
- Eye, ear, nose & throat
- Female reproductive
- Gastrointestinal tract and abdomen
- Musculoskeletal/spine
- Peripheral vascular
- Psychiatric
- Respiratory/chest
- Skin/connective tissue
- Substance abuse
- Urinary tract (includes male reproductive)

Each of these categories are further divided into three criteria subsections:

SI = Severity of Illness

SI criteria are objective and measurable clinical indications (InterQual & Tennant, 1993a). How sick is the patient? The data are gathered from a thorough patient assessment and include any signs or symptoms the patient is exhibiting that reflect a need for acute hospitalization. Some SI criteria use *time of onset* of the symptoms as part of the definition. These criteria are

Acute/sudden onset = with 24 hours (InterQual & Tennant, 1993b)

Recent onset = within 1 week (1993b)

Recently or newly discovered = greater than 1 week (1993b).

Newly discovered = new findings during this episode of illness (InterQual & Tennant, 1993a)

The last two times of onset reflect the pace of change in the InterQual criteria. Either one may be used, depending on the revision of the criteria being used, although both are from 1993 manuals.

So that the reader may get a feel for how ill a patient must be for an acute hospital authorization, Display 6–1 lists some examples of SI criteria. Time of onset is not listed, but this might further prevent some patients from meeting SI criteria. Note also that if a patient almost meets an aggregate of three SI criteria, clinical rationale for hospital admission may be approved (InterQual & Tennant, 1993b).

IS = Intensity of Service

IS criteria define the diagnostic and therapeutic services for each category (InterQual & Tennant, 1993a). Essentially, IS constitutes the physician orders: what is being done for this patient in terms of diagnosis identification and treatment.

Some IS criteria may be preceded by an asterisk (*). This is to alert the reviewer to be mindful that these criteria may reflect a treatment that can be safely accomplished at a nonacute level of care (1993a). This would be the expected plan of care if the patient is not meeting severity of illness screens but is demonstrating discharge readiness (1993a). Display 6–2 lists some examples of Intensity of Service criteria.

Discharge Screens

Discharge screens are parameters indicating the patient's readiness and stability for either discharge home, or transfer to another level of care (InterQual, 1993b). Discharge screens have two components:

DISPLAY 6–1
Examples of InterQual's Severity of Illness Criteria

- Oral temperature 104 °F (40 °C) (Note: Other temperature criteria are offered but with further delineating factors.)
- Sustained pulse ≥ 160 bpm
- Respiratory rate ≥ 26 with a pulse oximeter reading ≤ 85% on room air
- Blood pressure Systolic ≥ 250 or below 80 mm Hg
- Blood pressure Diastolic ≥ 120 or below 40 mm Hg
- Hgb below 7 g
- HCT below 21 g (note: Hgb and HCT criteria may change in future ISSI revisions.)
- Pneumothorax/hemothorax
- Acute myocardial infarction
- Gross blood in vomitus, stool, or gastric aspirant
- Open wound to bone
- Sudden loss of vision
- Block or filling defect of major blood vessel
- Gross and persistent hemoptysis

(Adapted from InterQual & Tennant, 1993a, 1993b)

1. *Clinical/functional*—These are like severity of illness data in that they are objective and measurable clinical indicators; only this time they denote clinical parameters showing the patient is stable for discharge or transfer (InterQual & Tennant, 1993a). These may include findings such as passing flatus/fecal material, therapeutic ranges for specified drugs, catheter removed for 8 hours, and postvoid residual is less than 140 mL. Social parameters include the patient/caretaker demonstrating willingness and ability to care for drainage tubes, prosthesis, wounds, and so on, or demonstrating refusal of treatment.

2. *Options*—This essentially prompts the reviewer into looking at potential options for alternative treatment/care (or medications that can be offered at a nonacute level of care (ie, observation unit, skilled nursing facility, subacute level, home, hospice). Some prompts include changing from IV to intramuscular or oral medication routes or changing to another level of care.

Rules for Applying ISSI Criteria

Some general rules for applying the ISSI criteria follow (InterQual & Tennant, 1993a, 1993b). For more specific usage, consult one of the InterQual manuals and attend a seminar that specifically teaches ISSI criteria.

DISPLAY 6-2
Examples of InterQual's Intensity of Service Criteria

- Intravenous fluids requiring ≥ 30 mL/kg of body weight in 24 hours (72 hours postoperatively)
- IV/IM analgesics at least 4 x / 24 hours or a continuous IV analgesic drip
- Ventilator assistance
- Initial tracheostomy care
- Chest tube suction/drainage
- IV antibiotics, antifungals, antidiuretics, steroids
- IV cardiac glycosides (eg, digitalis)
- IV insulin
- IV anticoagulants
- Protective isolation
- Skin care requiring professional nursing care at least 6 x /24 hours (eg, major burn care)
- Intermittent bladder irrigation
- Initial training for functional mobility with prosthesis, orthosis, assistive device and/or splint

(From InterQual & Tennant 1993a, 1993b).

1. Either SI *or* the specified number of IS criteria must be met on admission.
2. *Both* SI and the specified number of IS criteria (from the same anatomic category) must be met within 24 hours of admission. Exception: The generic category may be used with other anatomic categories, but apply the body system criteria first and add the generic screen if needed.
3. In general, a patient who is admitted to the hospital for an elective procedure such as a nonemergent hysterectomy or cholecystectomy will not meet SI criteria.
4. If a patient is admitted through the emergency room on an emergency basis, both SI *and* the specified number of IS criteria must be met at the time of admission.
5. When IS screens are no longer met and discharge screens are met, discharge should be planned for that day (1993a). In an earlier revision of 1993 (1993b), the reviewer had 24 hours to obtain the discharge. This is an example of the changing pace of healthcare. Please note that some patients with severe, chronic illnesses may never meet the discharge screens and usually require intensive case management from the day of admission.
6. When the IS criteria are met (with an asterisk *) but severity of illness criteria are no longer applicable, an alternative level of care should be explored. For example, if a patient has been diagnosed with osteomyelitis requiring 6 weeks of IV antibiotics and is medically stable, the antibiotics could be provided for at home or at an ECF (depending on social support and insurance coverage).
7. Discharge screens must be matched with the same category as IS and SI.
8. Review should be obtained at least every 3 days or more often if a patient is nearing medical stability, discharge, or transfer to another level of care.

InterQual's Review Process

There are four potential types of review in InterQual's review process: preadmission review, admission review, subsequent reviews, and discharge reviews.

Preadmission Review

Preadmission review is initiated prior to an admission (InterQual & Tennant, 1993b). The reviewer determines whether the diagnostic services and therapeutic modalities are appropriate and match the level of care. As noted earlier, elective admissions may not meet SI criteria.

Admission Review

Admission review may often be the initial chart review on a patient. If a patient is admitted directly from a physician's office or from the emergency room, no reviewer may have seen the chart. More progressive hospitals are placing social workers and utilization management nurses or NCMs in the emergency room level of care. In general, admission reviews are done within 24 hours of admission. This review also determines medical necessity and appropriateness of the level of care (InterQual & Tennant, 1993b).

Subsequent Reviews

Subsequent reviews are done intermittently throughout the hospitalization with a 3-day interval between reviews considered maximum (InterQual & Tennant, 1993a). The frequency is determined by the level of care, the severity of the patient's illness, and other factors. An experienced reviewer has a feel for when the next review needs attention. As a patient nears discharge or transfer to another level of care, these reviews become more frequent, usually daily.

Discharge Reviews

Discharge reviews use the discharge screens from the same category as were used to assess IS and SI. This review is used to determine stability for treatment and services at a lesser level of care (InterQual & Tennant 1993b). Documentation discussions of why a patient does not meet discharge screens are important; documentation of discharge planning is equally important.

If a patient is not meeting discharge screens and a discharge is initiated and that patient is readmitted to an acute care facility within 15 to 30 days, Medicare may look at the first hospitalization for quality of care issues or premature discharge indications. If the patient was discharged without documentation of passing discharge screens and had a bad outcome connected to the discharge, it could mean a risk management issue for the hospital. Discharge documentation should also include improvements noted from previous reviews. If the patient was initially admitted with a temperature of 39.8° C, a chest x-ray showing a right middle lobe infiltrate, and a white blood cell count of 25.5 TH/UL, and is on IV antibiotics every 4 hours, then discharge documentation might reflect that the patient is afebrile, off IV antibiotic (ie, on oral antibiotics) for 24 hours, the white blood cell count is 9.6 TH/UL, and the chest x-ray is now clear.

NOTE

This overview of InterQual will provide the NCM with a basic understanding of the ISD-A criteria and examples of the ISSI Criteria are included in chapter Appendix 6–B. If your organization or hospital does not have an InterQual manual or review system to look at, call or write one of the main branches for materials and possible teaching seminars.

InterQual, Inc
44 Lafayette Road
North Hampton, NH 03862-0988
(603) 964-7255

InterQual, Inc
293 Boston Post Road West
Suite 180
Marlborough, MA 01752
(508) 481-1181

Clinical Pathways

Of all utilization modalities, Clinical Pathways most completely takes into account the total multidisciplinary aspects of the patient's care. Various names and formats for these pathways are being used throughout the country, such as clinical pathways, critical pathways, Care MAP (Zander, 1992), progress pathway, progress map. Although we look at pathways as a 90s medical tool, the methodologies have been around for decades in the construction and engineering fields. The healthcare field researched them as early as the 1970s, but the environment was unreceptive at that time (Coffey et al., 1992).

Clinical pathways are a multidisciplinary management tool that proactively depicts important events that should take place in a day-by-day sequence. Throughout the entire episode of illness, the key events change daily and move the patient and the healthcare team toward discharge. The overall goal is to achieve optimal quality of care while minimizing delays and resource utilization (Coffey et al., 1992); they are also written to stay within the DRG allotted LOS. Pathways can be used by all team members to coordinate, plan, deliver and monitor care, and document and perform UR activities concurrently. Clinical pathways have been written for various patient populations. Some are based on DRG-related diagnoses such as pneumonia or myocardial infarction. Other pathways were written for patient conditions such as ventilator dependency weaning. Surgical procedures such as total knee replacements or lumbar laminectomies comprise many pathways.

Clinical pathways can also be written for various timelines of care. The most common scope of care is the inpatient hospital pathway (Coffey et al., 1992). Other pathways extend until postdischarge follow-up is completed. Places such as New York University Hospital and Vanderbilt University Hospital and Clinic are using pathways for more chronic conditions (1992). Patients with end-stage renal disease (ESRD), chronic obstructive pulmonary disease (COPD), benign prostatic hypertrophy (BPH), or Crohn's disease could benefit from these pathways in the ambulatory setting.

Visually, many pathway formats are set up very similarly. In chart form, the hospital days stretch across horizontally, and the key categories line down vertically (see Display 6–3). The medical events are cross-referenced by category and hospital day; these events may differ: for example, a clinical path for a total hip replacement alters from that for congestive heart failure.

Treatments include interventions that must be performed by the healthcare team, such as tube and site care, telemetry, daily weights, Foley catheter care, vital signs, neurochecks, suture removal, IV site changes, small volume nebulizer (SVN) treatments. *Consults/referrals* bring in other members of the healthcare team, such as those in ostomy care, social service, diabetic education, rehabilitation, physical therapy, or dietary services. *Diagnostic tests* include measurable data, such as radiology, x-rays, lab tests, electrocardiography (ECG), urine or stool studies, and blood sugar monitoring. *Medications* include the drugs ordered with dosage, times, and route. IV antibiotics may be ordered on Days 1 and 2,

DISPLAY 6–3
Critical Pathway Chart

	Day 1	Day 2	Day 3	Day 4	Day 5
Treatments					
Consults/referrals					'
Diagnostic tests					
Medications					
Activities/safety mobility					
Diet/nutrition					
Discharge planning					
Teaching/education					

whereas oral antibiotics may be charted for the following hospital days. Medications may include anything from anticoagulants to stool softeners. Pain control is also documented along with route of medications (oral, intramuscular, IV, or epidural). *Activities/mobility* outlines the patient's allowable activities. Across the days, this may progress from bed rest to chair to ambulation or sitting up in chair or head of bed elevations. Document length of time that the patient sat in the chair or how far he or she ambulated. *Diet/nutrition* defines the patient's dietary needs and may advance from nothing by mouth (NPO) to a regular or specialty diet, depending on the patient's requirements. Chart the percentage of diet taken and how well the patient tolerated it. *Discharge planning* optimally starts prior to admission. Since this is not always possible, a social service referral may be charted for Day 1 or 2. Insurance eligibility or ECF placement referrals may be recommended. *Teaching/education* are interactions necessary to help the patient/family become more independent and self-sufficient. Teaching may include physical therapy safety modalities, proper administration of medications with possible side effects, insurance explanations, tube-feeding administration, or post-transplantation lifestyle. All events are tailored to the needs of the diagnosis and hospital day.

The above clinical pathways leave unanswered questions and signal limitations. They are not ideally suited to patients with multiple concurrent medical problems, although many healthcare professionals are working on solutions to this problem. In general, it is recommended that the staff use the clinical pathway matching the most immediate problem (Zander, 1991). For example, if a postop patient is having a difficult time weaning from ventilator assistance, change the pathway to a ventilator pathway until the patient can get back on the original path. In less extreme circumstances, the patient may deviate from the pathway and smaller adjustments may need to be made; pathways are an outline and a tool, and it may not always be possible to follow them exactly.

Other problems may arise if one patient has multiple physicians with multiple practice patterns. If an agreement cannot be reached, the pathway may cause additional stress and defeat its purpose.

Although not a limitation per se, the event changes are not standing orders (Zander, 1992). A few facilities have concurrent standing orders that coincide with each day's events. If an attending physician has already visited the patient that day and the nurse has been prompted by the clinical pathway that a change to oral (from IV/IM) medication may be recommended, the nurse can call the physician for clarification. Perhaps the doctor had a reason to keep the patient on IV medication (eg, the patient is NPO); but perhaps it was an oversight and the phone call could save resources and possibly an extra day in the hospital.

Reactions to clinical pathways have been mixed, especially from physicians. Although doctors have been essential to their development, underlying fears include increased liability (Zander, 1992). Some physicians feel that clinical pathways are a road map for a plaintiff's attorney and a loss of their own autonomy. To remedy this, some hospitals have more than one pathway for the same DRG diagnoses to accommodate the different practice patterns of various physicians (Coffey et al., 1992). Many physicians appreciate the at-a-glance multidisciplinary charting. They have also received positive feedback from their patients.

When a patient's care does not meet the changes as outlined in the clinical pathway, a *variance* has occurred, that is, a detour off the path. These detours can be positive or negative, avoidable or unavoidable (Coffey et al., 1992). A positive variance may show a patient progressing more quickly than the pathway anticipated. Negative variances usually result in an extended LOS, and the patient takes longer to reach desired outcomes (see Lag Days and Variances earlier in chapter).

Proponents of clinical pathways say that because a variance can be sighted almost immediately (through the prompting inherent in the clinical pathways system), lag days can be reduced. The goal is to recognize and resolve the variance as quickly as possible and get the care back on the path in a timely manner (Sinnen & Schifalacqua, 1991). Variance sheets are filled out and the causes of the deviation are explored immediately, allowing corrective action to be taken. Analysis of variance data is directly related to quality improvement activities, allowing less fragmentation of hospital systems.

Benefits and Goals of Clinical Pathways

A summation of some of the benefits and goals of clinical pathways follows:

- The utilization management and quality improvement activities, as well as the multidisciplinary activities are all-inclusive.
- Of all the various utilization modalities, the patient (not only symptoms or doctor's orders) is the primary focus in clinical pathways. Therefore, the patient is the common denominator of all activities, and the patient/family satisfaction is improved. It has been noted that patients who have been

made aware of the day-by-day changes in their clinical pathway have a decreased level of anxiety—they know approximately what to expect—and an increased sense of involvement and control. Hence, the patients use the changes as goals to attain (Coffey et al., 1992). Some facilities have even written a patient's version of each pathway using lay, rather than technical, terminology.

- Clinical pathways are an effective tool for decreasing LOS and resource utilization, since they efficiently move the patient toward discharge goals. Last-minute oversights are avoided.
- Quality of care is enhanced with continuous, concurrent attention to variances.
- Satisfaction and communication among the multidisciplinary team members are enhanced. It is case management "at a glance."
- Clinical pathways are compatible with other utilization modalities.
- Clinical pathways are easy to use.
- When clinical pathways are used as a documentation tool, nurses report less time spent on charting and improved shift reports.
- Clinical pathways serve as excellent guidelines for novice nurses who may be unsure of the course a patient should be taking for a particular DRG or diagnosis. They can be used as education tools and orientation models, delineating expected outcomes. One case manager commented that what had taken her 2 years to know and understand through constant experience with a case type, a new clinician could now master within 6 weeks (Etheredge, 1987).
- Clinical pathways provide cues to the staff for all aspects of care.
- Clinical pathways lend themselves as a tool for an applied research process, whereby algorithms are embedded within the pathway itself (Zander, 1992). Examples of clinical pathways can be found in chapter Appendix 6–C.

Milliman & Robertson Guidelines

Milliman & Robertson's *Healthcare Management Guidelines* (HMGs) resemble a combination of LOS criteria and mini clinical pathways. Their goal LOS are very tight, resembling the upper 10th percentile in the PAS books. The authors explain in their guidebook that they feel typical LOS programs are too liberal and most acuity criteria are too permissive. Critics feel the Milliman & Robertson guidelines are extremely optimistic and perhaps unrealistic (Milliman & Robertson, 1992). Where Milliman & Robertson guidelines emphasize alternative care settings, critics feel that they rely on an overuse of emergency room services (1992). As with all utilization management tools, these guidelines are an attempt to eliminate nonproductive days while maintaining quality of care.

The minipathways are called Optimal Recovery Guidelines (ORGs) and depict daily protocols for procedures and patient conditions that require hospitalization. They are categorized into five groups: medical, surgical, pediatric, mental health, and psychoactive substance abuse. As the title implies, these are optimal scenarios and are meant for routine, uncomplicated cases. For the insurance companies that use these criteria for hospital authorization, the NCM may need to put on the patient advocate hat, especially when the insurance company attempts to squeeze more complex patients into these guidelines. Even the Milliman & Robertson Guidelines recognize some limitations in the Optimal Recovery Guidelines:

> The Optimal Recovery Timetables describe patterns for recovery and care for those patients who do as well as one hopes without complications. They are not inflexible expectations for all patients, but should be considered possible standards for initial authorization and review schedule. (Milliman & Robertson, p. 2.44, 1992).

In addition to the Optimal Recovery Guidelines, Milliman & Robertson also include alternative setting criteria and sets of criteria describing "adequate" and "inadequate" reasons for hospital admission. Some find the inclusion of ICD-9-CM, CPT-4, and DSM-IIIR codes very helpful. As mentioned, the LOS goals are very compact, perhaps adequate under the best circumstances. Milliman & Robertson (1992) believe that by actively managing healthcare, rationing will not be necessary. Examples of goal LOS follow:

- Coronary artery bypass graft—LOS = 4 days (newer criteria are expected to reduce this to a goal LOS of 3 days)
- Hip arthroplasty—LOS = 4 days (may soon be changed to 3-day goal LOS)
- Craniotomy—LOS = 4 days
- Asthma (even with an intensive care unit admission for respiratory failure)—LOS = 1 day
- Seizures including new onset—LOS = ambulatory (ie, no hospital admission)
- Pneumonia, community-acquired, admitted to ICU—LOS = 2 days
- Septicemia with ICU admission—LOS = 2 days
- Lysis of adhesions (with Day 1 being the day of surgery)—LOS = 4 days

Alternative levels of care are encouraged, since Milliman & Robertson (1992) feel that unnecessary admissions of medical cases are common. Two general types of alternative settings to hospital admissions include the following:

1. *Home care*—This can be provided with necessary nursing and equipment. Here nurses stay in close contact with the primary physician. Office visits or even house calls are suggested as part of this alternative setting. One Milliman & Robertson spokesperson suggested that laparoscopic cholecystectomies may not need the usual 23-hour observation stay *if* prior arrangements could be made for home preparations such as RN supports, IVs, patient-controlled anesthesia (PCA) pump for pain control.
2. *More prolonged observation and treatment in the emergency room setting*—If a physician is uncomfortable with the home care option for reasons such as uncertainty about a diagnosis or response to initiation of treatment protocols, perhaps several hours in an emergency room would alleviate this hesitation. The patient could then go home with the aforementioned home support if clinical improvement is assessed through various evaluation parameters, thus

avoiding admission. These alternative levels of care also include recommendations for transferring patients to an ECF, hospice, or other level of care.

Examples of Milliman & Roberts ORGs can be found in chapter Appendix 6–D.

NOTE

There are approximately 25 Milliman & Robertson offices throughout the United States. The corporate headquarters could put you in touch with an office near you for further information.

Milliman & Robertson, Inc
1301 Fifth Avenue
Suite 3800
Seattle, Wasington 98101-2605
(206) 624-7940

CASE STUDY

Mr. Timmer, age 76, arrived at the emergency room on a Thursday evening complaining of chest and abdominal pain. Although generally a poor historian, he did manage to convey to the staff that he had suffered gunshot and bayonet wounds and malaria as a POW during World War II. He also stated that he has had pneumonia.

The ECG taken in the emergency room showed an acute anterolateral myocardial infarction. Tissue plasminogen activator was immediately started with effective results. His chest x-ray revealed cardiomegaly and questionable congestive heart failure. His breath sounds were described as tubular; no pedal pulses could be appreciated.

In questioning Mr. Timmer, ER personnel found his living situation to be transient: currently he was residing in a motel. He had two children but didn't know where they were or how to get in touch with them.

Mr. Timmer was admitted to the intensive care unit, where tissue plasminogen activator was continued along with heparin, tridil, and lidocaine drips, and IV methylprednisolone (Solu-medrol). An echocardiogram, abdominal ultrasonography, and cardiac catheterization were ordered.

On hospital Day 2, the ultrasound examination showed cholelithiasis. On Day 3, Mr. Timmer was moved to a telemetry floor level of care. A cardiac catheterization, originally scheduled for Monday (Day 5), was rescheduled for Tuesday (Day 6) because of catheterization lab scheduling conflicts.

The cardiac catheterization revealed the need for a triple coronary artery bypass graft (CABG). Surgery was performed the following day, Day 7.

Mr. Timmer was on an intra-aortic balloon pump until Day 9 (2 days postop) and went to the telemetry floor on Day 10 (postop Day 3).

Day 11. Mr. Timmer complained of being too weak to ambulate; cardiac rehabilitation was ordered. His oxygen was reduced from 4 to 2 L per nasal cannula. Small-volume nebulizer treatments were added for diminished breath sounds and egophony in the left base.

Day 12. Mr. Timmer again refused to leave his room to ambulate.

Day 13. Still refused to work with cardiac rehab. A social service consultation was ordered.

Day 14. Complaints of weakness continued. A chest x-ray revealed atelectasis and small pleural effusions. A multigated acquisition (MUGA) scan was performed.

Day 15. Arterial blood gases with patient on 2 L of oxygen showed an oxygen saturation of 95%; therefore, Mr. Timmer's oxygen was discontinued. He still refused to leave his room for cardiac rehab.

Day 16. The MUGA scan taken 2 days previously was read and revealed an adequate ejection fraction of 48%. A transfer for the following day to an ECF was requested. Social service personnel saw the patient and began working on a transfer to a veterans' facility.

Day 17. On the planned day of transfer, Mr. Timmer complained again of chest pain. Because of the patient's sedentary postop course, physicians felt the need to rule out pulmonary emboli and ordered a ventilation/qualification (V/Q) scan.

Day 20. V/Q scan was negative. An adenosine cardiolite stress test was performed; it showed no myocardial infarction or ischemia. Still the patient complained of chest pain. The chest x-ray showed atelectasis without any change from the last x-ray. Mr. Timmer began to ambulate 40 feet with a minimum assistance of two people. He was told he would be transferred the next day. On hearing this news, the patient expressed suicide ideation, but refused to speak to a psychiatrist for a consult.

Day 21. Patient was transferred to a respite center.

CASE STUDY QUESTIONS

1. Discuss the social service support both in content and in time responsiveness. When should discharge planning have begun? What and when was the first clue that social service was needed?
2. Discuss the use of hospital days prior to the patient's postop day for the coronary artery bypass graft (CABG).
3. Discuss solutions to problems assessed in question 2.
4. Compare this hospital course and LOS with the utilization modalities in this chapter. (Milliman & Robertson CABG ORG, a CABG clinical pathway, and InterQual's Screens for a coronary care unit are included in the chapter Appendix).
5. Discuss the legal and ethical implications of the discharge plan.
6. Discuss options to tighten the LOS starting from postop Day 3 (hospital Day 10.)
7. Evaluate this case for "nonacute" days.
8. Would a multidisciplinary team meeting have been appropriate? Who should attend? When would the NCM call for one?

References

Anonymous. (1989). Managed care: Integrating "Q.A." in everyday practice. *Definition, 4*(3), 1–2.

Bueno, M. M., & Hwang, R. (1993). Understanding variances in hospital stay. *Nursing Management, 24*(11), 51–57.

California Medical Review, Inc. (CMRI). (1990). *Utilization review seminar workbook.* San Francisco: Author.

Coffey, R. J., Richards, J. S., Remmert, C. S., LeRoy, S. S., Schoville, R. R., & B Baldwin, P. J. (1992). An introduction to critical paths. *Quality Management in Healthcare, 1*(1), 45–54.

Etheredge, M. L. (Ed.). (1987). Critical paths: Marking the course. *Definition, 2*(3), 1–4.

Healthcare Knowledge Resources. (1991). *Length of stay by diagnosis and operation.* Ann Arbor: Author.

InterQual & Tennant, T. (Ed.). (1993b). *The ISD-A (TM) review system with adult ISD (TM) criteria.* North Hampton: Author.

InterQual & Tennant, T. (Ed.). (1993a). *Utilization review and management training manual.* North Hampton: Author.

Kongstvedt, P. R. (1993). *The managed health care handbook.* Gaithersburg, MD: Aspen Publishers.

Milliman & Robertson. (1992). *Healthcare management guidelines.* Seattle: Author.

Sederer, L. I. (1987). Utilization review and quality assurance: Staying in the black and working with the blues. *General Hospital Psychiatry, 9,* 210–219.

Sinnen, M., & Schifalacqua, M. (1991). Coordinated care in a community hospital. *Nursing Management, 22*(3), 38–42.

Zander, K. (1991, January). Profile. *The Case Manager,* 48–50.

Zander, K. (1992), Physicians, Care Maps (TM) and collaboration. *Definition, 7*(1), 1–4.

APPENDIX 6–A
272 Hospitals, Western Region, January–December 1990, by Diagnosis

3: Respiratory tuberculosis (010–012)

Type of Patient	Total Patients	Avg. Stay	Vari-ance	Percentiles						
				10th	25th	50th	75th	90th	95th	99th
1. Single DX										
A. Not Operated										
0–19 yrs	12	7.8	220	1	1	3	6	23	50	54
20–34	36	5.4	13	1	3	5	7	10	13	16
35–49	28	6.3	16	1	4	6	8	12	14	19
50–64	6	5.5	14	<1	1	6	8	10	10	10
65+	4	8.3	38	3	4	6	12	17	17	17
B. Operated										
0–19 yrs	1	11.0		11	11	11	11	11	11	11
20–34	11	7.5	12	2	5	9	10	11	12	12
35–49	13	9.2	61	4	6	6	9	18	30	33
50–64	3	5.3	1	4	4	6	6	6	6	6
65+	3	7.3	32	1	3	9	11	12	12	12
2. Multiple DX										
A. Not Operated										
0–19 yrs	17	7.3	27	1	3	6	12	15	16	16
20–34	72	7.2	59	2	3	5	9	13	17	50
35–49	73	8.5	141	2	3	5	10	20	24	77
50–64	58	7.5	35	2	3	6	11	17	19	27
65+	46	9.4	30	4	5	8	12	18	21	23
B. Operated										
0–19 yrs	8	7.6	12	4	5	7	9	13	15	15
20–34	38	11.0	150	4	7	8	11	19	21	78
35–49	36	14.8	107	7	9	11	18	35	46	99+
50–64	35	12.2	98	3	7	8	16	26	30	49
65+	31	14.8	107	3	8	13	20	24	43	44
Subtotals:										
1. Single DX										
A. Not Operated	86	6.2	42	1	3	5	8	11	14	41
B. Operated	31	8.1	32	3	6	6	10	13	14	33
2. Multiple DX										
A. Not Operated	266	8.0	69	2	3	6	11	17	21	30
B. Operated	148	12.8	113	4	7	10	17	24	35	78
1. Single DX	117	6.7	40	1	3	6	8	12	14	40
2. Multiple DX	414	9.7	90	2	4	7	12	19	24	54
A. Not Operated	352	7.6	63	2	3	6	10	16	19	31
B. Operated	179	12.0	102	4	6	9	14	23	33	70
Total										
0–19 yrs	38	7.6	80	1	3	6	10	15	16	54
20–34	157	7.7	70	2	4	6	9	13	18	56
35–49	150	9.7	110	2	4	6	11	21	31	91
50–64	102	8.9	59	2	4	7	11	19	25	39
65+	84	11.3	65	3	5	10	16	21	23	44
Grand Total	531	9.1	80	2	4	7	11	18	23	52

(Continued)

Length of Stay data included in this publication are provided with permission from HCIA, Inc., Baltimore, MD.

4: Nonrespiratory tuberculosis (013–018)

Type of Patient	Total Patients	Avg. Stay	Vari-ance	Percentiles						
				10th	25th	50th	75th	90th	95th	99th
1. Single DX										
A. Not Operated										
0–19 yrs	0									
20–34	3	8.7	16	5	6	8	12	13	13	13
35–49	1	4.0		4	4	4	4	4	4	4
50–64	3	4.3	10	2	2	3	7	8	8	8
65+	1	2.0		2	2	2	2	2	2	2
B. Operated										
0–19 yrs	10	3.5	17	<1	1	2	3	10	14	14
20–34	5	3.8	9	1	2	3	5	9	9	9
35–49	2	16.0	2	15	15	16	17	17	17	17
50–64	1	2.0		2	2	2	2	2	2	2
65+	1	15.0		15	15	15	15	15	15	15
2. Multiple DX										
A. Not Operated										
0–19 yrs	6	8.5	117	1	2	5	7	28	30	30
20–34	18	15.1	271	2	4	9	16	46	55	58
35–49	12	7.3	61	<1	2	5	8	22	25	26
50–64	7	10.9	65	3	5	8	17	23	24	24
65+	5	9.0	55	1	3	7	15	19	19	19
B. Operated										
0–19 yrs	10	27.8	718	7	12	15	52	93	99+	99+
20–34	20	14.9	75	4	7	16	20	27	30	32
35–49	8	30.8	618	8	9	22	55	65	65	65
50–64	14	22.8	420	6	7	13	40	51	67	72
65+	9	25.0	356	3	12	20	41	53	56	56
Subtotals:										
1. Single DX										
A. Not Operated	8	5.6	15	2	3	4	8	12	13	13
B. Operated	19	5.4	31	1	2	3	8	15	16	17
2. Multiple DX										
A. Not Operated	48	11.1	149	2	4	7	15	25	37	58
B. Operated	61	22.4	376	4	9	16	32	57	68	99
1. Single DX	27	5.5	26	1	2	3	8	15	16	17
2. Multiple DX	109	17.4	306	3	6	12	22	47	58	93
A. Not Operated	56	10.3	133	2	3	7	13	24	33	58
B. Operated	80	18.4	346	2	4	14	24	49	65	97
Total										
0–19 yrs	26	14.0	416	1	2	7	15	53	91	99+
20–34	46	13.3	150	3	4	10	17	28	38	58
35–49	23	16.1	354	1	4	8	19	49	65	65
50–64	25	16.4	304	3	6	9	21	40	55	72
65+	16	17.9	278	2	4	15	20	48	54	56
Grand Total	136	15.0	272	2	4	9	19	40	57	90

(Continued)

Length of Stay data included in this publication are provided with permission from HCIA, Inc., Baltimore, MD.

147: Acute myocardial infarction (410)

Type of Patient	Total Patients	Avg. Stay	Vari-ance	Percentiles						
				10th	25th	50th	75th	90th	95th	99th
1. Single DX										
A. Not Operated										
0–19 yrs	0									
20–34	5	6.0	39	1	1	3	11	15	15	15
35–49	82	4.9	7	1	2	5	7	8	9	13
50–64	195	5.3	7	2	4	5	7	8	9	13
65+	172	5.4	7	2	4	6	7	8	9	13
B. Operated										
0–19 yrs	0									
20–34	11	6.0	12	1	4	6	8	11	12	12
35–49	110	5.2	6	2	3	5	7	8	9	10
50–64	134	5.6	7	2	4	5	7	9	11	12
65+	146	6.1	11	2	4	6	7	10	12	17
2. Multiple DX										
A. Not Operated										
0–19 yrs	2	6.0	8	4	4	6	8	8	8	8
20–34	26	5.0	7	2	3	5	6	8	11	12
35–49	435	5.9	9	2	4	6	7	10	12	16
50–64	1371	6.3	12	3	4	6	8	10	12	19
65+	4687	7.4	13	4	5	7	9	11	14	20
B. Operated										
0–19 yrs	0									
20–34	67	6.9	11	3	4	7	9	11	14	17
35–49	1105	7.0	26	3	4	6	8	11	13	27
50–64	2564	8.1	36	3	5	7	9	13	17	34
65+	2998	9.7	44	4	6	8	12	17	21	34
Subtotals:										
1. Single DX										
A. Not Operated	454	5.3	7	1	4	5	7	8	9	13
B. Operated	401	5.7	8	2	4	6	7	9	11	16
2. Multiple DX										
A. Not Operated	6521	7.0	13	3	5	7	8	11	13	20
B. Operated	6734	8.6	39	3	5	7	10	15	19	33
1. Single DX	855	5.5	8	2	4	5	7	9	10	13
2. Multiple DX	13255	7.8	27	3	5	7	9	13	16	27
A. Not Operated	6975	6.9	13	3	5	7	8	11	13	19
B. Operated	7135	8.4	37	3	5	7	10	14	18	32
Total										
0–19 yrs	2	6.0	8	4	4	6	8	8	8	8
20–34	109	6.3	12	2	4	6	8	11	13	16
35–49	1732	6.5	20	3	4	6	8	10	12	22
50–64	4264	7.3	27	3	5	6	9	12	15	27
65+	8003	8.2	26	4	5	7	10	14	17	27
Grand Total	14110	7.7	26	3	5	7	9	13	16	26

(Continued)

Length of Stay data included in this publication are provided with permission from HCIA, Inc., Baltimore, MD.

148: Angina pectoris (413)

Type of Patient	Total Patients	Avg. Stay	Vari-ance	Percentiles						
				10th	25th	50th	75th	90th	95th	99th
1. **Single DX**										
A. Not Operated										
0–19 yrs	0									
20–34	11	1.5	1	1	1	1	2	3	3	3
35–49	75	1.7	2	1	1	1	2	3	3	9
50–64	159	1.9	1	1	1	2	2	3	4	6
65+	151	1.9	1	1	1	2	2	3	4	6
B. Operated										
0–19 yrs	0									
20–34	0									
35–49	22	2.5	6	<1	1	2	3	3	7	13
50–64	44	2.1	2	<1	1	2	2	4	5	8
65+	64	2.8	11	1	1	2	3	7	10	19
2. **Multiple DX**										
A. Not Operated										
0–19 yrs	0									
20–34	32	2.3	2	1	1	2	3	5	5	6
35–49	418	2.2	3	1	1	2	3	4	6	8
50–64	1258	2.4	3	1	1	2	3	4	6	9
65+	2902	2.9	5	1	2	2	3	5	7	10
B. Operated										
0–19 yrs	0									
20–34	8	3.8	7	1	2	3	6	8	8	8
35–49	300	3.0	6	1	1	2	4	7	8	12
50–64	891	3.8	15	1	1	2	5	9	11	16
65+	998	4.6	20	1	2	3	7	10	12	20
Subtotals:										
1. **Single DX**										
A. Not Operated	396	1.8	1	1	1	2	2	3	4	6
B. Operated	130	2.5	7	1	1	2	3	5	8	14
2. **Multiple DX**										
A. Not Operated	4610	2.7	4	1	1	2	3	5	6	10
B. Operated	2197	4.1	16	1	1	3	6	9	11	17
1. **Single DX**	526	2.0	3	1	1	2	2	3	4	11
2. **Multiple DX**	6807	3.1	9	1	1	2	4	6	9	13
A. Not Operated	5006	2.6	4	1	1	2	3	5	6	10
B. Operated	2327	4.0	16	1	1	2	5	9	11	17
Total										
0–19 yrs	0									
20–34	51	2.4	3	1	1	2	3	5	6	8
35–49	815	2.5	4	1	1	2	3	5	7	11
50–64	2352	2.9	8	1	1	2	3	6	8	13
65+	4115	3.3	9	1	2	2	4	7	9	13
Grand Total	7333	3.0	8	1	1	2	4	6	8	13

(Continued)

Length of Stay data included in this publication are provided with permission from HCIA, Inc., Baltimore, MD.

159: Subarachnoid hemorrhage without paralysis (430)

Type of Patient	Total Patients	Avg. Stay	Vari-ance	Percentiles						
				10th	25th	50th	75th	90th	95th	99th
1. Single DX										
A. Not Operated										
0–19 yrs	2	4.0	2	3	3	4	5	5	5	5
20–34	1	4.0		4	4	4	4	4	4	4
35–49	5	5.8	25	2	3	3	9	14	14	14
50–64	0									
65+	3	5.7	12	2	3	6	8	9	9	9
B. Operated										
0–19 yrs	3	12.3	6	10	10	12	14	15	15	15
20–34	17	8.5	19	2	5	9	12	14	15	16
35–49	28	9.3	37	2	3	9	14	18	19	22
50–64	18	14.6	58	4	8	14	22	25	26	26
65+	0									
2. Multiple DX										
A. Not Operated										
0–19 yrs	1	7.0		7	7	7	7	7	7	7
20–34	3	11.0	19	6	8	13	14	14	14	14
35–49	4	10.0	21	6	6	10	14	14	14	14
50–64	10	8.5	107	<1	1	4	11	25	34	34
65+	33	11.2	54	3	5	11	14	22	27	31
B. Operated										
0–19 yrs	8	17.1	364	2	5	9	29	48	49	49
20–34	17	14.2	73	4	7	12	19	27	30	32
35–49	76	21.8	299	7	10	15	28	50	64	94
50–64	79	22.4	306	6	12	16	29	51	72	99+
65+	68	18.9	172	5	9	17	24	35	48	64
Subtotals:										
1. Single DX										
A. Not Operated	11	5.3	13	2	3	4	7	11	14	14
B. Operated	66	10.7	42	2	5	11	14	21	22	26
2. Multiple DX										
A. Not Operated	51	10.5	57	2	5	10	14	20	28	34
B. Operated	248	20.5	255	5	10	16	27	46	58	99+
1. Single DX	77	9.9	41	2	4	9	14	18	22	26
2. Multiple DX	299	18.8	235	5	9	14	25	41	54	95
A. Not Operated	62	9.5	53	2	4	8	14	17	26	34
B. Operated	314	18.4	226	4	9	14	24	41	53	93
Total										
0–19 yrs	14	13.5	222	3	5	9	12	46	48	49
20–34	38	11.2	50	3	6	11	14	20	27	32
35–49	113	17.6	248	3	8	13	23	45	55	85
50–64	107	19.8	265	3	10	15	26	42	59	99+
65+	104	16.0	145	4	7	14	21	31	37	63
Grand Total	376	17.0	208	3	8	13	22	37	51	86

(Continued)

Length of Stay data included in this publication are provided with permission from HCIA, Inc., Baltimore, MD.

160: Subarachnoid hemorrhage with paralysis (430 plus 342 or 344)

Type of Patient	Total Patients	Avg. Stay	Vari-ance	Percentiles						
				10th	25th	50th	75th	90th	95th	99th
1. **Single DX**										
A. Not Operated										
0–19 yrs	0									
20–34	0									
35–49	0									
50–64	0									
65+	0									
B. Operated										
0–19 yrs	0									
20–34	0									
35–49	0									
50–64	0									
65+	0									
2. **Multiple DX**										
A. Not Operated										
0–19 yrs	0									
20–34	1	13.0		13	13	13	13	13	13	13
35–49	0									
50–64	3	4.3		4	4	4	5	5	5	5
65+	8	17.1	50	8	13	16	22	27	28	28
B. Operated										
0–19 yrs	2	31.0	50	26	28	36	84	99+	99+	99+
20–34	1	13.0		13	13	13	13	13	13	13
35–49	9	20.7	94	9	12	22	30	33	33	33
50–64	6	30.7	702	6	14	19	56	69	71	71
65+	6	32.2	533	8	16	36	63	94	99+	99+
Subtotals:										
1. **Single DX**										
A. Not Operated	0									
B. Operated	0									
2. **Multiple DX**										
A. Not Operated	12	13.6	64	4	6	13	18	27	28	28
B. Operated	24	26.6	339	8	14	23	36	71	99+	99+
1. **Single DX**	0									
2. **Multiple DX**	36	22.3	282	5	12	18	32	65	88	99+
A. Not Operated	12	13.6	64	4	6	13	18	27	28	28
B. Operated	24	26.6	339	8	14	23	36	71	99+	99+
Total										
0–19 yrs	2	31.0	50	26	28	36	84	99+	99+	99+
20–34	2	13.0		13	13	13	13	13	13	13
35–49	9	20.7	94	9	12	22	30	33	33	33
50–64	9	21.9	612	4	5	14	31	65	71	71
65+	14	23.6	292	7	14	19	34	69	92	99+
Grand Total	36	22.3	282	5	12	18	32	65	88	99+

(Continued)

Length of Stay data included in this publication are provided with permission from HCIA, Inc., Baltimore, MD.

187: Bacterial pneumonia (481–482.9)

Type of Patient	Total Patients	Avg. Stay	Vari-ance	Percentiles						
				10th	25th	50th	75th	90th	95th	99th
1. Single DX										
A. Not Operated										
0–19 yrs	156	3.5	6	2	2	3	4	7	8	14
20–34	111	3.5	3	2	2	3	4	6	7	9
35–49	102	4.2	8	2	3	4	5	7	8	18
50–64	66	4.1	4	2	2	4	5	7	8	11
65+	97	4.7	6	2	3	4	6	8	10	12
B. Operated										
0–19 yrs	1	3.0		3	3	3	3	3	3	3
20–34	3	12.3	42	6	7	12	17	19	19	19
35–49	5	5.4	8	3	3	4	8	9	9	9
50–64	5	6.8	29	2	3	6	9	16	16	16
65+	2	7.5	1	7	7	7	8	8	8	8
2. Multiple DX										
A. Not Operated										
0–19 yrs	551	5.8	37	2	3	4	8	11	14	21
20–34	440	5.7	22	2	3	4	7	11	15	24
35–49	617	5.9	19	2	3	5	7	10	13	26
50–64	1000	6.6	20	3	4	6	8	12	15	22
65+	4804	7.5	22	3	4	6	9	13	16	25
B. Operated										
0–19 yrs	63	15.3	259	4	7	11	18	28	82	99+
20–34	93	15.4	164	5	7	13	21	34	46	99+
35–49	154	13.8	121	4	6	10	18	31	40	99+
50–64	189	14.0	145	5	7	11	16	25	36	72
65+	721	15.2	123	6	8	12	19	28	38	66
Subtotals:										
1. Single DX										
A. Not Operated	532	3.9	6	2	2	3	5	7	8	12
B. Operated	16	7.3	23	3	4	6	9	16	18	19
2. Multiple DX										
A. Not Operated	7412	7.0	23	3	4	6	9	12	15	24
B. Operated	1220	14.9	136	5	8	12	18	29	39	79
1. Single DX	548	4.0	6	2	2	3	5	7	8	12
2. Multiple DX	8632	8.1	46	3	4	6	10	15	19	38
A. Not Operated	7944	6.8	22	3	4	6	8	12	15	24
B. Operated	1236	14.8	135	5	8	12	18	28	39	78
Total										
0–19 yrs	771	6.1	57	2	2	4	8	12	15	41
20–34	647	6.7	53	2	3	5	7	14	20	50
35–49	878	7.1	45	2	4	5	8	13	19	44
50–64	1260	7.6	45	3	4	6	9	14	18	36
65+	5624	8.5	41	3	5	7	10	15	20	36
Grand Total	9180	7.9	45	3	4	6	10	14	19	37

(Continued)

Length of Stay data included in this publication are provided with permission from HCIA, Inc., Baltimore, MD.

188: Other pneumonia (480; 483–486)

Type of Patient	Total Patients	Avg. Stay	Vari- ance	Percentiles						
				10th	25th	50th	75th	90th	95th	99th
1. **Single DX**										
A. Not Operated										
0–19 yrs	1611	3.2	4	1	2	3	4	5	7	10
20–34	296	3.6	4	2	2	3	4	6	6	11
35–49	255	3.9	5	2	2	3	5	6	7	10
50–64	139	3.7	4	2	3	3	5	6	7	12
65+	253	5.0	8	2	3	4	6	8	11	14
B. Operated										
0–19 yrs	16	5.2	17	<1	2	4	7	12	13	14
20–34	10	8.3	16	4	5	7	13	14	15	15
35–49	17	7.3	15	3	4	7	10	13	16	17
50–64	9	6.6	13	1	3	7	9	11	12	12
65+	4	7.5	8	5	5	7	10	10	10	10
2. **Multiple DX**										
A. Not Operated										
0–19 yrs	5161	4.0	12	1	2	3	5	7	10	18
20–34	850	4.6	8	2	3	4	6	8	10	14
35–49	1204	5.0	13	2	3	4	6	9	11	18
50–64	1892	5.7	15	2	3	5	7	10	12	19
65+	9132	6.7	17	3	4	6	8	11	14	22
B. Operated										
0–19 yrs	182	11.1	150	3	4	8	13	25	58	99+
20–34	122	11.7	146	3	5	8	15	22	34	70
35–49	213	11.6	107	3	6	9	15	22	26	60
50–64	295	11.2	71	4	6	9	14	20	29	45
65+	920	12.1	74	5	7	10	14	22	28	45
Subtotals:										
1. **Single DX**										
A. Not Operated	2554	3.5	5	1	2	3	4	6	7	12
B. Operated	56	6.8	15	2	4	6	10	13	14	17
2. **Multiple DX**										
A. Not Operated	18239	5.6	16	2	3	5	7	10	13	20
B. Operated	1732	11.7	90	4	6	9	14	22	30	58
1. **Single DX**	2610	3.6	5	1	2	3	4	6	7	12
2. **Multiple DX**	19971	6.2	25	2	3	5	8	11	15	25
A. Not Operated	20793	5.4	15	2	3	4	7	10	12	20
B. Operated	1788	11.6	89	4	6	9	14	22	29	56
Total										
0–19 yrs	6970	4.0	15	1	2	3	5	7	10	19
20–34	1278	5.0	25	2	3	4	6	9	12	23
35–49	1689	5.7	29	2	3	4	7	10	14	25
50–64	2335	6.2	25	2	3	5	8	11	15	28
65+	10309	7.2	24	3	4	6	9	12	16	26
Grand Total	22581	5.9	24	2	3	5	7	11	14	25

(Continued)

Length of Stay data included in this publication are provided with permission from HCIA, Inc., Baltimore, MD.

217: Intestinal obstruction without mention of hernia (560.0–560.2; 560.8–560.9)

Type of Patient	Total Patients	Avg. Stay	Vari- ance	Percentiles						
				10th	25th	50th	75th	90th	95th	99th
1. Single DX										
A. Not Operated										
0–19 yrs	124	1.8	2	1	1	1	2	3	4	7
20–34	132	3.5	10	1	2	3	4	6	9	21
35–49	206	3.1	4	1	2	3	4	6	7	10
50–64	219	3.1	4	1	2	3	4	5	7	10
65+	235	3.1	3	1	2	3	4	5	7	9
B. Operated										
0–19 yrs	107	5.6	31	2	3	4	7	10	11	32
20–34	71	7.1	12	3	5	7	9	11	15	18
35–49	92	7.5	12	4	5	7	9	12	14	20
50–64	82	7.8	8	5	6	8	9	11	13	17
65+	69	7.8	7	4	6	7	9	12	12	14
2. Multiple DX										
A. Not Operated										
0–19 yrs	144	3.9	13	1	2	3	5	8	11	20
20–34	200	3.8	7	1	2	3	5	8	9	13
35–49	424	4.1	7	1	2	3	5	7	9	14
50–64	699	4.2	14	1	2	3	5	8	9	15
65+	2174	5.1	15	2	3	4	6	9	12	19
B. Operated										
0–19 yrs	206	9.8	135	4	5	6	9	17	33	91
20–34	177	10.2	38	4	6	9	12	20	23	31
35–49	377	11.9	109	5	7	9	13	21	28	86
50–64	486	12.4	89	6	7	10	14	22	30	52
65+	1338	13.7	75	6	8	11	16	24	31	48
Subtotals:										
1. Single DX										
A. Not Operated	916	3.0	4	1	2	2	4	5	7	10
B. Operated	421	7.0	16	3	5	7	9	11	13	18
2. Multiple DX										
A. Not Operated	3641	4.7	13	2	2	4	6	8	11	17
B. Operated	2584	12.7	86	5	7	10	15	23	30	52
1. Single DX	1337	4.3	12	1	2	3	6	8	10	15
2. Multiple DX	6225	8.0	59	2	3	6	10	16	21	39
A. Not Operated	4557	4.3	12	1	2	4	5	8	10	17
B. Operated	3005	11.9	80	5	7	9	14	21	29	49
Total										
0–19 yrs	581	5.8	67	1	2	4	7	10	16	53
20–34	580	6.1	27	2	3	4	8	12	17	24
35–49	1099	6.9	56	2	3	5	8	13	18	38
50–64	1486	6.9	52	2	3	5	9	13	19	36
65+	3816	8.0	53	2	3	6	10	16	21	36
Grand Total	7562	7.3	53	2	3	5	9	15	20	36

(Continued)

218: Noninfectious gastroenteritis and colitis (558)

Type of Patient	Total Patients	Avg. Stay	Vari- ance	Percentiles						
				10th	25th	50th	75th	90th	95th	99th
1. Single DX										
A. Not Operated										
0–19 yrs	563	1.9	2	1	1	2	2	3	4	6
20–34	329	1.8	1	1	1	2	2	3	4	7
35–49	198	1.9	1	1	1	2	2	3	4	6
50–64	86	2.2	2	1	1	2	3	4	4	8
65+	47	2.3	2	1	1	2	3	5	6	6
B. Operated										
0–19 yrs	33	3.2	3	1	2	3	4	5	6	9
20–34	47	3.7	5	2	2	3	4	5	9	13
35–49	29	3.7	3	2	3	3	4	6	7	8
50–64	8	4.1	8	<1	1	4	7	8	8	8
65+	6	3.7	3	<1	3	4	4	6	6	6
2. Multiple DX										
A. Not Operated										
0–19 yrs	1790	2.5	5	1	1	2	3	4	6	12
20–34	618	2.4	5	1	1	2	3	4	6	9
35–49	559	2.9	7	1	1	2	3	6	7	14
50–64	521	3.1	6	1	2	2	4	6	8	12
65+	1324	4.1	16	1	2	3	5	8	10	16
B. Operated										
0–19 yrs	53	7.1	95	2	3	4	6	17	24	61
20–34	72	4.8	15	2	2	4	6	9	14	19
35–49	112	6.6	55	2	3	5	7	10	25	43
50–64	86	6.4	28	1	3	5	9	15	22	72
65+	239	8.9	77	3	4	7	10	17	23	52
Subtotals:										
1. Single DX										
A. Not Operated	1223	1.9	2	1	1	2	2	3	4	7
B. Operated	123	3.6	4	2	2	3	4	6	7	11
2. Multiple DX										
A. Not Operated	4812	3.1	9	1	1	2	4	6	8	14
B. Operated	562	7.4	61	2	3	5	8	15	22	49
1. Single DX	1346	2.1	2	1	1	2	3	4	5	8
2. Multiple DX	5374	3.5	16	1	2	2	4	7	9	19
A. Not Operated	6035	2.8	8	1	1	2	3	5	7	13
B. Operated	685	6.7	52	2	3	5	7	14	20	46
Total										
0–19 yrs	2439	2.5	6	1	1	2	3	4	6	13
20–34	1066	2.4	5	1	1	2	3	4	6	13
35–49	898	3.2	14	1	1	2	4	6	8	19
50–64	701	3.4	10	1	2	3	4	7	9	17
65+	1616	4.8	28	1	2	3	6	9	12	23
Grand Total	6720	3.2	13	1	1	2	4	6	8	17

(Continued)

Length of Stay data included in this publication are provided with permission from HCIA, Inc., Baltimore, MD.

239: Acute pyelonephritis (590.1)

Type of Patient	Total Patients	Avg. Stay	Vari-ance	Percentiles						
				10th	25th	50th	75th	90th	95th	99th
1. Single DX										
A. Not Operated										
0–19 yrs	140	3.0	2	1	2	3	4	5	6	7
20–34	174	3.0	2	2	2	3	4	4	5	7
35–49	45	3.2	2	2	2	3	4	5	6	8
50–64	17	3.1	2	1	2	3	4	5	5	5
65+	19	2.9	2	1	2	3	4	5	5	5
B. Operated										
0–19 yrs	8	4.5	4	2	3	4	6	7	8	8
20–34	2	4.0	2	3	3	4	5	5	5	5
35–49	2	5.5	5	4	4	5	7	7	7	7
50–64	1	6.0		6	6	6	6	6	6	6
65+	1	7.0		7	7	7	7	7	7	7
2. Multiple DX										
A. Not Operated										
0–19 yrs	450	3.5	3	2	2	3	4	6	7	9
20–34	719	3.7	3	2	3	3	5	6	7	9
35–49	362	4.2	4	2	3	4	5	7	8	12
50–64	298	4.8	6	2	3	4	6	8	9	13
65+	652	5.3	10	2	3	5	7	9	11	18
B. Operated										
0–19 yrs	41	6.5	14	2	4	6	8	12	14	16
20–34	41	8.1	34	2	4	7	11	19	20	24
35–49	39	9.2	60	3	5	7	12	15	27	41
50–64	48	9.1	52	4	5	7	10	15	28	39
65+	87	9.5	49	3	5	8	12	15	25	40
Subtotals:										
1. Single DX										
A. Not Operated	395	3.0	2	1	2	3	4	5	5	8
B. Operated	14	4.9	4	3	3	5	6	7	8	8
2. Multiple DX										
A. Not Operated	2481	4.3	6	2	3	4	5	7	8	12
B. Operated	256	8.7	44	3	4	7	11	15	22	39
1. Single DX	409	3.1	2	1	2	3	4	5	6	8
2. Multiple DX	2737	4.7	11	2	3	4	6	8	10	17
A. Not Operated	2876	4.1	6	2	3	4	5	7	8	12
B. Operated	270	8.5	42	3	4	7	10	14	22	38
Total										
0–19 yrs	639	3.6	4	2	2	3	4	6	7	11
20–34	936	3.8	5	2	2	3	4	6	7	12
35–49	448	4.5	11	2	3	4	5	8	9	15
50–64	364	5.3	14	2	3	5	7	9	11	21
65+	759	5.7	16	2	3	5	7	10	12	23
Grand Total	3146	4.5	10	2	3	4	5	8	10	16

(Continued)

Length of Stay data included in this publication are provided with permission from HCIA, Inc., Baltimore, MD.

240: Miscellaneous kidney infections (590.0; 590.2–590.9)

Type of Patient	Total Patients	Avg. Stay	Vari-ance	Percentiles						
				10th	25th	50th	75th	90th	95th	99th
1. Single DX										
A. Not Operated										
0–19 yrs	120	3.3	3	1	2	3	4	6	7	10
20–34	125	3.0	2	2	2	3	4	5	5	7
35–49	49	3.8	3	2	3	4	5	6	7	8
50–64	17	2.9	2	<1	2	3	4	5	6	6
65+	12	2.9	5	<1	1	2	4	6	8	8
B. Operated										
0–19 yrs	4	6.5	17	2	3	7	10	10	10	10
20–34	4	5.3	7	3	3	4	7	9	9	9
35–49	4	5.0	19	<1	1	4	8	11	11	11
50–64	2	4.5	5	3	3	4	6	6	6	6
65+	2	3.0		3	3	3	3	3	3	3
2. Multiple DX										
A. Not Operated										
0–19 yrs	300	3.7	4	2	2	3	5	7	8	10
20–34	353	3.8	4	2	2	3	5	6	8	11
35–49	193	4.8	9	2	3	4	6	8	10	17
50–64	157	5.1	9	2	3	4	7	9	11	15
65+	250	5.4	10	2	3	5	7	9	10	17
B. Operated										
0–19 yrs	68	6.6	17	3	4	6	8	12	16	86
20–34	44	7.0	24	2	4	6	8	14	16	24
35–49	40	13.1	126	2	6	10	17	35	39	43
50–64	44	9.9	36	3	5	8	14	18	21	27
65+	47	10.0	45	3	6	8	13	21	25	30
Subtotals:										
1. Single DX										
A. Not Operated	323	3.2	3	1	2	3	4	5	6	8
B. Operated	16	5.1	10	2	3	4	7	10	11	11
2. Multiple DX										
A. Not Operated	1253	4.4	7	2	3	4	6	8	9	13
B. Operated	243	9.0	50	3	4	7	12	17	24	41
1. Single DX	339	3.3	3	1	2	3	4	5	7	10
2. Multiple DX	1496	5.2	17	2	3	4	6	9	12	23
A. Not Operated	1576	4.2	6	2	2	4	5	7	9	13
B. Operated	259	8.8	48	3	4	7	11	17	23	41
Total										
0–19 yrs	492	4.0	7	2	2	3	5	7	9	14
20–34	526	3.9	6	2	2	3	5	7	8	14
35–49	286	5.8	33	2	3	4	7	10	15	37
50–64	220	5.9	18	2	3	5	7	11	15	22
65+	311	6.0	18	2	3	5	7	10	14	25
Grand Total	1835	4.8	15	2	3	4	6	8	11	21

(Continued)

Length of Stay data included in this publication are provided with permission from HCIA, Inc., Baltimore, MD.

501: Incision, excision of skull, brain, and cerebral meninges (01.0–01.15; 01.3–01.6)

Type of Patient	Total Patients	Avg. Stay	Vari- ance	Percentiles						
				10th	25th	50th	75th	90th	95th	99th
1. **Single DX**										
0–19 yrs	121	6.7	27	2	3	5	8	13	20	25
20–34	113	7.6	31	3	4	6	9	14	19	30
35–49	106	6.0	14	1	3	6	8	11	13	17
50–64	107	6.8	22	2	4	6	9	13	15	27
65+	102	7.5	20	2	5	7	9	14	17	22
2. **Multiple DX**										
0–19 yrs	352	14.2	226	2	5	10	17	35	51	99+
20–34	221	14.5	186	3	5	9	18	36	45	65
35–49	378	12.8	141	4	6	9	15	28	41	82
50–64	374	12.6	188	3	6	9	15	23	36	93
65+	634	13.6	97	5	7	11	17	25	33	54
Total Single DX	549	6.9	24	2	4	6	9	13	17	25
Total Multiple DX	1959	13.5	157	4	6	10	17	28	40	83
Total										
0–19 yrs	473	12.2	186	2	4	8	15	30	46	99+
20–34	334	12.2	145	3	5	8	15	31	38	54
35–49	484	11.3	121	3	5	8	13	24	35	69
50–64	481	11.3	157	3	5	8	13	22	28	87
65+	736	12.8	92	4	7	10	16	24	31	53
Grand Total	2508	12.0	135	3	5	9	15	24	36	71

502: Craniotomy and craniectomy (01.2)

Type of Patient	Total Patients	Avg. Stay	Vari- ance	Percentiles						
				10th	25th	50th	75th	90th	95th	99th
1. **Single DX**										
0–19 yrs	89	4.9	7	3	3	4	6	8	10	17
20–34	32	8.9	75	3	4	5	11	21	25	42
35–49	30	7.4	24	2	3	6	11	15	18	19
50–64	22	9.7	95	4	5	6	10	20	31	47
65+	15	6.5	14	4	5	6	7	8	16	19
2. **Multiple DX**										
0–19 yrs	147	14.6	255	3	5	10	20	49	97	99+
20–34	104	15.0	196	4	6	10	19	35	47	61
35–49	102	13.8	131	4	6	9	19	31	35	53
50–64	88	22.0	357	6	8	18	28	47	68	99
65+	99	14.6	146	6	8	11	17	28	34	97
Total Single DX	188	6.7	35	3	4	5	7	14	18	36
Total Multiple DX	540	15.7	224	4	6	11	21	36	54	99+
Total										
0–19 yrs	236	10.9	184	3	4	6	14	27	55	99+
20–34	136	13.5	174	4	5	9	16	32	43	61
35–49	132	12.4	114	4	5	8	15	26	34	53
50–64	110	19.5	328	5	7	14	25	46	64	98
65+	114	13.5	136	5	7	11	16	26	32	96
Grand Total	728	13.4	190	3	5	9	17	30	47	99+

(Continued)

Length of Stay data included in this publication are provided with permission from HCIA, Inc., Baltimore, MD.

503: Cranioplasty (02.0)

Type of Patient	Total Patients	Avg. Stay	Vari-ance	Percentiles						
				10th	25th	50th	75th	90th	95th	99th
1. Single DX										
0–19 yrs	262	3.7	2	2	3	3	5	5	6	8
20–34	31	3.5	4	1	2	3	4	6	10	10
35–49	17	4.6	15	1	2	3	6	11	14	15
50–64	9	4.4	6	1	3	4	5	8	10	10
65+	4	4.0	11	2	2	3	6	9	9	9
2. Multiple DX										
0–19 yrs	202	6.3	68	2	3	4	6	13	22	81
20–34	107	8.8	109	2	3	6	10	18	33	81
35–49	53	10.3	156	2	3	6	10	34	42	55
50–64	29	8.4	153	2	4	5	8	15	20	69
65+	29	6.1	33	1	2	3	10	16	18	22
Total Single DX	323	3.7	4	2	3	3	5	6	7	12
Total Multiple DX	420	7.6	95	2	3	5	8	16	30	68
Total										
0–19 yrs	464	4.8	33	2	3	4	5	7	11	43
20–34	138	7.6	91	2	3	5	9	16	30	71
35–49	70	8.9	127	1	3	5	9	24	38	53
50–64	38	7.4	120	2	4	5	8	13	17	69
65+	33	5.8	31	2	2	3	9	15	18	22
Grand Total	743	5.9	59	2	3	4	6	11	17	55

504: Ventricular shunt (02.2–02.3)

Type of Patient	Total Patients	Avg. Stay	Vari-ance	Percentiles						
				10th	25th	50th	75th	90th	95th	99th
1. Single DX										
0–19 yrs	81	5.2	39	1	2	3	5	11	22	30
20–34	17 .	6.2	9	3	4	6	9	11	12	13
35–49	16	7.3	33	2	4	6	8	14	22	25
50–64	11	3.7	4	1	2	4	5	7	7	7
65+	20	6.3	16	2	4	5	8	12	15	18
2. Multiple DX										
0–19 yrs	287	11.2	211	2	3	6	14	36	65	99+
20–34	58	13.2	160	3	5	8	16	38	46	95
35–49	54	13.9	240	3	5	8	17	37	64	98
50–64	81	16.5	184	3	7	13	22	39	49	87
65+	142	13.7	128	4	6	9	20	32	42	53
Total Single DX	145	5.6	30	2	2	4	6	11	19	30
Total Multiple DX	622	12.9	189	2	4	8	17	36	49	99+
Total										
0–19 yrs	368	9.8	180	2	3	5	12	30	56	99+
20–34	75	11.6	134	3	4	7	13	33	44	86
35–49	70	12.4	199	3	4	8	15	29	62	93
50–64	92	15.0	180	2	6	11	21	37	48	83
65+	162	12.8	120	3	5	8	17	30	39	49
Grand Total	767	11.5	167	2	4	7	14	31	43	99+

(Continued)

Length of Stay data included in this publication are provided with permission from HCIA, Inc., Baltimore, MD.

565: Lobectomy and complete pneumonectomy (32.4–32.5)

Type of Patient	Total Patients	Avg. Stay	Vari-ance	Percentiles						
				10th	25th	50th	75th	90th	95th	99th
1. Single DX										
0–19 yrs	8	5.5	13	3	4	4	6	12	14	14
20–34	0									
35–49	18	9.8	128	5	6	6	7	17	39	53
50–64	42	8.9	180	4	5	7	8	9	15	92
65+	38	7.1	4	5	6	7	8	11	12	12
2. Multiple DX										
0–19 yrs	24	9.7	68	4	5	8	10	14	32	41
20–34	23	16.5	275	6	7	9	22	34	50	78
35–49	82	10.5	30	5	7	9	12	19	21	30
50–64	343	10.0	36	6	6	8	11	16	21	37
65+	514	11.2	53	6	7	9	13	18	23	49
Total Single DX	106	8.1	95	4	6	6	8	11	14	70
Total Multiple DX	986	10.8	52	6	7	9	12	18	23	42
Total										
0–19 yrs	32	8.6	57	4	4	7	9	13	27	41
20–34	23	16.5	275	6	7	9	22	34	50	78
35–49	100	10.3	47	5	6	9	12	18	21	42
50–64	385	9.8	52	5	6	8	11	16	21	39
65+	552	10.9	51	6	7	9	12	18	22	48
Grand Total	1092	10.5	57	6	7	8	12	17	22	43

566: Bronchoscopy (33.22–33.23)

Type of Patient	Total Patients	Avg. Stay	Vari-ance	Percentiles						
				10th	25th	50th	75th	90th	95th	99th
1. Single DX										
0–19 yrs	187	1.9	5	<1	1	1	2	4	7	14
20–34	18	6.7	35	<1	1	5	11	17	19	19
35–49	19	9.5	59	1	4	8	14	17	26	33
50–64	22	4.5	19	1	1	3	6	11	14	18
65+	9	4.2	7	1	2	4	6	9	9	9
2. Multiple DX										
0–19 yrs	290	8.2	133	<1	1	4	10	25	49	99+
20–34	224	11.8	84	3	6	10	15	23	31	48
35–49	226	11.6	84	3	5	9	15	22	30	49
50–64	287	11.3	135	2	4	8	14	25	34	63
65+	549	11.1	70	3	6	9	14	21	27	42
Total Single DX	255	3.1	18	<1	1	1	3	8	12	18
Total Multiple DX	1576	10.8	99	2	4	8	14	22	31	65
Total										
0–19 yrs	477	5.7	92	<1	1	2	7	17	31	99+
20–34	242	11.5	82	3	6	9	15	22	29	47
35–49	245	11.4	82	3	5	9	15	22	30	48
50–64	309	10.8	130	2	4	8	14	24	33	61
65+	558	11.0	71	3	6	9	14	21	27	42
Grand Total	1831	9.7	95	1	3	7	13	21	29	60

(Continued)

567: Miscellaneous operations on lung (32.6–32.9; 33.1; 33.3; 33.43; 33.49; 33.5; 33.93; 33.99)

Type of Patient	Total Patients	Avg. Stay	Vari-ance	Percentiles						
				10th	25th	50th	75th	90th	95th	99th
1. Single DX										
0–19 yrs	7	5.3	18	1	2	4	9	12	12	12
20–34	14	4.0	1	3	3	4	5	5	6	6
35–49	10	4.8	18	1	2	3	6	11	16	16
50–64	8	9.1	86	2	3	5	12	25	30	30
65+	7	6.0	9	2	4	6	9	10	10	10
2. Multiple DX										
0–19 yrs	27	10.4	108	3	5	9	10	18	28	56
20–34	34	10.2	124	2	3	6	11	24	41	48
35–49	34	8.4	85	2	3	5	11	16	24	50
50–64	45	9.6	76	2	4	6	12	23	26	46
65+	53	10.3	98	3	4	7	15	20	27	60
Total Single DX	46	5.6	24	2	3	4	6	11	14	30
Total Multiple DX	193	9.8	95	3	4	7	12	20	26	53
Total										
0–19 yrs	34	9.4	93	2	4	8	10	15	22	56
20–34	48	8.4	96	2	3	5	10	18	27	48
35–49	44	7.6	72	2	3	4	9	16	20	50
50–64	53	9.5	77	2	4	6	12	23	27	46
65+	60	9.8	89	3	4	6	14	19	25	58
Grand Total	239	9.0	84	2	4	6	11	19	25	51

568: Thoracotomy (34.0)

Type of Patient	Total Patients	Avg. Stay	Vari-ance	Percentiles						
				10th	25th	50th	75th	90th	95th	99th
1. Single DX										
0–19 yrs	111	4.4	7	2	2	4	5	9	10	13
20–34	285	4.5	13	2	3	4	5	8	10	18
35–49	106	5.0	15	2	3	4	6	10	14	20
50–64	35	4.7	9	1	3	4	6	9	11	15
65+	20	4.4	3	2	3	4	6	7	8	9
2. Multiple DX										
0–19 yrs	267	9.5	100	3	4	7	11	19	31	67
20–34	548	7.5	54	2	4	5	9	15	19	39
35–49	448	8.2	63	2	4	6	10	16	22	43
50–64	456	8.7	41	3	4	7	11	17	22	34
65+	843	10.0	69	3	5	7	12	21	26	41
Total Single DX	557	4.6	12	2	3	4	5	9	10	19
Total Multiple DX	2562	8.9	64	3	4	7	11	18	24	43
Total										
0–19 yrs	378	8.0	79	2	3	5	9	15	22	64
20–34	833	6.4	42	2	3	5	8	12	17	30
35–49	554	7.6	56	2	3	5	9	15	20	40
50–64	491	8.4	40	3	4	7	11	16	22	34
65+	863	9.9	68	3	5	7	12	21	26	41
Grand Total	3119	8.1	58	2	4	6	10	16	22	40

(Continued)

Length of Stay data included in this publication are provided with permission from HCIA, Inc., Baltimore, MD.

573: Cardiac catheterization (37.21–37.23)

Type of Patient	Total Patients	Avg. Stay	Vari- ance	Percentiles						
				10th	25th	50th	75th	90th	95th	99th
1. Single DX										
0–19 yrs	178	1.8	3	<1	<1	1	1	5	7	9
20–34	64	2.8	13	1	1	2	3	5	9	24
35–49	346	2.6	4	1	1	2	3	6	8	11
50–64	504	2.5	6	1	1	2	3	5	7	12
65+	314	2.7	6	1	1	2	4	6	7	13
2. Multiple DX										
0–19 yrs	504	3.6	61	<1	<1	1	2	10	16	46
20–34	196	5.2	27	1	2	4	7	12	15	25
35–49	1918	4.3	20	1	1	3	6	9	11	24
50–64	4693	4.4	20	1	1	3	6	9	12	21
65+	5733	5.1	23	1	2	4	7	10	13	24
Total Single DX	1406	2.5	6	<1	1	1	3	6	7	12
Total Multiple DX	13044	4.7	24	1	1	3	6	9	12	23
Total										
0–19 yrs	682	3.1	47	<1	<1	1	2	8	13	36
20–34	260	4.6	25	1	1	3	6	11	15	26
35–49	2264	4.1	19	1	1	3	6	8	10	23
50–64	5197	4.2	19	1	1	3	6	9	11	20
65+	6047	4.9	23	1	2	4	7	10	13	24
Grand Total	14450	4.4	22	1	1	3	6	9	12	23

574: Pacemaker insertion, replacement, removal, and repair (37.70–37.78; 37.8; 37.94–37.98)

Type of Patient	Total Patients	Avg. Stay	Vari- ance	Percentiles						
				10th	25th	50th	75th	90th	95th	99th
1. Single DX										
0–19 yrs	10	3.6	5	1	2	3	5	7	8	8
20–34	12	2.9	13	1	1	2	3	7	13	14
35–49	14	4.6	55	1	1	2	3	12	25	29
50–64	47	2.7	4	1	1	2	3	6	8	8
65+	239	2.4	3	1	1	2	3	5	7	10
2. Multiple DX										
0–19 yrs	84	6.4	105	1	2	3	6	14	23	55
20–34	37	5.8	45	1	2	3	7	11	14	39
35–49	100	5.7	27	1	2	4	8	12	19	25
50–64	439	6.6	41	1	2	5	9	14	19	36
65+	2895	6.0	31	1	2	4	8	13	16	27
Total Single DX	322	2.6	7	1	1	2	3	5	8	12
Total Multiple DX	3555	6.1	34	1	2	4	8	13	16	29
Total										
0–19 yrs	94	6.1	96	1	2	3	6	13	22	55
20–34	49	5.1	39	1	2	3	6	11	14	39
35–49	114	5.6	31	1	2	4	8	11	19	28
50–64	486	6.3	39	1	2	5	8	14	18	36
65+	3134	5.7	30	1	2	4	7	12	15	27
Grand Total	3877	5.8	33	1	2	4	7	13	16	29

(Continued)

Length of Stay data included in this publication are provided with permission from HCIA, Inc., Baltimore, MD.

575: Miscellaneous operations on heart (35.0; 35.52; 36.03; 36.2–36.9; 37.0–37.1; 37.24–37.25; 37.3–37.4; 37.91–37.93; 37.99)

Type of Patient	Total Patients	Avg. Stay	Vari-ance	Percentiles						
				10th	25th	50th	75th	90th	95th	99th
1. Single DX										
0–19 yrs	24	5.6	24	<1	1	5	8	11	18	18
20–34	22	4.2	9	1	2	3	6	7	11	15
35–49	16	5.1	53	1	1	2	6	13	24	29
50–64	12	4.3	8	1	2	3	6	9	10	10
65+	5	9.0	28	5	5	8	11	18	18	18
2. Multiple DX										
0–19 yrs	68	7.7	42	<1	3	6	10	15	20	33
20–34	75	8.8	41	2	4	7	11	18	19	36
35–49	113	9.0	61	2	4	7	11	18	27	37
50–64	168	11.0	81	3	5	9	14	22	27	47
65+	179	12.2	91	3	7	10	15	23	33	52
Total Single DX	79	5.1	24	1	2	4	7	10	16	26
Total Multiple DX	603	10.3	73	2	5	8	13	19	26	43
Total										
0–19 yrs	92	7.1	39	<1	2	6	9	15	19	31
20–34	97	7.7	38	2	4	6	10	15	19	35
35–49	129	8.5	61	1	3	6	11	18	27	37
50–64	180	10.6	79	2	5	8	14	21	26	46
65+	184	12.1	90	3	6	10	15	23	32	52
Grand Total	682	9.7	70	2	4	8	12	18	25	42

576: Other diagnostic and therapeutic procedures on larynx, trachea, bronchus, lungs and heart (for ICD-9-CM codes, see Appendix)

Type of Patient	Total Patients	Avg. Stay	Vari-ance	Percentiles						
				10th	25th	50th	75th	90th	95th	99th
1. Single DX										
0–19 yrs	150	2.3	17	<1	1	1	2	4	7	15
20–34	81	3.9	16	1	1	2	5	9	11	20
35–49	55	3.6	12	1	1	3	5	8	11	19
50–64	53	3.5	9	1	1	2	5	9	10	11
65+	28	3.9	11	1	2	3	5	8	12	14
2. Multiple DX										
0–19 yrs	360	7.6	121	1	2	5	9	18	34	99+
20–34	251	7.9	87	1	3	5	10	15	23	56
35–49	415	8.8	60	2	4	7	11	18	25	39
50–64	774	8.1	53	2	3	6	10	17	24	38
65+	2103	9.2	48	3	4	7	12	18	22	35
Total Single DX	367	3.1	15	<1	1	2	4	7	10	17
Total Multiple DX	3903	8.7	61	2	4	7	11	18	23	40
Total										
0–19 yrs	510	6.0	97	1	1	3	7	13	22	94
20–34	332	7.0	73	1	2	5	9	14	19	45
35–49	470	8.2	58	1	3	6	10	17	25	38
50–64	827	7.8	52	2	3	6	10	16	23	38
65+	2131	9.2	48	3	4	7	12	18	22	35
Grand Total	4270	8.2	59	1	3	6	11	17	23	40

(Continued)

Length of Stay data included in this publication are provided with permission from HCIA, Inc., Baltimore, MD.

737: Total knee replacement (81.54)

Type of Patient	Total Patients	Avg. Stay	Vari-ance	Percentiles						
				10th	25th	50th	75th	90th	95th	99th
1. Single DX										
0–19 yrs	2	7.0		7	7	7	7	7	7	7
20–34	12	8.8	25	4	6	7	11	16	21	22
35–49	70	6.9	4	4	5	7	9	10	10	12
50–64	363	7.0	6	4	5	7	8	10	12	14
65+	1060	7.7	19	5	6	7	9	11	12	14
2. Multiple DX										
0–19 yrs	3	9.3	5	8	8	8	11	12	12	12
20–34	18	6.9	10	4	4	6	9	12	14	14
35–49	101	8.4	15	5	6	8	10	13	14	25
50–64	857	7.9	9	5	6	7	9	11	13	18
65+	3628	8.4	9	5	7	8	10	12	14	20
Total Single DX	1507	7.5	16	5	6	7	9	10	12	14
Total Multiple DX	4607	8.3	10	5	6	8	10	12	14	19
Total										
0–19 yrs	5	8.4	4	7	7	8	9	12	12	12
20–34	30	7.7	17	4	5	6	10	13	14	22
35–49	171	7.8	11	4	6	7	9	11	14	19
50–64	1220	7.7	9	4	6	7	9	11	13	17
65+	4688	8.2	12	5	6	8	9	12	13	18
Grand Total	6114	8.1	11	5	6	8	9	11	13	18

738: Arthroplasty of knee, except total replacement (81.42–81.47; 81.55)

Type of Patient	Total Patients	Avg. Stay	Vari-ance	Percentiles						
				10th	25th	50th	75th	90th	95th	99th
1. Single DX										
0–19 yrs	395	2.5		1	2	2	3	4	4	5
20–34	855	2.6	1	1	2	3	3	4	4	6
35–49	340	2.8	1	1	2	3	3	4	5	9
50–64	69	5.9	11	2	3	6	8	10	12	17
65+	84	6.2	6	3	4	6	8	9	10	11
2. Multiple DX										
0–19 yrs	546	2.7	1	1	2	3	3	4	5	9
20–34	1613	2.9	1	2	2	3	3	4	5	8
35–49	793	3.2	3	2	2	3	4	5	6	11
50–64	202	6.1	19	2	3	5	9	11	13	25
65+	372	7.9	21	4	6	7	9	11	13	22
Total Single DX	1743	2.9	3	1	2	3	3	4	6	9
Total Multiple DX	3526	3.6	8	2	2	3	4	7	9	13
Total										
0–19 yrs	941	2.6	1	1	2	3	3	4	4	7
20–34	2468	2.8	2	2	2	3	3	4	5	7
35–49	1133	3.0	3	2	2	3	3	4	6	10
50–64	271	6.1	18	2	3	5	8	10	13	24
65+	456	7.6	19	4	5	7	9	11	13	21
Grand Total	5269	3.4	6	2	2	3	4	6	8	12

(Continued)

739: Prosthetic replacement of joint, except hip and knee (81.56–81.59; 81.71; 81.73–81.74; 81.80–81.81; 81.84)

Type of Patient	Total Patients	Avg. Stay	Vari-ance	Percentiles						
				10th	25th	50th	75th	90th	95th	99th
1. Single DX										
0–19 yrs	4	2.0		1	1	2	3	3	3	3
20–34	13	2.6	3	1	1	2	4	5	6	6
35–49	37	2.6	2	1	1	2	3	5	6	8
50–64	83	2.8	3	1	1	2	4	5	7	9
65+	98	4.0	7	1	2	3	6	8	9	13
2. Multiple DX										
0–19 yrs	3	2.0	1	1	1	2	3	3	3	3
20–34	22	4.6	16	1	2	4	6	10	14	18
35–49	64	3.3	10	1	2	2	4	6	9	19
50–64	172	3.9	10	1	2	3	5	8	10	15
65+	323	5.1	14	2	3	4	6	9	12	16
Total Single DX	235	3.2	5	1	2	2	4	6	8	10
Total Multiple DX	584	4.5	13	1	2	4	6	8	11	17
Total										
0–19 yrs	7	2.0	1	1	1	2	3	3	3	3
20–34	35	3.9	12	1	1	3	6	7	10	18
35–49	101	3.1	8	1	1	2	4	6	8	18
50–64	255	3.6	8	1	2	3	5	8	9	14
65+	421	4.8	13	1	2	4	6	8	11	16
Grand Total	819	4.2	11	1	2	3	6	8	10	16

740: Miscellaneous repair of other joint, except hip and knee (81.49; 81.72; 81.75–81.79; 81.82–81.83; 81.85; 81.93–81.96; 81.99)

Type of Patient	Total Patients	Avg. Stay	Vari-ance	Percentiles						
				10th	25th	50th	75th	90th	95th	99th
1. Single DX										
0–19 yrs	285	1.7		1	1	2	2	3	3	4
20–34	667	1.7		1	1	2	2	3	3	4
35–49	419	1.8		1	1	2	2	3	3	5
50–64	236	2.0	1	1	1	2	2	3	4	6
65+	118	2.3	1	1	1	2	3	4	5	7
2. Multiple DX										
0–19 yrs	118	1.8		1	1	2	2	3	3	5
20–34	386	2.0	1	1	1	2	2	3	4	7
35–49	461	2.2	5	1	1	2	2	3	4	13
50–64	443	2.1	1	1	1	2	3	3	4	6
65+	313	2.8	4	1	1	2	3	5	6	13
Total Single DX	1725	1.8	1	1	1	2	2	3	3	5
Total Multiple DX	1721	2.2	3	1	1	2	3	4	5	9
Total										
0–19 yrs	403	1.7	1	1	1	2	2	3	3	4
20–34	1053	1.8	1	1	1	2	2	3	3	5
35–49	880	2.0	4	1	1	2	2	3	4	7
50–64	679	2.1	1	1	1	2	3	3	4	6
65+	431	2.6	4	1	1	2	3	5	6	13
Grand Total	3446	2.0	2	1	1	2	2	3	4	7

Length of Stay data included in this publication are provided with permission from HCIA, Inc., Baltimore, MD.

APPENDIX 6–B
Generic

Intensity of Service

Special Unit

See special unit criteria, pp 48 to 59

Rule

Physician evaluation ≥ **1x/24h**

and

- **Two** from Monitoring

and

- **One** from Treatments/Medications

or

- Scheduled Procedure

Monitoring

Pulse, resp. rate, BP ≥ **6x/24h**

Temp ≥ **6x/24h**

Neurovital signs ≥ **6x/24h**

Urine output ≥ **3x/24h**

Pulse oximetry ≥ **3x/24h**

Treatments/Medications

(*At Least Daily*)

- **IV** fluids (postoperative) requiring ≥ **30** *ml/kg* of body weight in **24h** (**72h** postoperative)
- **IV fluids (excluding KVO) requiring ≥ 30** *ml/kg* **of body weight in 24h**
- **IV/IM analgesics ≥ 4x/24h**
- **IV analgesics/Continuous drip**
- **IV chemotherapy (eg, cyclophosphamide)**
- **IV/IM antiemetics (eg, metoclopramide HCI)**

Scheduled Procedure

- To be performed same day as admission

and

- Requiring general/regional anesthesia

and

- Not on ambulatory procedure guidelines, pp 117–123

Discharge Screens

Clinical/Functional

Oral T ≤ **100°F** (37.8°C) for last **24h w/o** antipyretic

Caloric/Fluid intake meets nutritional needs

Passing flatus/fecal material

Voiding/Draining urine (≥ **400** *cc*) for last **8h**

Serum drug levels within acceptable range

Patient/Caretaker demonstrates willingness ***and*** ability to:

- Administer prescribed medications
- Assist ***with***/Perform activities of daily living
- Meet patient's physical ***and*** medical needs in a nonacute setting

Treatment refused

Options

Treatment/Care/Medications could be rendered in an alternate setting

- Observation unit
- Skilled nursing facility
- Subacute level
- Rehabilitation unit/Hospital
- Intermediate care facility
- Home care
  - -DME
  - -IV infusion
- Hospice
- Outpatient
  - -Diagnosis
  - -Treatment
- Residence

(Continued)

Generic

Severity of Illness

Special Unit
See special unit criteria, pp 48 to 59

Rule
- **One** from any category

Clinical Findings
(*Recent Onset*)

Sight loss

Aphasia

Paresis/Paralysis

Unconsciousness

Incapacitating pain

Vomiting/Diarrhea/Inadequate oral intake
   ***and* one:**
- Serum Na ≥ **150**
- Hct ≥ **60%**/Hgb ≥ **20** *gm/dL*
- Urine specific gravity ≥ **1.030**
- BUN ≥ **45**/Creatinine ≥ **3** *mg/dL*
- Absent bowel sounds
- Postural systolic BP drop ≥ **30**
- Pulse ≥ **100**/*min* at rest

Vital Signs
(*Newly Discovered*)

Oral T ≥ **104°F** (40°C)

Oral T ≥ **102°F** (38.9°C) ***and* one:**
- WBC ≥ **18,000** *cu.mm*
- WBC ≥ **15,000** *cu.mm* **with** ≥ **7%** bands

Oral T ≥ **100.4°F** (38°C) ***with*** neutrophil count ≤ **1,000** *cu.mm*

Sustained pulse ≥ **160**/*min*

Resp. rate ≥ **26**/*min* **and** pulse oximetry ≤ **85%** on room air

Systolic BP ≥ **250**

Diastolic BP ≥ **120**

Postural systolic BP drop ≥ **50**

Hematology
(*Newly Discovered*)
Blood
Hct ≤ **15%**/Hgb ≤ **5** *gm/dL*
WBC ≤ **2,000** *cu.mm*

Chemistry
(*Newly Discovered*)
Blood
Serum Na ≤ **123**
Serum Na ≥ **150**
Serum K ≤ **2.5**
Serum K ≥ **6.0**
Arterial pH ≤ **7.30**
Arterial pH ≥ **7.50**
Arterial pO_2 ≤ **60** *torr* on room air
Arterial pCO_2 ≥ **50** *torr* on room air
Presence of toxic level of drugs/chemicals

Microbiology
Blood
Smear/Culture positive for bacteria/fungi

(Continued)

Reprinted with permission of InterQual, Inc,. 44 Lafayette Road, North Hampton, NH, 03862. The above criteria were developed exclusively by InterQual, Inc. The above criteria were developed exclusively by InterQual, Inc.

Respiratory/Chest

Intensity of Service

Special Unit

See special unit criteria, pp 48 to 59

Rule

- Physician evaluation ≥ **1x/24h**

  and
- **Two** from Monitoring

  and
- **One** from Treatments/Medications

Monitoring

Pulse, resp. rate, BP ≥ **6x/24h**

Temp ≥ **6x/24h**

Neurovital signs ≥ **6x/24h**

Urine output ≥ **3x/24h**

Pulse oximetry ≥ **3x/24h**

PT/APTT ≥ **1x/24h**

Treatment/Medications
(*At Least Daily*)

Pulmonary lavage

Chest tube suction/drainage

Initial tracheostomy care

Respiratory medications by nebulizer ≥ **6x/24h (initial)**

Emergency radiation

IV antituberculous agents (eg, ethambutol)

IV anticoagulation (eg, heparin)

- **Ventilator assistance**
- IV/Equivalent oral antibiotics (eg, po ciprofloxacin HCl)
- IM antibiotics
- IV antifungal agents (eg, amphotericin B)
- IV antiviral agents (eg, acyclovir)
- IV antiprotozoal agents (eg, pentamidine, metronidazole)
- IV corticosteroids
- IV chemotherapy (eg, cyclophosphamide)
- IV bronchodilators (eg, theophylline)
- IV diuretics (eg, furosemide)

Discharge Screens

Clinical/functional

Last PT within therapeutic range **with** anti-coagulants

Clinical/Radiological evidence of improvement **with** documented plan for OP treatment/follow-up

Patient/Caretaker demonstrates willingness **and** ability to:

- Clean/Care for tracheostomy
- Administer medical gases

Options

Treatment/Care/Medications could be rendered in an alternate setting

- Observation unit
- Skilled nursing facility
- Subacute level
- Rehabilitation unit/Hospital
- Intermediate care facility
- Home care

  -DME

  -IV infusion
- Hospice
- Outpatient

  -Diagnosis

  -Treatment
- Residence

(Continued)

Respiratory/Chest

Severity of Illness

Special Unit
See special unit criteria, pp 48 to 59

Rule
One from any category

Clinical Findings
(*Recent Onset*)

Gross **and** persistent hemoptysis

Penetrating wound of chest cavity

Pulmonary burns

Wheezing **with** dyspnea unresponsive to bronchodilators/steroids

Severe crush injury, chest

Paroxysmal/Continuous/Uncontrollable cough unresponsive to outpatient therapy for ≥ **1** wk

Vital Signs
(*Newly Discovered*)

Oral T ≥ **102°F** (38.9°C) **and** bacteria by smear (sputum)

Imaging
(*Newly Discovered*)

Hemo/Pneumothorax

Pulmonary edema

Pleural effusion

Empyema

Lung abscess

Air in mediastinum

Pulmonary embolus/infarct

Bi-/Multi-lobar pneumonia

Mono-lobar pneumonia in immunosuppressed patient

Diffuse alveolar infiltrate

Alveolar hemorrhage

Mediastinal shift

ECG

Acute tachyarrhythmias ≥ **160**/*min*

Transient/Unsustained ventricular tachycardia

Hematology
(*Newly Discovered*)
Blood

Hct ≤ **27%**/Hgb ≤ **9** gm/dL **with** active bleeding

PT ≥ **1.5x normal with** active bleeding

APTT ≥ **1.5x normal with** active bleeding

Platelets ≤ **50,000** *cu.mm* **with** active bleeding

Platelets ≥ **1,000,000** *cu.mm* **with** thrombosis/bleeding

Chemistry
(*Newly Discovered*)
Blood

Arterial pO_2 ≤ **60** *torr* on room air

Arterial pCO_2 ≥ **50** *torr* on room air

Arterial pCO_2 ≥ **45** *with* asthma attack

Arterial pH ≤ **7.30**

Arterial pH ≥ **7.50**

Presence of toxic level of drugs/chemicals

Microbiology
(*Newly Discovered*)
Sputum
Smear/Culture positive for:

- Tubercle bacillus
- Gram negative bacillus
- Staphylococci
- Streptococci—Group A
- Fungi
- *Legionella pneumophila*
- *Pneumocystis carinii*

(Continued)

Coronary Care Unit

Intensity of Service

Rule

- Cardiac Monitoring (Continuous Telemetry)

and

Physician evaluation ≥ **2x/24h**

and

- **Three** IS criteria

Monitoring
(*At Least Hourly*)

Blood pressure

Urine output/Specific gravity

Arterial line

Pulmonary artery/wedge pressure (Swan-Ganz)

Central venous pressure

Pulse oximetry

Treatment/Medications
(*At Least Daily*)

Concentrated potassium drip ≥ **60** *mEq/L*

Balloon pump

Temporary pacemaker insertion

IV cardiac inotropics (eg, dobutamine)

IV vasopressors (eg, dopamine)

IV vasodilators (eg, nitroprusside)

IV nitroglycerine

IV thrombolytic agents (eg, streptokinase)

- Ventilator assistance
- Chest tubes
- IV antiarrhythmics (eg, xylocaine)
- IV cardiac glycosides (eg, digoxin)
- IV beta blockers (eg, propranolol)
- IV calcium channel blockers (eg, verapamil)
- IV anticoagulation (eg, heparin)
- IV diuretics (eg, furosemide)
- IV antibiotics

Discharge Screens

Clinical/Functional

Absence of unstable ventricular arrhythmias for last **12h**

Resp. status stable for last **12h**

Absence of Swan-Ganz

Absence of arterial line

Chest pain controlled by oral, sublingual *or* topical medication for last **12h**

Options

Treatments/Care/Medications could be rendered safely and effectively in an alternate setting

- Monitored bed (telemetry)
- General unit
- Outpatient
- Subacute level/facility

(Continued)

Coronary Care Unit

Severity of Illness

Rule

- **One** from any category

Clinical Findings
(Acute Onset)

Chest pain of suspected cardiac origin

Hypertensive crisis as evidenced by systolic BP $\geq$ **250**/diastolic BP $\geq$ **120** *with* **one:**

- BUN $\geq$ **45**/Creatinine $\geq$ **3** *mg/dL*
- Dyspnea/Anasarca
- Altered level of consciousness/Paresis

Dyspnea *and* **one:**

- Rales
- Distended neck veins
- Peripheral edema
- Tachycardia $\geq$ **130**/*min*

Syncope in presence of **one:**

- Aortic stenosis
- Known coronary artery disease
- Valve disease

Vital Signs
(Newly Discovered)

Pulse $\leq$ **40**/*min*

Pulse $\geq$ **180**/*min*

Resp. rate $\leq$ **8**/*min*

Resp. rate $\geq$ **30**/*min*

Systolic BP $\leq$ **70**

Diastolic BP $\geq$ **120**

Postural systolic BP drop $\geq$ **50**

Imaging
(Newly Discovered)

Pulmonary edema

Vessel occlusion

Cardiac tamponade

Hemo/Pneumothorax *with* circulatory/respiratory compromise

Pleural effusion *with* respiratory compromise

ECG

Post MI unstable arrhythmia, eg:

- Unsustained ventricular tachycardia
- R *on* T ventricular premature beats
- Multi-focal ventricular premature beats
- Torsade phenomenon

Myocardial ischemia

Myocardial infarction

Sustained ventricular tachycardia

Ventricular fibrillation

Complete/**2nd/3rd** degree heart block

Sustained atrial tachyarrhythmia $\geq$ **160**/*min*

Hematology
(Newly Discovered)

Hct $\leq$ **28%** *with* unresponsive angina

Chemistry
(Newly Discovered)
Blood

CPK/CK **2x $\geq$ upper limits of normal** *and* positive MB isoenzyme **>5%** total

LDH **2x $\geq$ upper limits of normal** *with* one:
    -Chest pain
    -Ischemia by ECG

ALT/SGOT **2x $\geq$ upper limits of normal** *with* **one:**
    -Chest pain
    -Ischemia by ECG

Serum Na $\leq$ **115**

Serum Na $\geq$ **160**

Serum K $\leq$ **2.0**

Serum K $\geq$ **6.0**

Serum Ca $\leq$ **7.5** *mg/dL* **with** ECG changes consistent *with* hypocalcemia

Serum Ca $\geq$ **15** *mg/dL*

Serum Mg $\leq$ ½ **lower limit** of lab value

Arterial pO_2 $\leq$ **50** *torr* on room air

Arterial pCO_2 $\geq$ **50** *torr* on room air

HCO_3 $\leq$ **16**

HCO_3 $\geq$ **40**

Arterial pH $\leq$ **7.30**

Arterial pH $\geq$ **7.50**

APPENDIX 6–C

DRG <u>89</u>   Estimated LOS: <u>4 days</u>
Admit Date_____
Payor_____
      (for DC planning purposes)

INTERDISCIPLINARY CLINICAL PATHWAY
Simple Pneumonia & Pleurisy with Comorbidity (≥ 17 yr)

	Day 1	Day 2
Assessment	TPR; resp system; O₂ sat; baseline mental status; psycho/social needs; consider TB screen	Mental status; O₂ sat; TPR; resp system
Diagnostic Studies	Sputum by RT (RT sputum induction policy); GS; C&S; *ABG; CXR-PA&LAT; Smac; *BCx2; UA; *C&S; *EKG; CBC with diff	Stool for C. diff if diarrhea; CBC; CXR-PA&LAT if condition warrants (evaluate for pleural effusion)
Treatments	I/O; saline lock/IV; O₂ as indicated; encourage po fluids; turn, deep breathe; suction prn; activity as tolerated in room.	Ambulate TID
Key Medications and IV Therapy	IV ABX; saline flushes as indicated; consider adrenergic beta-2 (bronchodilator) via SVN/MDI; Prns: antipyretic; NSAID/narcotic prn pleuritic pain; antacid; antiemetic BCOC; hypnotic	
Nutrition and Fluids	Advance DAT; encourage po fluids.	
Consults/ Multidisciplinary Education	*Pulmonary; Case Management; *Dietary consult; assess educational needs	Discuss postdischarge options with family/S.O.
Key Outcomes/Goals	IV ABX started in ED or within 2 hrs if direct admit; sputum collected	Patient afebrile; tolerates ambulation without respiratory complications; note GS result

* = if indicated

Date Adopted Medical Department/Committee _____ Date to MEC _____
Clinical Pathways are guidelines only and do not preempt the independent judgment of the physician.

Day 3	Day 4	Day 5
Same as Day 2	Same as Day 3	Same as Day 4
*CBC		
D/C saline lock/IV, evaluate need for O$_2$ by spot check O$_2$ sat (RT O$_2$ Therapy Policy)	D/C I&O (evaluate need for O$_2$)	Discharge
Consider switch to MDI; consider D/C IV ABX after 24-hour afebrile period and start po ABX; D/C saline flushes	Consider switch to MDI	D/C on po ABX; consider adrenergic beta-2 INH; NSAID/narcotic prn pleuritic pain
Contact: Primary Home Caregiver, Home Health, ECF; MDI Instruction	Initiate transfer form if applicable; disease process education	Home care management/discharge instruction
Sputum cult report in patient record; po ABX started if criteria met; normal rate, rhythm and depth of resp	Independent ADLs; afebrile	Discharge

(Continued)

DRG <u>209</u>   Estimated LOS: <u>4 days</u>
Admit Date_____
Payor_____
      (for DC planning purposes)

INTERDISCIPLINARY CLINICAL PATHWAY
Total Hip Replacement

	Day 1 (Surgery)	Day 2 (POD 1)
Assessment	Neurovascular checks q 2 hrs, vital signs and hemovac checks q 4 hrs	Neurovascular checks and vital signs q 4 hrs if stable, hemovac check q 8 hrs
Diagnostic Studies	Post-op x-ray	H/H, protime if on coumadin
Treatments	Hemovac, antiembolic hose, cough and deep breathe, I&O, abduction pillow, straight cath/foley*, bedrest, HOB up 30°, turn q 2 hrs	Hemovac, up in chair × 30 min × 1, HOB up 60° maximum, ambulate 10′ × 1
Key Medications and IV Therapy	IVF as ordered, IV antibiotics, PCA/epidural/IM pain medication, anticoagulants, routine medications as ordered	IV - saline lock, discontinue IV antibiotics, PCA/IM/epidural/pain meds, stool softeners, BCOC
Nutrition and Fluids	Regular diet, clear liquid if no bowel sounds or N/V	Diet as tolerated
Consults/ Multidisciplinary Education	Respiratory Therapy*, Internal Medicine/Family Practice physician*	Social Services*, Physical Therapy
Key Outcomes/Goals	Pain Management, stabilize post-op	Begin activity, afebrile

* = if indicated

Date Adopted Medical Department/Committee _____ Date to MEC _____
Clinical Pathways are guidelines only and do not preempt the independent judgment of the physician.

Day 3 (POD 2)	Day 4 (POD 3)	Day 5 (POD 4)
Routine vital signs	Assess bowel function	System discharge assessment
H/H, protime if on coumadin	Protime if on coumadin	
Hemovac discontinued, dressing changed, foley discontinued*, straight cath*, up in chair × 2 × 30 min, HOB up 75° maximum, ambulate 20' × 2, bedside commode	Dressing change per orders, up in chair × 2 × 45 min, ambulate 40'/BRP, minimum assist I & OOB	Enema/suppository if no BM
Saline lock discontinued, IM/PO pain medication, anticoagulants	PO analgesics	PO pain meds/instructions
I&O discontinued		
HHC/ECF liaisons/DME, OT for ADL training		Follow-up Social Services/HHC/DME, physician as needed, review home exercise protocol, dislocation precautions, discharge medications
Increase activity level, switch to PO pain meds	Establish plan for discharge needs, bowel movement	Discharge

(Continued)

DRG <u>209</u>　　　Estimated LOS: <u>4 days</u>
Admit Date_____
Payor_____
　　　(for DC planning purposes)

INTERDISCIPLINARY CLINICAL PATHWAY
Total Knee Replacement

	Day 1 (Surgery)	Day 2 (POD 1)
Assessment	Hemovac checks q 4 hrs, vital signs q 4 hrs, neurovascular checks q 4 hrs	Vital signs/neurovascular checks q 4 hrs
Diagnostic Studies	Post-op x-ray	H/H, Protime if on coumadin
Treatments	Antiembolic device, dressing and neurovascular checks q 2 hrs, cough and deep breathe, I&O, hemovac, straight cath/foley*, turn q 2 hrs, HOB up for comfort, CPM machine if ordered, advance per orders	Up in chair × 2 × 30 min, stand, ambulate 10′ × 1, CPM
Key Medications and IV Therapy	IVF per orders, IV antibiotics, epidural/PCA/IM pain meds, anti-coagulants, routine medications as ordered	Anticoagulants, IV - saline lock, IV antibiotics discon-tinued, PCA/IM/PO pain meds*, stool softeners, BCOC
Nutrition and Fluids	Regular diet - clear liquids if no bowel sounds or N/V	Diet as tolerated
Consults/ Multidisciplinary Education	Internal Medicine/Family Practice physician*, Respiratory Therapy*	Social Services*, Physical Therapy
Key Outcomes/Goals	Pain management, stabilize post-op	Begin activity, afebrile

* = if indicated

Date Adopted Medical Department/Committee _____ Date to MEC _____
Clinical Pathways are guidelines only and do not preempt the independent judgment of the physician.　　　ſ

Day 3 (POD 2)	Day 4 (POD 3)	Day 5 (POD 4)
Routine vital signs	Assess bowel function	System discharge assessment
H/H, protime if on coumadin	Protime if on coumadin	
Hemovac discontinued, dressing changed, up in chair × 2 × 45 min, ambulate 25' × 2, CPM 0–50°	Dressing change per orders, up in chair × 1 hr × 3/BRP, ambulate 50' × 2, minimum assist I & OOB	Assure BM prior to discharge, minimum assist needed for BRP, COPM
PO pain meds, anticoagulants as ordered	Anticoagulants as ordered	PO pain meds/instructions
Discontinue I&O		
HHC/ECF liaison, DME		Follow-up with Social Services, HHC, DME, physician*, review exercise protocol for home, discharge medications
Switch to PO pain meds, increase activity level	Established plan for discharge needs	Discharge

(Continued)

DRG <u>80.51</u>   Estimated LOS: <u>4 days</u>
Admit Date_____
Payor_____
      (for DC planning purposes)

INTERDISCIPLINARY CLINICAL PATHWAY
Post-op Lumbar Laminectomy Without Fusion, Without Complications, Non-traumatic, Non-CA

	Day 1	
	Preop/Surgery	Postop
Assessment	H&P; initial anesthesia assessment; VS; neuro exam (LOC, motor & sensory); systems assessment	VS and neuro exam q 4 hr; assess lumbar drsg q 4 hr; systems assessment
Diagnostic Studies	CBC, CMAC, coags, EKG, CXR, type and screen	
Treatments	Activity as tolerated; refer to standard surgical protocol; Teds	Up OOB to chair/commode in evening; Teds; PAS*; inc spirometer*; Foley*; TCDB q 2 hr
Key Medications and IV Therapy	Preop meds	IVF as ordered; pain meds IV/IM*; antibiotics IV × 24 hrs; steroids*; antiemetics*; muscle relaxers*
Nutrition and Fluids	NPO except for meds	NPO until fully awake and bowel sounds active; clear liquids then ADAT
Consults/ Multidisciplinary Education	BNI Education Guide; preop teaching; informed consent; special consents (i.e., blood); medical consults*	Resp Therapy*; Social Services*; Case Manager*
Key Outcomes/Goals	Verbalize understanding of preop teaching; discharge planning initiated	Stabilize patient

* = if indicated

Date Adopted Medical Department/Committee _____ Date to MEC _____
Clinical Pathways are guidelines only and do not preempt the independent judgment of the physician.

Day 2	Day 3	Discharge Day
VS and neuro exam q shift; assess drsg/incision line q shift; assess last bowel movement; systems assessment	VS and neuro exam q shift; incision line q shift; assess last BM; systems assessment q shift	VS and neuro exam q shift; assess incision line q shift; assess ability to care for self
CBC*; CP*		
Up in chair TID; ambulate in hall w/help; D/C foley; straight cath if unable to void; bowel care; temp >38°C; start inc spirometer; Teds	Ambulate in halls TID; ADLs with minimal assist (i.e., shower); remove drsg if not done already	Ambulate independent; bowel care (i.e., BM prior to discharge); ADLs done independently; Discharge
S.L. IV until completion of antibiotics, if no nausea and tolerating PO; bowel care meds; switch to PO pain meds	D/C S.L.; PO pain meds*; steroid taper*	PO pain med Rx; other Rx* (i.e., steroids, muscle relaxers, stool softeners)
ADAT	Regular diet	Regular diet
PT/OT C/S* if patient reluctant or weak; teach patient bed mobility and proper body mechanics; Home Health*		"Laminectomy discharge instruction sheet"; follow-up with Social Services, contact outpt therapies for any necessary arrangements for home; follow-up with neurosurgeon for suture/staple removal; review prescriptions; review proper body mechanics and activities allowed
Continue discharge planning; patient will ambulate in halls with assistance	Patient prepared for discharge	Meet discharge criteria; patient will verbalize understanding of discharge instructions and teaching

(Continued)

DRG <u>107</u>   Estimated LOS: <u>4 days</u>
Admit Date_____
Payor_____
      (for DC planning purposes)

INTERDISCIPLINARY CLINICAL PATHWAY
CABG

	Day 1		Day 2
	Pre-op Testing	Admission - Day 1 - Surgery	(POD 1)
Assessment	Admission assessment	Complete assessment; H&P on chart	Vital signs q 1–2 hrs; complete assessment q 2 hrs
Diagnostic Studies	CBC, CXR, EKG, CP-SMAC, T&C, Coag profile, ABG-RA, bedside PFT	H&H, K +, EKG, ABG, CXR, cardiac output, PTT *	CPK - MB x 1, H&H, chem panel, EKG, CXR, ABG
Treatments	Daily weight; permit signed; surgical shower; up ad lib	IV, art line, PA cath; pacemaker/wires; foley, chest tubes, NGT ETT-ventilator, pulse oximetry, end-tidal; wean -> extubated; I.S.; SVN *; bedrest	Dressing change; D/C; CT; D/C PA cath; I.S.; daily weight; heplock; evaluate for transfer; SVN *; dangle A.M., chair P.M, ROM x 5
Key Medications and IV Therapy	Continue present meds; bowel prep	Antibiotic - pre & post; KCl, analgesic, heparin, ASA, O_2, Inotrope *, anti-arrhythmic *, vasopressors *, MgSo4 *	Antibiotic, analgesic, O_2, ASA, stool softener
Nutrition and Fluids	Regular; NPO following MN	NPO	Clear liquids - > advance to soft
Consults/ Multidisciplinary Education	Pre-op teach, Cardiac Rehab, Anesthesia, Case Management		
Key Outcomes/ Goals	Ready for surgery	Stabilized post-op, extubate 12 hrs post-op	Hemodynamically stable, initiate activity, pain management

* = if indicated

Date Adopted Medical Department/Committee _____ Date to MEC _____
Clinical Pathways are guidelines only and do not preempt the independent judgment of the physician.

Day 3 (POD 2)	Day 4 (POD 3)	Day 5 (POD 4)	Day 6 (POD 5)
Vital signs q 4 hrs	Routine vital signs	Routine vital signs	Routine vital signs
CPK - MB × 1, H&H *, chem panel *, EKG *, CXR *, ABG *		CBC, CP, CXR, EKG, check RA O_2 sat - if > 92, D/C O_2	
Transfer to tele; D/C art line; D/C foley; restart heplock; I.S.; daily weight; dressing change; SVN *; ambulate up to 100′ × 1, ROM × 5	Telemetry; I.S.; daily weight; dressings off; ambulate 100–300' BID; active ROM	Telemetry; daily weight; I.S.; up ad lib; ambulate 1–2 laps TID, O_2	Daily weight; I.S.; up ad lib; ambulate 2–3 laps QID
Analgesic - PO, ASA, stool softener, O_2	Stool softener, ASA, routine home meds, analgesic, laxative, O_2	ASA, routine home meds, analgesic	ASA, home meds, analgesic
Regular	Regular diet	Regular diet	Regular diet
	Discharge teaching, Cardiac Rehab	Attend Cardiac Rehab class	
Transfer to tele floor, switch to PO pain meds	Increased activity	Established plan for discharge needs	Discharge

APPENDIX 6–D:
Milliman & Robertson, Inc.
Optimal Recovery Guidelines

M-83   Cerebral Thrombosis, Completed Stroke in a Patient With a Major Deficit With Severely Impaired Cognitive Function and/or Swallowing Function in Addition to Dense Hemiparesis (ICD-9: 434.0, 434.9)

Day 1: Admitted to regular floor care after CT from outpatient or emergency setting has excluded hemorrhage, hemiparesis with impaired speech, and/or swallowing. Incapable of ambulation. Parenteral hydration. Physical therapy evaluation. Possible neurologic consultation or occupational or speech therapy evaluations. Possible echocardiogram.

Day 2: Dense hemiparesis, swallowing difficulty and cognitive impairment continue. Continue parenteral fluids. Physical therapy for passive range of motion and other therapies as appropriate. Sinus rhythm and normal echocardiogram suggest no need for anticoagulation.

Day 3: Physical therapy, nursing care, limited chair activity with constant supervision. Speech therapy for swallowing. Rehabilitation consultation suggests that the patient will not be a good candidate for an acute rehabilitation facility.

Day 4: Dense hemiparesis, cognitive, and swallowing difficulties persist. Physical therapy, nursing care. Discharge planning to assess appropriateness of custodial care at home or a nursing home.

Day 5: Dense hemiparesis, major cognitive impairment and swallowing difficulties continue. Physical therapy, nursing care, parenteral feeding.

Day 6: Dense hemiparesis, major cognitive impairment and swallowing difficulties continue. Physical therapy, nursing care, parenteral feeding. Decision regarding nutritional support.

Day 7: Dense hemiparesis, major cognitive impairment and swallowing difficulties continue. Physical therapy, nursing care, parenteral feeding. Insertion of feeding tube if swallowing is unimproved.

Day 8: Dense hemiparesis, major cognitive impairment and swallowing difficulties continue. Physical therapy, nursing care, parenteral feeding. Tube feedings.

Day 9: Dense hemiparesis, major cognitive impairment and swallowing difficulties continue. Physical therapy, nursing care. Tube feedings tolerated. Discharge to custodial care at appropriate site.

Goal Length of Stay: 8 days

M-178   Gastrointestinal Bleeding
(ICD-9:578)

Adequate Reasons for Admission

- Significant continuing active bleeding
- Hemodynamic instability or major drop in blood count
- Recurrent bleeding from unknown site

Inadequate Reasons for Admission

(Continued)

- Rectal or lower GI bleeding except continuous colon hemorrhage
- Mallory-Weiss hematemesis
- Bleeding which has stopped with hemodynamic stability and known source

Alternatives

- Outpatient care in an emergency room, holding bed, urgent care, clinic, or office
    Transfusion and fluid replacement
    Endoscopy
    Angiography
    Hold for prolonged observation, repeat labs
    Initiation of diet and/or pharmacotherapy
- Home Care
    Nursing visits, office visits or house calls
    Diagnostic work-up

Goal Length of Stay: Ambulatory

Reprinted with permission from Milliman & Robertson, Inc
Healthcare Management Guidelines
Milliman & Robertson, Inc
Seattle, WA 98101

M-324   Renal Failure, Chronic
           (ICD-9:585, 586)

Adequate Reasons for Admission

- Pulmonary edema
- Dangerous electrolyte imbalance unable to be corrected in an outpatient setting
- Intractable vomiting
- Continuing gross hemorrhage
- Recurrent seizures
- Septicemia, due to infected vascular access
- Peritonitis
- Pericarditis with effusion
- Uremic complications unable to be corrected in an outpatient setting

Inadequate Reasons for Admission

- Uremic complications able to be corrected in an outpatient setting
- Initiation of dialysis
- Establishment of permanent surgical vascular access
- Declotting of vascular access

Alternatives

- Outpatient care in an emergency room, holding bed, urgent care, ambulatory surgery center, dialysis center, clinic, or office
    Parenteral fluid or medication
    Test to rule out obstructive uropathy
    Initation and maintenance of dialysis

(Continued)

Establishment or declotting of long term vascular access
Insertion of temporary access in stable patients

- Home Care
  House call by physician
  Nursing visit for assessment
  Laboratory testing
  Parenteral fluid

Goal Length of Stay: Ambulatory

M-327   Seizure
         (ICD-9:345, 345.3)

Adequate Reasons for Admission

- Status epilepticus

- Increased intracranial pressure

- Meningitis

- Sedative, hypnotic, anxiolytic agent withdrawal

- Metabolic predisposition, eg, prolonged hypoglycemia

Inadequate Reasons for Admission

- First seizure

- Focal neurological finding

- Fever, if lumbar puncture negative

- Inadequate control by medication unless status epilepticus is present

- Neurodiagnostic work-up

Alternatives

- Outpatient care in an emergency room, holding bed, urgent care, clinic, or office
  Neurological consultation and evaluation including EEG and imaging
  Lumbar punction, if indicated
  Observe with change in medication

- Home Care
  Nursing visit
  Outpatient work-up

Goal Length of Stay: Ambulatory

Reprinted with permission from Milliman & Robertson, Inc
Healthcare Management Guidelines
Milliman & Robertson, Inc
Seattle, WA 98101

S-390   Coronary Artery Bypass Graft (CABG)
         (CPT-4:33510, 33511, 33512, 33513, 33514, 33516, 33520, 33525, 33528)
         (ICD-9:36.10, 36.11, 36.12, 36.13, 36.14, 36.15, 36.16, 36.19)

Day 1: Operating room, ICU, intubated, chest tube, central lines, pacer wires, parenteral fluids, medications, and antibiotics. Possible PCA or epidural analgesics.

Day 2: Extubated, hemodynamically stable. Discontinue chest tube and central lines. Step-Down Unit for monitoring, oxygen, parenteral fluids, parenteral or

(Continued)

oral medications, light diet, chair and minimal ambulatory activity. Possible PCA or epidural analgesics.

Day 3: Step-Down Unit with monitoring, oxygen, parenteral fluids. Oral medications, increased ambulation and diet. Rhythm stable. Discontinue pacer wires. Change IV to heparin lock. Possible PCA or epidural analgesics.

Day 4: Routine floor care with telemetry. Oral medications, advanced diet and increased activity. Discontinue PCA or epidural analgesics.

Day 5: Discontinue heparin lock. Afebrile, increased activity without cardiac symptoms, oral medications, regular diet. Discharge.

Goal Length of Stay: 4 days

Reprinted with permission from Milliman & Robertson, Inc
Healthcare Management Guidelines
Milliman & Robertson, Inc
Seattle, WA 98101

S-700   Knee: Arthroplasty (Total)
         (CPT-4: 27440, 27441, 27442, 27443, 27445, 27446, 27447, 27486, 27487, 27488)
         (ICD-9: 81.54, 81.55)

Day 1: Prior home and physical therapy assessment/gait training. Operating room, parenteral fluids, medications, and antibiotics. Anticoagluation. Continuous passive motion. Possible PCA.

Day 2: Parenteral fluids, medications, and antibiotics. Continuous passive motion. Physical therapy for assisted ambulation. Diet as tolerated. Change IV to heparin lock. Possible PCA.

Day 3: Oral medications, regular diet. Continuous passive motion, physical therapy. Discontinue heparin lock. Discontinue PCA.

Day 4: Oral medications, regular diet. Continuous passive motion, physical therapy.

Day 5: Discharge.

Goal Length of Stay: 4 days

Reprinted with permission from Milliman & Robertson, Inc
Healthcare Management Guidelines
Milliman & Robertson, Inc
Seattle, WA 98101

CHAPTER 7

Legal Issues for Case Managers

IMPORTANT TERMS AND CONCEPTS

Adult Protective Services (APS)
advance directives
AMA (against medical advice)
anatomical gifts/organ donation
autopsies
child abuse
Child Protective Services (CPS)
competency
confidentiality
coroners' cases
danger to others
danger to self
death definition
discoverable
Do Not Resuscitate (DNR)
Durable Power of Attorney
    for Health Care
elder abuse

extraordinary treatment
implied consent
incompetency
informed consent
involuntary admissions
Living Wills
Medical Power of Attorney
    (Medical POA)
neocortical death
ordinary treatment
Patient Self-Determination Act of 1990
Prehospital Medical Care Directive
reportable events
"slow code"
statute of limitations
surrogate
voluntary admissions
Wickline Case

Volumes have been written on medical law. This section covers legal issues that are critical for nurse case managers (NCMs) to understand. Each of the following issues repeatedly surfaces in the course of nursing case managers' responsibilities; I am often asked about them from both staff nurses and patients:

Documentation

The Medical Record

Discharge Planning

Restraints & Falls

Informed Consent

Confidentiality

Special HIV Issues

Special Mental Health Issues

Advance Medical Directives & Surrogate Decision Makers

Reportable Events

Do Not Resuscitate—No Code Blue

Death—Anatomical Gifts—Autopsy

Laws change and vary from state to state. It is strongly recommended that NCMs learn the legal statutes for the state they are working in, because this material cannot be specific for each state.

Some nursing law books are broken down into clinical areas (eg, medicine, surgery, mental health, obstetrics, perinatal care, and cardiac care). They contain actual court cases in these areas, many of which are enlightening and can help the NCM to avoid mistakes. Also, it is important to be current on your institution's policies and procedures. If you have any doubt about a proper course, call your risk management department. Many institutions retain lawyers who can answer questions.

Two themes repeat themselves throughout this section: documentation and communication. The fact that our society is becoming more litigious is no secret. However, studies have shown that good communication and clear, factual, complete documentation make litigation less likely.

A study of lawsuits reveals that often the underlying cause of litigation is lack of information, lack of patient understanding, discourtesy, and other communication failures. Patients with chronic illnesses, for which the medical profession can only temporarily abate the symptoms and distress, are especially prone to frustration. These patients and often family members should be updated frequently—and especially with any treatment changes—and should be fully informed about both the treatment plan and any possible alternative treatment (Saue, 1988). Honesty about the limitations of the care received should also be communicated; patients sue when a complication occurs and no one has told them that it *could* occur.

Documentation recommendations are cited throughout this section. Often, from a legal standpoint, the documentation is the deciding factor in a case. More and more, courts are holding nurses (and NCMs) to professional nursing standards of care. If a case goes to court, precise documentation can show whether standards of care were met (Northrop & Kelly, 1987).

Documentation

The JCAH manual (1985) gives an excellent overview of the main points to document. Although it was originally written for staff nursing, much of the following quote is important for the NCM.

> Documentation of nursing care shall be pertinent and concise and shall reflect the patient's status. Nursing documentation should address the patient's needs, problems, capabilities and limitations. Nursing intervention and patient response must be noted. When a patient is transferred within or discharged from the hospital, a

nurse shall note the patient's status in the medical record. As appropriate, patients who are discharged from the hospital requiring nursing care should receive instructions and individualized counseling prior to discharge, and evidence of the instructions and the patient's or family's understanding of these instructions should be noted in the medical record. Such instructions and counseling must be consistent with the responsible medical practitioner's instructions (pp. 98–99).

In most states, the statute of limitations (time in which a patient has to file a lawsuit) is 2 years for adults and up to 21 years for a minor, depending on the age of the minor when the incident took place (Perin, 1992). Since few people remember details from years ago and courts in general believe what is written, proper documentation is critical if a lawsuit is to be filed. Some general criteria for documentation follow:

1. Chart the facts. Be objective. Subjective complaints are acceptable if a patient states them (ie, "my pain is much worse"). Subjective statements by the nurse or NCM should be considered carefully. For example, unless the occurrence was actually witnessed, the NCM would write "patient found on floor" (with details), not "patient fell out of bed." Documentation should be complete and correct.
2. Use JCAHO or the institution's approved abbreviations. This discourages ambiguity and prevents potentially harmful misunderstandings.
3. Use legible penmanship. It would be embarrassing for you to have your own charting on a giant screen in court and *you* yourself can't decipher it. Fortunately, more hospitals are changing to computer charting, which eases this issue.
4. Record as promptly as possible so that details are not lost. Use actual times accurately. Attorneys later use these times to reconstruct the case, as in a play. For example, if you called a physician at 5-minute intervals or gave sublingual nitroglycerine according to protocol, providing the times will be to your advantage.

Documentation in medical records is discoverable, meaning it can be requested for use in court (Perin, 1992).

More documentation recommendations are discussed under specific issues.

The Medical Record

The medical record is created through documentation. The quality and completeness of the documentation determines the effectiveness of the record. The purpose of the medical record is threefold:

1. It is a communication tool facilitating team interactions among the healthcare team, which in turn facilitates patient care (Northrop & Kelly, 1987). It contains a complete and accurate reflection of the whole episode of care including:

   • Medical history and physical
   • Psychosocial assessment

- Diagnostic tests/labs
- Nursing assessments
- Patient choices about treatment options
- Patient education
- Discharge planning
- Therapies and treatments ordered
- Patient response to treatments & therapies
- Complications
- Consults
- Diagnosis
- Discharge summary
- Other information pertinent to individual cases

A complete medical record enhances continuity and coordination of patient care.

2. This medical record then becomes both a medical history and a legal record for the patient (1987).
3. The medical record is used for third party (insurance) reimbursement (1987). Insurance companies scrutinize patient charts for several reasons:

- To determine whether services billed for were actually provided. All orders, tests and their results, medication administration, supplies, and other procedures will be looked at. Insurance companies may not reimburse if the evidence for the billed items is not in the chart.
- To determine whether this hospitalization or procedure was medically necessary. Nursing and physicians documentation should support admitting diagnosis completely and factually, with symptoms, vital signs, and treatment listed.
- To establish length of hospital stay. Any changes in the patient's condition may lend support to an increased length of stay; therefore, it is important for nurses to help identify and document complications and additional problems. NCMs should emphasize to staff nurses the importance of accurate charting in this arena. Usually, it is the NCM's role to ask for additional hospital days; the charting is necessary to support the NCM's claim of need for extra days. There have been cases in which insurance companies refused to pay for parts of hospitalizations if they felt that complications were caused by something that the institution could have prevented. Therefore, complete and accurate documentation is the wisest course legally. The hospital can negotiate with the insurance company for a few days' reimbursement, whereas a legal proceeding can be much more expensive.
- To look for evidence in the record regarding whether the patient is truly homebound, since most insurance companies will provide home nursing services in this circumstance. If the patient is not homebound, the insurance company will expect the patient to go to doctor's offices, outpatient physical therapy, occupational therapy, or speech therapy facilities, or free-standing clinics for posthospital care.

> **NOTE**
>
> Patients should be made aware that insurance companies will probably deny payment if the patient refuses to sign release authorizations for their reviews (Anonymous, 1990).

The importance of a complete and accurate patient medical record cannot be emphasized too strongly. Its role is primary when a hospitalization turns into a lawsuit. The Joint Commission (JCAHO) also places great emphasis on evaluating the completeness of patient records when determining whether the agency will pass accreditation status (Feutz-Harter, 1991). Medical records can legally be used for billing, auditing, utilization review, quality assurance studies, and research.

Patients often ask NCMs for copies of their medical charts, and staff nurses frequently do not know whether the patient is entitled to see the chart. Who owns the medical chart? The actual physical document belongs to the institution that created it; the institution is the custodian of the hard copy. The information, however, belongs to the patient (Anonymous, 1990). The patient is entitled not only to this information but to other items, such as actual x-rays, computed tomography (CT) scans, pathology slides, gallstones, and others. In most cases, failure to provide a patient with requested records is grounds for a civil suit.

If the attending physician feels that it is not in the patient's best interest to see the chart, the physician can deny the request (Anonymous, 1990). However, this could be deemed "withholding of medical information," and the patient could initiate litigation for disclosure. Any decision to veto a request for information from the patient should be well documented and should be done only when there is evidence that it could cause the patient severe harm. Documentation should support reasons for the denial, since this violates a basic patient right to information and may interfere with informed consent.

The aforementioned also applies when a request is made while the patient is still in the hospital. If there is no harm assessed to the patient, the record should be produced within a "reasonable time." However, note the following:

- Charges for copying materials may apply.
- A written, signed, and witnessed release form should be completed.
- The attending physician should be notified for approval.
- The NCM should document that the attending physician was notified, that the release was signed and by whom, the date when the records were released, and to whom the records were released.

Sometimes patient/family requests for charts demonstrate that they are harboring an underlying concern. Many times the NCM can explore these concerns with the family. Did the physician not explain everything fully? Was the talk too technical? Do they feel that the medical staff is hiding something from them? I have read portions of charts to the patient (with family members present if patient agrees); often this disclosure, along with clear explanations and answers to questions, alleviates their concerns and the request for the chart is dropped.

The patient can also authorize the release of medical records to others. Since the institution is responsible for the safety of these records, a signed release form is usually required. In fact, it would be legally unwise to disclose patient information without a signed consent form. In most states, even family members are not necessarily entitled to the records unless the patient has died. Here are some special situations:

- Most states allow the legal guardian of minors access to records. A noncustodial, divorced parent may not have rights to the chart (Perin, 1992). Consult your institution's attorney or risk management department.
- A subpoena *may* be a valid reason to release records, but not always (Perin, 1992). Checking with hospital counsel is suggested. A court order may be required to release information.
- Some records are protected by law. Drug and alcohol records from a drug/alcohol detoxification program and mental health records may need a court order before information is released (Anonymous, 1990). It is suggested that NCMs be familiar with their own state laws in these instances. Sometimes a true emergency, in which the person is in imminent danger, is a reason to release records.
- Many states have enacted confidentiality statutes for HIV patients (Anonymous, 1990). See the section on Special HIV Issues.

Custodians of medical records must balance confidentiality with the many requests for records from insurance companies, billing departments, quality assurance people, attorneys, and the courts. Also they need to be aware that computerized charting, although wonderfully efficient, exposes the risk for potential privacy abuses.

Discharge Planning

Discharge planning is one of the most important responsibilities of the NCM and the social worker. An effective social worker is an extremely valuable asset to a healthcare team; the accuracy of the psychosocial assessment can make or break the discharge plan.

The stage at which discharge planning begins depends on the type of case being managed. For example, for a patient requiring an elective total hip replacement, the discharge assessment and plan can begin with preoperative teaching. For a patient who fell and requires the same operation, but emergently, the planning should commence as soon as possible, usually within 24 hours of admission. In either case, NCMs, social workers, and discharge planners are no longer afforded the liberty of waiting until the last minute to start planning posthospital care.

The healthcare cost containment atmosphere requires safe and efficient planning. At the same time, there is pressure to discharge ailing patients earlier. Because of this, the likelihood of allegations such as abandonment or premature discharge is increased.

The Wickline Case (see discussion of Length of Stay in Chapter 5: Insurance) was based on allegations of harm done due to premature discharge (Anonymous, 1987). The court ruled that no physician may shift legal responsibility for a patient's medical welfare to a third party by complying with a cost containment program (Saue, 1988). In other words, a patient cannot be discharged merely because insurance stops payment. Still, the pressure for quick discharges is on. The following recommendations stress accurate and complete documentation. If the discharge plan is evaluated in a court of law, thorough documentation may show good faith and appropriate intentions.

The Health Care Financing Administration (HCFA) generic screens in the Quality Assurance section reveal the importance of discharge planning in two critical aspects: the adequacy of the discharge plan and the medical stability of the patient within 24 hours of discharge.

Adequacy of Discharge Planning

The adequacy of discharge planning describes the discharge plan for posthospital care, with the NCM as the link between the patient and the community resources. The questions to be addressed are: Is the plan appropriate and adequate for this individual? Does the plan consider physical, emotional, social, mental health, and safety needs? The following are guidelines to help the NCM with discharge planning:

1. Before any referrals are made, obtain consent from patient, family/significant other, and physician.
2. Document all communications with patient and family. Record direct quotes, if possible. Note whether the responses are inappropriate, which may signal a need for a guardian if the patient remains confused.
3. Document the patient's limitations and refusals in an objective manner. For example, Mr. Grant is 82 years old. He refuses an extended care facility (ECF). You feel that he needs one. Chart: "Patient refuses ECF at this time. Patient states he lives alone with intermittent visits from one neighbor. Physical therapy charts patient can walk 10 feet with front-wheeled walker and maximum assist of two." Now your discharge work begins. This shows that the patient is unsafe for discharge home alone. Many times patients later agree to a short stay in an ECF for the purpose of gathering strength. Before discharge, an appropriate discharge agreement must be reached and documented. Without further discharge consideration, the patient can go home, fall, break a hip, and file a lawsuit.
4. If the discharge plan changes, as is often the case, document the change, who requested the change, the reasons for the change, and your activities now. Mr. Grant in #3 may agree to home healthcare with aides and private

duty nursing. Before actual discharge, he may decide that an ECF is the best alternative at this time. Sometimes deterioration of the patient's condition or an unexpected improvement deems the plan change appropriate. Document the medical status of the patient to substantiate the necessary change in the discharge plan.

5. Document all interventions and the patient's *responses* to them.

6. On the day that a patient is transferred to another facility or discharged home, communication with family must be documented. This is especially important when the patient is going home with many discharge needs.

7. Document contacts with other agencies and institutions, and times, dates, whom you spoke with, and what was said and agreed on.

8. Documentation of patient/family education and teaching is extremely important. If anything goes wrong postdischarge, the family can sue; documentation can show proper and adequate teaching. Also, if documentation is inadequate, and the patient is readmitted, insurance companies may attempt to deny reimbursement, based on a supposition that the member was inadequately taught or prepared for discharge. Chart how much time was spent teaching, what was taught, to whom the information was given (eg, caretaker, patient), and how well the "student" did. If follow-up teaching is necessary, include plans for that and, when completed, add notations. If someone other than yourself did the teaching, identify the person in your notes, then encourage the person to document his or her results thoroughly.

9. Whenever possible, provide written as well as verbal instructions and provide demonstrations. Document teaching tools used.

10. It is critical to chart confirmation of the patient/caretakers's understanding of what is being told, such as special diets, treatments, potential complications, follow-up doctor visits, wound care, medications and side effects, and activity level.

11. It is not enough to explain and document potential side effects and complications of medicines and treatments. The patient or caretaker must also know what to do if complications arise; that is, *seek medical attention.* Some people, hearing from a doctor about a possible side effect, may wrongly interpret that side effect as being normal and expected and may continue with whatever caused the problem. Document that the patient and caretaker were told what to do if anything unusual occurs.

12. Many patients go home with durable medical equipment, such as oxygen, suction machines, Bipap ventilators, feeding pumps, and IV pumps. Document arrangements for ordering equipment, verifications from insurance companies, all the teaching that was done, and who was taught and their comprehension. Documentation of coordination—that the equipment will be available when the patient arrives home—is also important.

13. Educational needs should be addressed as soon as possible. Peer review organization (PRO) reviewers feel that last-minute teaching is not always indicative of acceptable discharge planning.

Medical Stability of Patient Within 24 Hours of Discharge

HCFA details six important stability markers to note during the last 24 hours of a patient's hospitalization (see also Chapter 6: Utilization Management):

1. Blood pressure (BP)—The patient may be considered unstable for discharge if:

   - The systolic BP is less than 85 or the systolic BP is over 180.
   - The diastolic BP is less than 50 or the diastolic BP is over 110.

2. Temperature—The patient may be considered unstable for discharge if the temperature is:

   - Over 101 °F (orally) (38.3 °C)
   - Over 102 °F (rectally) (38.9 °C)

3. Pulse—The patient may be considered unstable for discharge if:

   - Pulse is less than 50 without beta-blockers.
   - Pulse is less than 45 when patient is taking beta-blockers.
   - Pulse is over 120.

   Documentation: If any of the above vital signs fall out of the range listed, notify the physician of findings and document the physician's response, that is, why the doctor still approves of the discharge.

4. Abnormal results of diagnostic services not addressed or explained in the medical record. This may include lab tests or other tests done on the day of discharge.

   Documentation: Notification of physician of abnormal tests and physician response. If tests are done on day of discharge, chart test results, notification of attending physician of those results, and doctor's response. If the patient is going home before test results are back, document follow-up instructions to the patient.

5. Intravenous fluids or drugs after 12:00 midnight or on day of discharge.

   Documentation: Notification of physician and response: why it is acceptable to discharge patient.

6. Purulent or bloody discharge of postoperative wounds within 24 hours before discharge. Other wounds may also be included in this screen.

   Documentation: Chart condition of wound and physician notification and the response. Appropriate follow-up treatment such as home healthcare, outpatient facility, or ECF should be in place and documented.

Restraints and Falls

Restraints and falls go together like stop signs and traffic accidents; even with the best of intentions, accidents happen. Falls and resulting injuries are one of the most frequent causes of lawsuits. Restraining patients also carries risks. Some may cry "false imprisonment," which is the inhibition of the right to come and go as one chooses or the unjustified infringement of a person's freedom of movement. The key word here is "unjustified." Documentation must supply the justification for restraints, whether chemical or physical; it should support that there is a foreseeable susceptibility of injury. Restraints should not be used for staff convenience, but for patient safety. The safety of others should also be taken into consideration.

As an example, note that Mr. Ketter was lucid during the day but at night would "sundown" and become confused. One night he was especially confused and continuously pulled out his IV. No matter how often the nurse replaced it, each time she went back to check on Mr. Ketter, the IV line was out and there was a fair amount of bleeding. At one point that night, Mr. Ketter decided to pay a visit to some of the other patients. With a blood-stained gown, he burst into several of the hospital rooms, hollering "axe murderer on the loose." Looking himself much the part of a deranged killer, he terrified three other elderly patients! The night nurse faced a choice—either a sitter or temporary restraints.

Another case involved a male patient with newly diagnosed tuberculosis. He wanted to leave before tests could prove his medication therapy effective. Since legislation exists in some states that prohibits individuals from deliberately expos-

DISPLAY 7–1
Guidelines for the Use of Restraints

- Use for patient safety—*not staff convenience*—and document reasons and incidents leading to restraint.
- Assess need thoroughly.
- Know your institution's policy regarding restraints. Many institutions require a doctor's order. If no physician order is required, then the nurse becomes more responsible in a court of law for the decision to restrain and the outcome of the restraint.
- Use the least restrictive restraint necessary to accomplish the desired purpose. Perhaps a one-hand, soft restraint or mild sedative is all that is needed. A "velvet-glove" approach can demonstrate good faith.
- Carefully observe and monitor chemical "restraints."
- Practice safety measures when using restraints:
  1. Apply restraints for a limited time frame.
  2. Document how frequently the patient is checked—should be every 30 minutes.
  3. Document how frequently the restraints are removed—should be off about 20 minutes every 2 hours.
  4. Document assessment of skin.
  5. Perform range of motion and document. Know your institution's policy and procedures on safe restraint maintenance.
- Discontinue restraints as soon as it is safe to do so.

(Adapted from Northrop & Kelly, 1987.)

ing others, physical restraining may have become necessary if this patient had not changed his mind and stayed a few more days.

Display 7–1 offers tips on the use of restraints when they are necessary.

It is hoped that the frequency of falls can be reduced, but sometimes even with the best of intentions and the most appropriate use of restraints, falls do occur. If the nurse has shown compliance with standards of care and that compliance has been carefully documented, then a fall may not end in litigation. If a fall does occur, completely document the following:

1. Assessment of the injury and what was done immediately after discovery of the fall. For example, "I helped patient back into bed with assist of two, covered patient with blanket, and immediately called house staff to further assess injuries."
2. Timely notification of doctor. Depending on the assessment, notify as soon as possible or immediately if the patient appears seriously hurt.
3. Any treatments initiated.
4. Patient observation for changes in condition that were not apparent immediately after the fall; observe frequently.
5. Safety precautions resumed.

Recent JCAHO guidelines recommend that restraints be used *only after exhausting all other reasonable alternatives* (Mion & Stumpf, 1994). Studies have shown that between 13% and 47% of older patients who fall *were* restrained and that the seriousness of the injury from the fall was greater in these restrained persons than when a nonrestrained patient fell (1994). Use of restraints is not risk-free. Other than the obvious anger and frustration caused by their use, restraints have been responsible for complications ranging from bedsores, new onset of bowel and bladder incontinence, joint contractures, and brachial plexus nerve injuries, to hypoxic encephalopathy and death from strangulation (1994). The JCAHO standard of practice—nonrestraint except under rare circumstances—warrants consideration.

Informed Consent

A long time ago and in a medical environment far, far away, before the advancement of technology with all its multiple potential complications, a doctor-to-patient handshake was all that was needed for a physician to proceed with patient care. Now we have informed consents, a quasilegal document that the courts frequently rule "invalid" (Curtin, 1993). The following discussion will reveal some reasons for invalid rulings and how to avoid them.

Informed consents are used specifically for the treatments and procedures that are invasive or that have potentially dangerous side effects or complications (Feutz, 1991). Depending on the institution's policies and procedures, state laws, and the emergent need of the procedure, a signed informed consent form may be required. "Implied" consent may be appropriate in an emergency situation in which lack of action may cause greater harm than the potential risks of the treatment (1991).

Before a patient is informed of anything, that patient must be capable of comprehending what is being said. It is important to document the patient's ability or inability to understand. *Incapacity* is based on a patient's ability to understand the information, to make choices, and to communicate—verbally or nonverbally (Feutz, 1991). A patient under chemical sedation may be only temporarily incapacitated. An *incompetent* patient must be so labeled in a court of law; these people cannot sign on their own behalf (see the section on Advanced Directives & Surrogate Decision Makers).

There are two basic steps to an informed consent process: the disclosure of information and the signature.

The Disclosure of Information

The following, at the minimum, need to be discussed with the patient (or surrogate):

- The patient's condition or problem (Feutz, 1991)
- The nature and purpose of the proposed tests, treatment, or procedure (1991)
- Any hazards, risks, or potential complications of the proposed test, therapy, or procedure (1991)
- Any feasible alternatives to the proposed tests, therapy, or procedure (1991)
- The expected outcome of the proposed test, therapy, or procedure (1991)
- The risks and prognosis if the proposed test is NOT done (1991)

Most litigation surrounding disclosure issues addresses the physician's failure to reveal "material" risks or dangers (Northrop & Kelly, 1987). When a complication arises and the patient was not aware of its possibility, the chance of a lawsuit increases. Yet there is a delicate balance between disclosing too little and too much. Patients can become so overwhelmed with frightening, potential dangers and risks that they are no longer capable of sifting out the important information and making appropriate choices.

Again, complete documentation is essential in case the patient claims he was not fully informed. If the NCM is performing the disclosure task, document the following:

- The information discussed—include the above list of topics (Feutz, 1991)
- Who the explanation was given to and who else was present (1991)
- How long the discussion took (1991)
- Teaching materials used such as videos, flip charts, booklets, or drawings (1991)
- That the opportunity to ask questions was offered (1991)
- Indication of comprehension, whether more thought, time, and discussion are needed before the decision can be made

Incomplete or inaccurate information could deem the dispenser of the information liable. Take time to chart completely.

Signing of the Informed Consent

Most of the time, the NCM or staff nurse presents the informed consent form to the patient sometime after the disclosure of information. Often, the NCM or staff nurse did not conduct—or even witness—the disclosure. Therefore, the NCM must be skilled in assessing the adequacy of the information and patient comprehension. As a patient advocate, the NCM has a legal and ethical responsibility to protect patients from misinformation, omissions, and errors (Northrop & Kelly, 1987). If lack of understanding is assessed about the treatment, hazards, alternatives, risks, expected outcomes, or prognosis if therapy is not performed, the NCM can fill in omissions and clarify misunderstandings if she feels qualified to do so. Notification to the physician regarding problem areas is advised, along with complete documentation. If you feel that the patient requires more explanation from the physician, communicate that to the physician and document your concerns in the chart.

Where informed consent for minors is concerned, parents and legal guardians must sign consent forms. If the patient is considered an emancipated minor, some states allow that patient to sign informed consent forms (Perin, 1992).

Some parents may refuse to sign permits or informed consents for lifesaving treatments. But in many states, the courts can overrule parents' wishes if the patient is not otherwise terminally ill. There is a difference between a patient who is of the Jehovah's Witness faith, which objects to blood transfusions, and a parent who borders on abuse or neglect of his child. The social situation must be considered. If a child's prognosis is poor and the patient is terminal, parents can decline conventional medicine and try alternative care.

Confidentiality

Confidentiality has been given statutory power to give legal clout to professional relationships. It is hoped that this creates trust between the individual and professional helper. The ANA Code for Nurses states: "The nurse safeguards the client's right to privacy by judiciously protecting information of a confidential nature" (ANA, 1985, p. 3).

Maintaining patient confidentiality is not an easy task. Consider some of those—the multidisciplinary medical team—who may access the patient's medical records: attending physicians, residents, interns, medical students, nurses, nursing students, physical therapists, occupational therapists, speech therapists, social workers, case managers, utilization review people, insurance company case managers, hospital utilization reviewers, auditors, coders, billers, PRO review teams, JCAHO accreditation teams, hospital quality assurance, researchers, the courts, and lawyers.

As an NCM, you will be speaking to many people on each case. Care must be taken in each conversation to reveal only what is necessary. Give only the portion of information that the other party requires. Social service needs are different from an insurance company's utilization review requirements. Home health agencies or ECFs require different information from the state health department. It is usually safer for the NCM to call the insurance company or home health agency than to risk getting a phone call from a stranger requesting confidential information. Calls from family and friends to the nurses station to find out how a patient is faring can be a "confidential" nightmare if the nurse is not careful.

Recently, I had a case involving a drug user who overdosed in a deliberate suicide gesture. Her "roommate and best friend" called a staff nurse to see how she was doing. A personal and detailed exchange of information followed. The "best friend" then called the patient's mother and filled her in. This mother then hopped on a plane and flew across the country to be at her daughter's bedside. Her mother was the last person this patient wanted to see, and she furiously accused the nursing staff of breaking confidentiality. Handle phone calls with extreme discernment!

Some situations outweigh confidentiality, but in each of these cases an agency may not be entitled to the entire patient record. Sometimes the good of the public is protected over confidentiality issues. In some states, failure to report certain situations may result in criminal liability (see the section on Reportable Events). A few exceptions to confidentiality laws include child and elder abuse, gunshot wounds, other wounds probably sustained during an illegal altercation, cancer and seizures (some states), and communicable diseases.

Records from drug and alcohol treatment programs, mental health records and HIV-positive patients have extra piggybacked protection with other federal and state laws (Anonymous, 1990). Unless a patient gives a valid, signed and dated release in these instances, caution is advised (see sections on Medical Records, Special HIV Issues, and Special Mental Health Issues).

Special HIV Issues

Since the late 1980s, more and more states have enacted legislation that specifically relates to HIV matters. However, these issues are still in debate in some states. It is wise to be familiar with the HIV laws in your state and your institution's policies and procedures. Some of the issues include confidentiality, guidelines for the disclosure of HIV information, requirements for consents for HIV testing and the exceptions (ie, where no consent is required), workers' compensation and HIV exposure, and disclosure of exposure to a close contact of an HIV-positive person.

Most states have some form of confidentiality protection for a person with an HIV-positive blood test result. Fines or civil action may be enforced if release of HIV information was not done in good faith. In the following situations, disclosure of information may be allowable, but it is still best to get a written consent signed, which states the purpose of the disclosure and the extent of the information to be released (Anonymous, 1990). Not all motives require the same sections (or all) of the medical record. When in doubt, call your risk manager. You may be able to release information:

- For discussions with the other healthcare professionals when the purpose is medical diagnosis and treatment (Perin, 1992)
- For state health departments which are required by federal mandates to trend and investigate certain communicable diseases. They may not need the whole

record, only portions relating to diagnosis, treatment, and control of the disease (1992).

- If the record is court ordered (1992)
- If the patient or patient's attorney requests the information—through a signed consent which allows HIV information to be included (1992)
- For purposes of billing, quality assurance, and utilization review (1992)
- For some adoption agencies or for foster care placement (1992)
- For worker's compensation claims (1992)
- For the death certificates (1992)

Disclosure of HIV information to people who were close contacts of an HIV-positive person is not absolute or specific in many states. The Department of Health and Human Services encourages those tested as HIV-positive to contact and voluntarily tell spouses, significant others, and those with whom they have shared needles about their HIV status. Physicians in many areas are told that it is within their professional scope of conduct to inform a healthcare worker of a patient's HIV positivity, if an exposure to blood or body fluids is significant. Victim's rights laws, where they exist, allow requests for HIV tests and the final results to be revealed to the victim of sexual crimes (Perin, 1992).

Before a person can have blood tested for the presence of HIV antibodies, many states require a written, signed consent. Many institutions also require pre-consent HIV counseling by trained counselors, often social workers or nurses. Some exceptions to written consents do exist:

- Emergency situations: when diagnosis is needed for treatment, when no surrogate can be found after an honest attempt, and when the patient cannot sign due to incapacity (Perin, 1992).
- Nonemergency situations with the same criteria as above. Here, the attending and a consultant must verify that it is in the patient's best interests to know the HIV status (1992).
- To determine cause of death (1992).
- For anonymous testing—oral consent is satisfactory (1992).
- For certain types of research—identity remains anonymous (1992).

Complete documentation is again stressed for all gray areas pertaining to HIV confidentiality, release of medical information, and HIV testing.

Special Mental Health Issues

Before the 1960s, mental health patients were offered few legal protections. They were cloistered away in institutions, sometimes for decades. Now, mental health patients are afforded basic rights mandated by state and federal laws called *mental health codes*. Mental health patients are not just in institutions; they can be at home, in emergency rooms or ICUs, on medical floors in hospitals, or on the streets, homeless. Sometimes these patients deteriorate quickly. Staff nurses often look to the NCM for protocol. It is recommended that NCMs working with mental health patients know the state's mental health codes, the agency's policy and procedure on all types of restraints, how to contact security, how to get a STAT psychiatry consultant, and all emergency contact numbers, such as for psychiatric RN specialists on staff and local emergency mental health agencies.

Admission procedures to psychiatric units or mental health hospitals are regulated by the mental health codes of each state. There are two basic types of admission: voluntary and involuntary or emergency admissions.

Voluntary Admissions

Obviously, voluntary admissions are smoother and preferable for the mentally unstable patient. The patient is deemed mentally ill and assessed as benefiting from further treatment through a psychiatric evaluation and specific behaviors. Often the patient is assessed as a danger to self or others, but if the patient is willing to sign commitment papers to a mental health facility, he or she is considered a voluntary admittance.

Those who have agreed to treatment voluntarily are often allowed more freedom to help with treatment decisions at the facility. They can also apply to sign out and be discharged. When such is the case, the facility has several days to either (a) discharge the patient or (b) initiate formal procedures to have the patient involuntarily committed (Northrop & Kelly, 1987). Documentation would include all contacts with mental health professionals, their responses, objective personal observation of the patient's behaviors, communications with patient, family, and friends, and any other events deemed important, such as a requirement for 24-hour sitters, responses to medication, and safety precautions initiated.

Involuntary or Emergency Admissions

Involuntary transfers to a mental health facility are not very gratifying, but if the patient is a danger to self or another human being and refuses further treatment or if irreversible deterioration of the mental illness is imminent, the NCM and mental health team have no other recourse. Involuntary/emergent admissions are usually initiated by someone other than the troubled individual: NCM, psychologist, police officer, psychiatric RN specialist, family, friend, or physician (Perin, 1992). This person must make an application on behalf of the individual, based on personal observation of the individual's specific behaviors. Documentation should demonstrate that the person is a danger to self or others and is in immediate need of assistance (1992). Psychology evaluations and court proceedings follow. States must adhere to standards and due process, because this type of admission results in more restrictions than does voluntary status. For example, petitions for discharge from the institution may be more tightly controlled.

After the petition is initiated, the individual can be immediately detained (Northrop & Kelly, 1987). (About now, the NCM is wishing and hoping that this individual will change his or her mind and agree to voluntary admission.)

Another possibility is that the involuntary proceedings go on quietly without the patient's knowledge, until the patient is picked up for transfer. This requires extremely careful documentation as to the reasons why the mental health professionals deemed the secrecy necessary.

Involuntary admission is a difficult event to witness. The worst-case scenario emphasizes "detainment." Around-the-clock sitters are usually in place for all mental health transfers: often that "detains" the patient throughout the episode. But sometimes the patient gets agitated and violent, necessitating four-point leather restraints and a call to the institution's security guard. Leather restraints are a last resort and require good reason and careful documentation of events leading up to their use. Confirmation of the patient's desire to leave after the involuntary petition is in progress may be demonstrated with a signed AMA (leaving against medical advice) form, although in reality a frightened, agitated patient rarely signs anything. Prior to the use of leather restraints, documentation also has to substantiate the need for such a rigorous type of restraint (Perin, 1992). Again, objective observation of the patient's behaviors, all communications with the patient, family, mental health professionals, and other important events need thorough documentation.

Advance Directives & Surrogate Decision Makers

Most nurses have at one time or another taken part in a resuscitation effort that they felt should never have been initiated. With regret and feelings of hopelessness, they try to "bring back" patients who will never come back to their baseline—however poor it was—and who remain ventilated for hours, days, or weeks in a vegetative state before they die. As a patient advocate, there may not be a more important task than the discussion of advance directives, that is getting a patient's wishes for care and treatment in writing—and fulfilled.

In compliance with the *Patient Self-Determination Act of 1990*, hospitals, ECFs, home health agencies, and hospices are federally mandated to counsel patients about their right to accept or refuse treatment and their right to the use of advance directives (Bosek & Fitzpatrick, 1992). *Advance directives* are legally executed documents, drawn up while the individual is still competent; they can **only** be used if that individual becomes incapacitated or incompetent. in this situation, patients are directing their own care in advance of the need (prior to incapacity). Individual autonomy is the end result, since the person is able to, without coercion, make some extremely important decisions about him or herself.

The two most recognized advance directives are the *Living Will* and the *Medical Power of Attorney* (also called the Durable Power of Attorney for Healthcare). A third advanced directive, which is being used more frequently, is a *Prehospital Medical Care Directive*. This directive focuses on several aspects of the resuscitation event such as defibrillation, chest compressions, assisted ventilation, intubation, and advanced life support medications (Perin, 1992). The individual can choose all, none, or any number of the above treatments.

Living Wills

Living wills are legal documents directing the healthcare team in holding or withdrawing life support measures. Death must be imminent prior to its use (Bosek & Fitzpatrick, 1992). Some living wills are vague and have not held up in court, but when used with a medical power of attorney or other form of surrogate decision maker, they do guide healthcare decisions with more definition.

Some states now require the appointment of an advocate in the living will document. This is similar to a medical power of attorney in that this advocate cannot make decisions unless the patient becomes incapacitated. It should also be noted that the appointed advocates cannot be billed for medical care (unless the person has financial responsibility for the debt), and death that follows a decision by the appointee will not be considered a homicide ("Living Wills," 1994).

Medical Power of Attorney

The medical power of attorney (POA) is also a legal/medical document (not to be confused with a standard durable POA, who can pay bills and complete transactions). This document has two important functions: first, it names the person who will act as surrogate in the event that the patient becomes incapacitated; second, it outlines specific instructions in many aspects of care (Bosek & Fitzpatrick, 1992). Although a living will focuses on the withholding and withdrawal aspects of care, the medical POA may have checklists that are very comprehensive, including everything from intravenous fluids, tube feeds, and initiation of hemodialysis, to organ donation. Many patients sign these documents after admission to the hospital, but they must be of sound mind when signing. In most states, the two witnesses cannot be anyone in the patient's estate or will, a relative, anyone involved in their direct care (as a staff nurse), or the person named medical POA (Perin, 1992).

Some of these documents are several pages long and have very specific instructions. The named medical POA may have only limited decision-making capacity. The NCM is responsible for knowing the extent and content of the directives. Advance directives can be revised or changed. Be sure the most up-to-date version is being used. There are also some state laws that limit the medical POA's ability to consent to certain aspects of healthcare: abortion, sterilization, psychosurgery, convulsive treatments, and commitment to a mental health facility.

Often much "advance directive" talk goes on between an NCM and the patient. These communications should be documented. As a patient advocate, the NCM can be alert to any differences that may arise between what the patient has told the NCM and the decisions of the surrogate. I usually give the original document back to the family and make a copy of it for the chart. But find out the policy and procedure at your institution.

A competent adult, one who can rationally make choices on his or her own behalf, can refuse even ordinary treatment. Ordinary treatment is considered any commonly used care modality. Extraordinary treatment is defined as elaborate or heroic. Discontinuing or refusing extraordinary treatment in a competent adult is often the case that goes to the ethics committee or the courts. These are, for example, the chronic COPD (chronic obstructive pulmonary disease) patients, who have ended up on a ventilator and want it discontinued; or the terminal cancer patient, who demands that her g-tube feedings be terminated.

The courts usually uphold a patient's right to choose. If a patient decides to withhold or withdraw treatment and that patient is of sound mind, the NCM should assess whether the patient's condition, prognosis, dangers of refusing or withdrawing the treatment and alternatives have been thoroughly explained. Also, assess whether the patient's choice was made without coercion or pressure from others. If further education or counseling is needed, provide it. And document all that was discussed and the final decisions that were made. Courts will not, however, give free rein, such as when suicide is involved, when the court must protect innocent third parties, or if it will damage the ethical standards of the healthcare profession.

It is the incapacitated or incompetent patient that requires surrogate decision makers. Incompetency can stem from mental illness, which requires legal definition; or, a patient may be *clinically* incompetent from a disease such as Alzheimer's. Legal guardianship proceedings are not usually required for clinically incompetent patients if someone is willing to be a surrogate. A surrogate is essentially a substitute, required to, in good faith, make reasonable efforts to duplicate the patient's wishes.

Display 7–2 lists surrogates in order of priority, which most states uphold if the patient becomes incompetent and no Medical POA or medical legal guardian has been appointed (Perin, 1992).

Note that the decision concerning artificial food and fluid cannot be made by surrogates (except a medical POA) in some states. This was well documented in the famous Cruzan v Director, Missouri Department of Health case (Kolodner, 1992).

Nancy Cruzan was a 25-year-old who was in a motor vehicle accident in 1983 and remained in a persistent vegetative state for years. In this landmark "right to die" case, the state of Missouri deemed (in 1990) that "substituted judgments" (of surrogates) is not clear and convincing evidence of the patient's intent (Kolodner, 1992). The state refused the request to remove artificial feedings and hydration. (Other states also do not recognize all aspects of "substitute judgment." It is best to know your state's laws on surrogate's authority.) Nancy's parents and friends knew her wishes, but without a written, signed document, her wishes could not be upheld.

Because of the AIDS epidemic, NCMs are working with greater numbers of very ill young adults. Many may know little about documents such as medical POA, but most have thought a lot about dying and feel very little control over it. Although no one controls the death process, people can sometimes maintain authority over the events surrounding death and can make sure their last wishes are carried out.

NCMs and social workers are often asked to initiate discussions about advanced directives; most institutions have on hand the forms to sign. It is recommended that NCMs understand advance directives and feel comfortable discussing the subject with their clients. Workshops about advanced directives and those addressing death and dying are helpful.

DISPLAY 7–2
Surrogates for Patients Who Become Incompetent or Lack a Medical Legal Guardian.

1. Legal parent, if patient is a minor, or patient's spouse (unless legally separated).
2. Adult child of patient. If there is more than one adult child, a majority consensus is usually (but not always) safe. Often disagreement among family members makes decision-making a battleground. Sometimes legal guardianship is the only way to avoid a lawsuit, for example, if one wants DNR and the other adamantly opposes that stance. A disadvantage of obtaining a legal guardianship is that guardianship proceedings often take several weeks.
3. Parent of adult patient.
4. If the patient is unmarried, the domestic partner/significant other.
5. Adult brother or sister.
6. Close friend of patient must desire to act on patient's behalf.
7. If none of the above is available, two physicians or a physician and a medical ethics committee.

(Adapted from Perin, R. L. [1992]. *Arizona Statutes Affecting Nursing Practice.* Wisconsin: Professional Education.)

Another way to learn about advanced directives is to choose a medical POA for yourself—or become a medical POA for a close family member. The process is enlightening.

Reportable Events

All states have laws that require mandatory reporting by healthcare professionals. Criminal penalties can be imposed if those events are not reported to the proper authorities, since the laws are generated for the protection and well-being of the public. Conversely, if the reporting was done with reason and in good faith, most states provide civil immunity to the reporter for possible repercussions of libel, slander, or invasion of privacy (Perin, 1992). Thoroughly document all objective data and personal observations, especially in abuse cases. In this section, five reportable events will be discussed: coroners' cases, communicable diseases, violent crimes, child abuse, and elder abuse.

Coroners' Cases

Deaths that may not be clearly and without question due to natural causes are coroners' cases; therefore, the coroner must provide investigation. Following are some types of coroners' cases (Perin, 1992):

- Death that is unusual or suspicious
- Sudden death in a previously healthy person
- Violent death
- Death during surgery or anesthesia
- Death of a prisoner (in a prison)
- Death of a fetus
- Death when the cause could have been due to a public danger
- Death associated with a person's employment or occupation
- Death in which no attending physician is available
- Death that may be from other than natural causes

Note: In some places a nurse may substitute for a medical attending, such as in a home hospice setting. This case then may not become a coroner's case.

Communicable Diseases

The Centers for Disease Control and Prevention (CDC) was created by Congress for the purpose of data collection, analysis, and surveillance of certain communicable diseases. All states have mandatory reporting of specific diseases to the local or state health departments, which reports regularly to the CDC. A few of the many reportable diseases are gonorrhea and other sexually transmitted diseases, tuberculosis, shigellosis, measles (rubella), HIV, chickenpox, hepatitis, salmonellosis, mumps, aseptic meningitis, scarlet fever, and typhoid fever.

Violent Injuries

Violent injuries include but may not be limited to the following: gunshot wounds, stab/knife wounds, and other miscellaneous wounds that were most likely caused by a fight, robbery, or unlawful act. When reporting, give the name of all involved, a wound description, and any other unusual observed circumstances or facts.

Child Abuse

Child abuse is an issue that can produce rage in the most nonjudgmental NCM. Child abuse has many variations and is not limited to any ethnic or socioeconomic group. It is estimated that more than 1 million children are abused or neglected each year; 90,000 cases of sexual abuse are reported. In this country, 5000 children die annually of abuse or neglect. Not only is reporting of suspected child abuse mandatory, but if a classic case is not reported and the child suffers further danger or even death, the nurse can be deemed criminally negligent. There will be little sympathy for the nurse (and much for the child) in a court of law. I have seen medical personnel reluctant to commit to this "diagnosis." However, certainty at this point about the abuse is not necessary; only reasonable cause that maltreatment occurred is required for reporting.

Definitions of child abuse speak of nonaccidental injuries from mistreatment, sexual abuse, or exploitation such as child prostitution and deprivation of necessities. The perpetrator can be a parent, legal guardian, uncle or aunt, grandfather or grandmother, babysitter, boyfriend—anyone. Many books and articles have been written on how to recognize child abuse. Some classic signs are certain types of bodily harm (especially with radiologic evidence of older, healing fractures), failure to attend to medical, physical, or hygiene problems, sexually transmitted diseases, apprehensiveness or secretiveness, bruising or bleeding near genitalia, overly compliant behavior, suicidal attempts or gestures, and failure to thrive (which can also be caused by medical problems, so a medical cause must first be ruled out).

Verbal reports are acceptable initially to a peace officer and child protective services (CPS) worker. Written reports are usually due within 48 hours. These reports include names and addresses of parents, guardians, and anyone else involved in the case; a description of injuries, including any evidence of older trauma; and the age of the child. If there is reasonable cause that a child's death was the result of abuse, the medical examiner or coroner must also be notified.

A child may be taken into protective custody by CPS if there is reason to suspect the child is in imminent jeopardy. The multidisciplinary team working with the child is accountable for cooperating with CPS in identification, reporting, and case management aspects of the case.

Adult/Elder Abuse

Elder abuse has many of the same characteristics as child abuse. It is also an event that brings with it mandatory reporting requirements. As with reporting child abuse, if done in good faith and with reasonable cause, the person reporting has state immunity against libel or slander claims. Adult abuse can also take many forms. Some include physical abuse, neglect, exploitation of property or pets, unreasonable confinement, sexual assault, medical neglect, psychological abuse, or failure to thrive not caused by medical conditions. Most definitions include the stipulation that the adult is incapacitated or vulnerable and helpless to defend him- or herself (Perin, 1992).

The NCM, on finding out to what state agency to report, can call in a summary of the situation and document completely what was discussed, who was spoken to, and what the response was. A written report should follow. Some states have an Adult Protective Services (APS) for reporting and investigation. APS takes priority emergency cases first. These investigators seldom visit hospital units because they feel that at the time the patient is hospitalized he or she is in a safe environment. The next step is usually a multidisciplinary team meeting for purposes of discussing a safe discharge. Sometimes a patient is safe enough to be discharged to the previous arrangement with APS making a same-day-as-release visit to the home. Other times, other discharge arrangements, such as to a foster home or ECF, must be made. An APS investigation should follow in the latter case, also.

Elder abuse in a long-term care facility is not unheard of, and it can cost the facility Medicare and Medicaid licensing. Some of the rights afforded patients in a long-term care institution by Omnibus Budget Reconciliation Act 1987 (OBRA) include the right to privacy, notice prior to a room change or change in roommate, voice grievances, meeting with other residents, participation in planning care or treatment, and *freedom from physical or mental abuse, involuntary seclusion, or the use of physical or chemical restraints for the purposes of (staff) convenience or punishment* (Northrop & Kelly, 1987). Like child abuse, elder abuse cannot be tolerated in any level of care; failure to report it can lead to the same criminal action and lack of sympathy (for the negligent reporter) from the courts.

Do Not Resuscitate (DNR)—No Code Blue

In 1988, JCAHO established standards that required hospitals to develop "do not resuscitate" policies. The intent was to provide assurances that patient rights will be respected. If a patient is competent, the right to choose or refuse resuscitation measures belongs solely to that person. Incapacitated patients need a prior signed advanced directive or a surrogate (see section on Advanced Directives & Surrogates Decision Makers). If family members disagree about whether they want their loved one resuscitated, the medical staff should think twice about making that decision for them; legally, doctors would be putting themselves in a vulnerable position if they were to write a DNR order; a legal guardianship may be necessary if agreement cannot be reached. Of course, if no DNR exists, a full code must commence, if needed.

"Slow codes" and "partial codes" have always made nurses uneasy. These codes are illegal in some states and carry potential legal complications because of their vagueness. Some hospitals are clearing up the uncertainty with Prehospital Medical Care Directives or DNR orders, which break down the Code Blue tasks: external pacing/cardioversion, chest compressions, defibrillation, mechanical ventilation, intubation, and advanced life support medications. Even refusal of blood products or transfers to intensive care units can be opted for or out. A competent patient can then chose all, none, or some of the "menu" in case the need arises. This is a form of advance directive, since it is decided on and signed in advance of the need.

It is important to note that families are often confused about what "do not resuscitate" means, feeling that their loved one will not get necessary treatment. It must be clearly explained that "do not resuscitate" is not the same as "do not treat"—that the patient will not be abandoned and that everything will be done for the patient up to the point of arrest.

In most institutions, the DNR order must be written (or at least cosigned) by the attending physician. The physician who discusses codes with the patient or family should document the prognosis estimate and reversibility of the patient's condition and with whom these were discussed. The NCM documents a summary of any additional counseling or teaching and states who was present. NCMs may find themselves "reminding" the medical staff that the 98-year-old patient in terminal condition does not have any code instructions written yet. It is best to consider this before a crisis (in a patient of any age, if the condition is labile). Know your institution's policy on telephone (verbal) DNR orders—not all institutions allow it. Also, many hospitals require a new DNR order written when levels of care have changed.

Death, Anatomical Gifts, Autopsy

Most states define death as an irreversible cessation of cardiopulmonary functions or an irreversible cessation of brain function (Feutz, 1991). Some have pushed for a third definition (so far unsuccessfully): neocortical death. This is essentially an irreversible loss of consciousness and function (1991). An example of this would be the persistent vegetative state, where there is seemingly no awareness of anyone or anything. These patients live at a primitive reflex level and often have eye-blink reflexes and react to noxious smells, sound, pain, or light. Although their prognosis is poor, diagnosis as a form of death strains the definition.

In most institutions, the physician must "pronounce" the patient and fill out the paperwork. As stated in the section on Coroner's Cases, under certain conditions such as home hospice care nurses may pronounce the patient and fill out paperwork. Often the NCM is tending to family or attempting to contact family. If the family is en route to the hospital after their loved one has died, every effort should be made to meet them before they reach the room.

The HCFA generic screens (see Chapter 9: Quality Improvement and Risk Management) stress the importance of thorough documentation when deaths (1) occur during or after elective surgery, (2) occur after returning to an ICU or within 24 hours of being transferred out of an ICU, or (3) occur unexpectedly. Documentation should include, but not be limited to, complete patient assessments, prompt responses to any changes in patient condition (lab results, vital signs, cardiac rhythms, breathing patterns, pain, bleeding, and drug reactions), timely physician notification, equipment malfunctions, and interventions. If the staff feels that an equipment malfunction played a significant role in the demise of the patient, the NCM may want to strongly suggest that the hospital hold on to the piece of equipment, whether it is ventilator or a pacemaker. The hospital would like to prove that it was equipment failure and not user failure; the manufacturer would like to prove that it was not "equipment failure."

Anatomical gifts can be voluntarily donated by anyone 18 years or older. Driver's licenses and durable medical POA for healthcare documents are two ways to check a person's wishes about organ donation. If there are no indications that the person had any objections, the following can approve donations, in order of legal priority: (1) spouse (or parent if under 18 years old), (2) adult child, (3) either legal parent, (4) adult siblings, (5) legal guardian, (6) the person responsible for burial (Perin, 1992).

Some states require a "request of organ donation" through the use of preestablished criteria. In these states, hospitals are mandated to make a request for organ donation upon the death of the patient.

Autopsies (postmortem examinations) are usually required in coroner's cases. In other cases, they may not be mandatory. The following can give authorization for autopsy: (1) spouse (or parent if patient is a minor), (2) adult child, (3) legal guardian, and (4) next of kin. If none of these is found, the person responsible for the burial can give consent (Perin, 1992).

A NCM may be asked about who pays for autopsies. I have never heard of a family being billed. Many hospitals perform autopsies as a courtesy to the medical staff. But often hospitals perform autopsies at no charge even when the patient has earlier left the hospital and subsequently dies. There is usually a time limit in this case; 6 months is average.

The issue of autopsies is very personal to some people. I will never forget the grief one woman suffered when she discovered that her husband was mistakenly autopsied against his wishes. If this is within your realm of job responsibilities, document to whom you spoke and the decision made concerning postmortem examination.

CASE STUDY

Michael is 24 years old with an extensive history of suicide attempts and substance abuse. Methods of suicide gestures have included one attempted hanging, one self-inflicted knife wound of a superficial nature, and several drug overdoses, some of which he claimed were accidental. His use of drugs includes alcohol, LSD, marijuana, cocaine, and amphetamines.

Precipitating factors focus on dysfunctional relationships and episodes of major depression. Each admission has lasted 2 to 3 days, since Michael quickly stabilizes medically and each time renounces any further plans to harm himself.

Michael is now readmitted after ingesting a handful of cold medicine tablets and the remainder of his prescription for fluoxetine (Prozac), about 22 pills. The precipitating event is a date with a man, which occurred 1 week ago. He enjoyed the experience and is feeling immensely distressed because of it.

After 24 hours in the ICU, Michael is medically stable and ready for another level of care. He has again been diagnosed with major depressive episodes and multidrug abuse. Because Michael is now stable and has been eager to go home for 2 days, discharge orders have been written. Discharge will occur pending a social service referral to appropriate outpatient counseling and support groups. (Outpatient care is limited for this patient because of inadequate psychiatric insurance coverage, which includes only 72 hours of emergency inpatient care for episodes such as suicide attempts.)

The social worker has assessed available options and is discussing with Michael the appointments that have been made and the support groups available. In a surprising turn of events, Michael now states that he wants to remain in the hospital and that if he cannot be an inpatient, he will do further harm to himself when he leaves.

The discharge is being held to allow psychiatrists to reevaluate the patient. While waiting for his psychiatric interviews, Michael again turns the tables, announcing that he wants to leave the hospital *immediately*, before any additional evaluation has taken place.

CASE STUDY QUESTIONS

1. What is the first action that should be taken?
2. What are the patient's rights?
3. What is the hospital staff's responsibility?
4. Is a signed AMA form adequate?
5. Discuss documentation issues for this case.
6. Discuss potential risk management issues in this case.
7. Discuss the possibilities of voluntary versus involuntary admission to an inpatient mental health unit.
8. Discuss the insurance issues of this case.

References

American Nurses Association (1985). *Code for nurses with interpretive statements.* Kansas City: Author.

Anonymous. (1990). Medical records access: Practical legal tips for the 1990s. *AGG Notes,* *4*(2), 1–4.

Anonymous. (1987, Fall). *Managing your risk: A primer on contractual liability.* St. Paul Fire & Marine Insurance Co., pp. 149–151.

Bosek, M. S. D., & Fitzpatrick, J. (1992). A nursing perspective on advance directives. *MEDSURG Nursing, 1*(1), 33–38.

Curtin, L. L. (1993). Informed consent: cautious, calculated candor. *Nursing Management, 24*(4), 18–19.

Feutz-Harter, S. A. (1991). *Nursing and the law.* Wisconsin: Professional Education Systems.

Joint Commission on Accreditation of Hospitals. *Accreditation Manual for Hospitals,* 1985, pp. 98–99.

"Living Wills" set limits of treatment. (1994, May). *The Arizona Republic,* p. F6.

Kolodner, D. E. (1992). Advance medical directives after Cruzan. *MEDSURG Nursing, 1*(1), 56–59.

Mion, L., & Stumpf, N. (1994). Use of physical restraints in the hospital setting: Implications for the nurse. *Geriatric Nursing, 15*(3), 127–131.

Northrop, C. E., & Kelly, M. E. (1987). *Legal issues in nursing.* St. Louis: C. V. Mosby.

Perin, R. L. (1992). *Arizona statutes affecting nursing practice.* Wisconsin: Professional Education Systems.

Saue, J. M. (1988, August). Legal issues related to case management. *Quality Review Bulletin,* JCAHO, Chicago, pp. 80–85.

CHAPTER 8

Ethical Issues and Dilemmas

IMPORTANT TERMS AND CONCEPTS

Advance Directives
ethical dilemma
ethics
ethics committees
Ethics Delphi Study
Guide for the Uncertain in Decision-
    Making Ethics (GUIDE)

"medical necessity"
NCM as gatekeeper
patient advocate
Patient Self Determination Act of 1990
rationing of healthcare
"unnecessary" treatment

Ethical issues shift as society, technology, and professional practice patterns change. Step back in time to 1950. Few of the prominent ethical issues of today were discussed: abortion, euthanasia (doctor-assisted suicide), genetic experimentation, or rationing of healthcare. At the time genetic research was not far enough advanced to cause major concern, and healthcare was basic enough—with little high-tech equipment—to be affordable. The 1950 American Nurses Association (ANA) code stated that a nurse's obligation was to carry out the physician's orders and to protect the physician's reputation (Wright, 1987). This code left little motivation for a nurse to assess an ethical dilemma concerning poor physician choices or practice patterns, if it were to come up. Professional life appeared more clearcut than it does now, but not necessarily more ethical.

Ethics in healthcare is about choices and morals and the basic rights of free choice and autonomy. Ethical dilemmas are more difficult; one must select a course of action in which more than one choice is available. Often each choice holds an undesirable prognosis (Wright, 1987).

Nurse case managers are frequently confronted with ethical dilemmas during the course of a day's work. Although there is a finite number of ethical dilemmas, each case can present a new twist to the problem. Like the turn of a kaleidoscope, each case necessitates a new perspective on the issue. The perspective we see is also influenced by our values and morals, both personal and professional; these are what shape our choices, helping to resolve conflict and come to a point of resolution.

Each NCM has a portfolio of ethical issues and dilemmas. Some are generic; others are case-specific. An NCM who works in the neonatal ICU grapples with issues different from those of a pediatric NCM, an oncology NCM, or a rehabilitation NCM. Here are some classic examples:

- A family member will not consent to DNR (do not resuscitate) status for a patient. The patient has multisystem failure, and a code blue is imminent. The code occurs, the patient survives, and the rest of the story is a nightmare. This scenario has been played out in thousands of hospitals.
- A patient, mentally competent to make decisions, insists on being discharged home—to a clearly unsafe situation.
- A patient reveals her dread of being discharged because she will return to serious abuse perpetrated by her husband on their young daughter. She has told you to keep this secret. What about confidentiality? What about the legal aspect? Child abuse is a reportable event. Can you put aside the judgment about a mother failing to protect her child? A choice—to tell or not to tell—must be made in this case.
- A husband makes it clear that he does not want to be placed on a respirator. His medical condition destabilizes, he becomes unconscious, but his wife insists on intubation.
- A patient with a medical condition incompatible with pregnancy refuses to have an abortion. Her condition deteriorates daily. In the seventh month, the baby dies in utero. Two days later, the mother dies.
- A 75-year-old man had cardiac bypass surgery in 1983, necessitating several blood transfusions. It is 8 years later, and he is admitted with a perplexing diagnosis. Tests show that he is positive for the HIV virus and has full-blown AIDS. He wants to know what is wrong, but his wife insists that no one tell him the diagnosis.

Some ethical dilemmas end up in the courtroom. But even court decisions may leave more ethical challenges than the original case appeared to have. They may resolve some aspects but don't always solve the original dilemma. Consider the case of Nancy Cruzan mentioned in the last chapter. Nancy's parents were aware of her wishes about not wanting to remain in a persistent vegetative state. Still, they waited several years, from 1983 to 1990, for her to regain even basic awareness of the world. When the parents finally asked the courts to allow withdrawal of artificial food and hydration, the court ruled that there was no clear and convincing evidence of Nancy's desires (Kolodner, 1992). Nancy *telling* her family and friends that she would never want to be a "vegetable" was not enough.

Other cases never make it to the courtroom but have more ominous overtones. In Chicago, when a father's pleas to have his brain-dead child removed from the ventilator was met with hospital insistence that he obtain a court order, he held the medical staff at gunpoint and discontinued the ventilator himself (Fiesta, 1992).

These two heartbreaking cases did not go by unnoticed and without consequence. The impact of Nancy Cruzan resulted in the Patient Self-Determination Act of 1990 (Kolodner, 1992). Every patient in every hospital in America is affected by this. Had Nancy written her own advance directive, no court would have questioned her wishes. The impact in the second case is more subtle, but the message is clear. Should we hold human beings on the threshold of death just because we have the technology to do so? Fewer hospitals now are resisting removal from life support if the family agrees to it when a patient is declared brain-dead.

As NCMs, we play important roles in helping the client understand what advance directives are all about and his or her choices concerning them. We are often privy to verbal statements about "no heroic measures." But without a written, signed document, the patient's wishes may go unfulfilled. Advance directives are about a patient making his or her own life choices. Explaining these important documents and helping to explore feelings about these life-directing decisions and life goals may be important advocacy roles.

Withholding and Withdrawing of Care

Both of the preceding cases brought up the dilemma of withdrawing some treatment that the patient was receiving: food and hydration in one case and respiratory support in the other case. Withholding and withdrawing of some aspect of care is a recurrent theme in many ethical dilemmas and is the reason for much debate, both ethically and legally.

In 1983, the President's Commission for the Study of Ethical Problems in Medicine and Biomedical and Behavioral Research discussed the withdrawing and withholding of treatment as follows:

> The distinction between failing to initiate and stopping therapy—that is, withholding versus withdrawing treatment—is not itself of moral importance. A justification that is adequate for not commencing a treatment is also sufficient for ceasing it.

The last sentence, written in 1983, is just catching on over a decade later. But these are ethical recommendations—not legal precedents—and they lead to further questions. Is withdrawal of withholding of lifesaving treatment a form of assisted suicide? Or, is there a difference between actively causing death (withdrawing) and allowing it to occur by not intervening (withholding)? Asking tough questions can lead to that resolution that lies somewhere between right and wrong—yet is neither: it is merely a best choice, hopefully made in good faith.

As in the Nancy Cruzan case, withholding or withdrawing of nutrition and hydration is still being debated, and legal and medical people often have differing viewpoints. NCMs play a pivotal role in helping patients and their families clarify and articulate their views in these difficult cases. Many medical conditions lend themselves to an inability to orally feed a patient. Often the placement of a permanent feeding tube is a very difficult decision for a family to make, even if the patient is alert.

One case involved an 84-year-old nursing home resident, who came in with pneumonia (probably aspiration pneumonia) and complaints that he was hungry.

He was alert but very confused and managed to pull out every line the nurses could get into him. Having a recent history of several bouts of pneumonia, a modified barium swallow was performed to evaluate his swallowing ability. The results showed a high probability for aspiration if fed orally, so the recommendation was for placement of a permanent feeding tube.

The patient's daughter was distressed by this option. Unquestionably caring, she didn't want to prolong her father's life "in this state." I discussed with her the fact that, although her father was frail, he was not showing signs of impending death. He had no end-stage organ diseases, and his vital signs were stable. In addition, he was telling the facility staff that he was hungry. After much deliberation the daughter agreed to the feeding tube. But what if this patient had been imminently dying? Would *not* feeding him be ethically appropriate? What about hydration with IV fluids? Is this a form of withholding life support?

Leah Curtin stresses the distinction between withdrawal of life support and withdrawal of nutritional support.: "It is one thing to decide not to resuscitate a terminally ill patient, it is quite another to starve a person to death whether or not he has some hope for survival" (Curtin, 1994, p. 14). To lump the question of withdrawal of nutritional support under the classification as the withdrawal of medical life support measures confuses the issue (1994). The aforementioned patient died suddenly and unpredictably soon after the insertion of the feeding tube. But the decision was sound for this set of circumstances.

Suppose death is imminent. Whether to initiate feeding depends on the patient's medical and mental condition. Simple hydration may be appropriate in some cases. A more alert patient should be able to choose. Consider that:

> In the face of inevitable death from some other source, nutrition is used to provide comfort—not to sustain life. Any means of feeding that produces more discomfort than comfort can be eliminated from an ethical perspective. In some cases, the patient can tell us clearly what he wants. In other cases, we must rely on our own assessment and judgments. In all cases, the goal is comfort not adequate nutrition (Curtin, 1994, p. 15).

Ethics Committee

The kaleidoscope turns; look at another case about nutritional dilemmas, similar to the last case but with a different perspective, which required the assistance of an ethics committee.

Mrs. Norris is a 79-year-old patient most recently hospitalized for pneumonia (probable aspiration pneumonia). Her medical history includes a cholecystectomy, hysterectomy, several surgeries for metastatic intestinal cancer including resections for small bowel obstructions, multiple strokes, congestive heart failure, end-stage cardiomyopathy, and, most recently, frequent bouts of pneumonia. Mrs. Norris was alert and oriented until 1 year ago. At that time she filled out an advance directives form stating her wishes not to be kept alive through artificial measures; this specified and included food and hydration as an artificial measure that she did not want if her condition became irreversible and the quality of life was poor. After signing her wishes, the series of strokes occurred. Mrs. Norris is now cognitively poorly responsive. She opens her eyes, has reflexes, but does not respond meaningfully. Her present bout of pneumonia is clearing up. Swallowing studies confirmed that Mrs. Norris has severe esophageal reflux and is a firm candidate for further aspiration pneumonia if fed orally. Nasal feeding tubes have been unsuccessful because they have been coughed up or repeatedly pulled out. Due to multiple intestinal resections and complicated by severe esophageal reflux, a permanent feeding tube could be a rather tricky procedure requiring general anesthesia. The medical team is leaning toward comfort care measures only. Mrs. Norris is an extremely poor surgical risk, but attempts at feeding her without an intestinal feeding tube could lead to further aspiration pneumonia, which could also cause her demise.

Mrs. Norris' daughter Marion is furious with the doctors' suggestions of comfort care and states, "If you let my mother starve to death, I'll sue you!" No other family member voiced an opinion.

Case Discussion

This case leaves several options open for the medical team:

- Opt for comfort care only on the guidance of their own judgment and the advance directives.
- Call for a family conference.
- Attempt a feeding tube.
- Ask for judicial intervention.
- Ask the institution's ethics committee for assistance.

For the purpose of illustration, let us say that the last option was chosen. Several institutions have organized ethics committees to guide healthcare workers through the quandary that some situations present. The core membership of these committees includes physicians, nurses, clergy, an attorney, and a lay person. At times these committees appear to have some kind of magical ethical compass. In actuality, the conclusions are drawn through a process that includes "Socratic dialogue and devil's advocacy" (Levenson & Pettrey, 1994, p. 87).

First, the ethics committee needs the medical facts including a medical history, the present status of the patient, and a realistic prognosis. All possible treatment options and alternatives are then explored, including the possible outcomes for each modality. Brainstorming for unthought-of treatment alternatives may occur in the hopes that another answer may relieve the dilemma. A psychosocial assessment is also pertinent. Often conflicting morals and values of family members are a main cause of ethical problems. In the case of Mrs. Norris, the patient's directions were challenged by the daughter, and the doctor's attempts at explanations did not seem to clarify the medical problems and concerns.

When dealing with ethical dilemmas, it is important to distill out any legal issues. In Mrs. Norris' case, the advance directives was an important document to consider. But judicial resolution has its consequences: it is expensive; it is time-consuming, which can disrupt patient care; it can cause a strained relationship between the medical team and the surrogate decision makers, and it can turn a private matter into a media circus (Curtin, 1994).

Next, the ethics committee may apply various ethical "tools." The first tool is the use of various *schools and theories of ethical thought,* which may help bring the case to a point of resolution. (*Note*: Although this chapter will not analyze the various theories, several excellent books have been written on the subject; see Bibliography.)

A second ethical tool some feel is important is the use of *humor* to gain or maintain a sense of perspective. Care must be taken not to "make fun of" the situation at the expense of anyone. But a moment of shared laughter did occur when one of Marion's sisters quipped, "That Marion, even as a child she had trouble following Mom's directions!"

A third tool that may be used is *contemporary thought* on a particular issue. According to an article in *Issues in Law and Medicine,* the recent consensus on the subject of withholding or withdrawing artificial food and hydration is as follows:

Unconscious, Imminently Dying Patient (Progressive and Rapid Deterioration). The dying process will (most likely) not be reversed, and therefore nutrition and hydration are an unreasonable burden.

Conscious, Imminently Dying Patient. The patient is conscious and can make the decision, but artificial nutrition and hydration may be an unreasonable burden.

Conscious, Irreversibly Ill, Not Imminently Dying Patient. Again, the patient can ultimately decide since he or she is conscious. The disease process may not be reversible or curable, but nutrition and hydration to sustain life are useful. As long as the patient wants it and doesn't feel it is an unreasonable burden, then it has use.

Unconscious, Nondying Patient. Nutrition and hydration should be supplied to this patient. In this case, if no provisions were made to feed and hydrate the patient, the physician could be a party to "starving the patient to death." Unless there are other indications to the contrary, nutrition and hydration is not an unreasonable burden and is justifiable.

A fourth tool is *effective communication skills.* The art of listening and well-placed questioning punctuated with a caring attitude can often defuse difficult situations.

A fifth tool is *honesty.* It has been said that "ethics is honesty in action" (Curtin, 1992, p. 20). This basic human value is especially important in the final stage—the deciding recommendations. These recommendations will be born out of all the tools, personal values and morals, and judgments of the committee.

Guide of the Uncertain in Decision-Making Ethics (GUIDE)

Our present ability to sustain life or prolong dying almost indefinitely is the basis for many painful ethical situations. Medical personnel know that a fairly healthy heart plus a ventilator—maybe with the addition of hemodialysis treatments—can keep a human body alive for a long time; never mind if the brain is fatally damaged. Fewer and fewer people are seeing the glory in this scenario, and Americans are changing their ideas about dying. In quick succession, Jacqueline Onassis and Richard Nixon both said "no" to futile care that merely postponed the inevitable. And several articles about technology, death and dying followed. A landmark study found that most dying patients or their families now decide against resuscitation efforts (Knox, 1994). Even with more public awareness and new attitudes, medical professionals—especially physicians and NCMs—are often asked to referee disagreements between the patient/family and the healthcare team. This is a difficult task. And some feel the "Guide for the Uncertain in Decision-Making Ethics (GUIDE) (see Display 8–1) to be concrete help, especially when an ethics committee is not readily available.

DISPLAY 8–1
Guide for the Uncertain in Decision-Making Ethics

Scenario	Guidelines
1. Healthcare team favors treatment, patient/family opposed to treatment	• Review options carefully to ensure that patient has complete understanding of prognosis and options; competent adult patient has right to refuse medical treatment if patient has adequate understanding of information.
	• If patient has made an advance directive, it should be reviewed. In Virginia the Health Care Decisions Act provides an optional formal advance directive procedure, which can be written or oral, that applies when the patient's death is imminent or the patient is in a persistent vegetative state.
	• Discussions and patient's decision(s) should be completely documented in chart.
2. Healthcare team favors treatment/patient not competent, family opposed	• Need to identify primary decision-maker among involved family/significant others.*
	• Review information carefully to ensure that family/significant others have full understanding of patient's prognosis, condition and options and can make an informed decision. This should include any advance directives made by the patient.
	• If other family member disagrees with primary decision-maker, see Scenario 5.
	• May consult ethics committee.
	*Surrogate Decision Maker: Virginia law recognizes the authority of a Surrogate Decision Maker to make treatment decisions for an individual who is incompetent or incapable of making an informed decision. If patient previously made an advance directive appointing someone as "agent to make healthcare decisions" for him/her, that individual is empowered as the proxy (equivalent to durable power of attorney for healthcare). In the absence of any advance directive, Virginia law establishes the following order of priority for proxies: 1. A legal guardian, if one already had been appointed 2. The spouse 3. An adult son or daughter 4. A parent 5. An adult brother or sister 6. Any other relative in descending order of blood relationship

(Continued)

DISPLAY 8–1 *(Continued)*
Guide for the Uncertain in Decision-Making Ethics

3. Patient and family in disagreement concerning treatment decisions	• An adult patient has the right to refuse or consent to any intervention if he or she has adequate understanding of all information and is competent to make an informed decision. • Family should be included in all discussions but final decision about resuscitation and other interventions is made by the competent adult patient. • Patient should consider an advance directive. • Provision for family support may be needed.
4. Healthcare team does not favor treatment/ patient (or family if incompetent patient) does favor treatment	• Healthcare team is not required to undertake interventions that cannot help. Engage in further conversation with patient/family; ensure that they have received adequate information about futility of treatment. Reinforce that intervention(s) in question is not being offered because no benefit (either cure or comfort) exists. • Encourage/arrange second opinion. • Give patient/family option to transfer patient's care to another physician/hospital. • May consult hospital ethics committee.
5. Patient is incompetent/ family in disagreement concerning treatment	• Attempt to identify primary decision-maker (see Scenario 2 for statutory priority). Under Virginia law, if two or more persons of same priority level (eg, adult children of patient) disagree, the physician may rely on authorization of a majority. • However, every effort should be made to bring family to agreement. Attempt to have family/significant others focus on what the patient's wishes would be. Ask questions such as: "What would the patient tell us himself if he could speak?" and "Has he ever discussed what he would want if this happened?" Any advance directive made by the patient should be reviewed with the family. • May consult ethics committee.
6. Healthcare team in disagreement concerning treatment (ie, physician vs nurse, attending physician vs medical director)	• Attempt to reconcile through discussion and justification of viewpoint. • Seek guidance from chief of service, nurse manager, or other appropriate administrative pathway. • If patient favors treatment, seek second opinion about appropriateness of treatment. If treatment is judged to be futile (offering no benefit), see Scenario 4.
7. Healthcare team and family favor treatment/incompetent patient not objecting	• See Scenario 2 for guidance. Should identify primary decision-maker, but parties essentially in agreement in this scenario.
8. Healthcare team and family favor treatment/incompetent patient objecting to treatment	• Under Virginia law, if an incompetent patient actively refuses treatment, a surrogate decision-maker cannot be used without judicial review. This may take the form of seeking the appointment of a legal guardian, or a judicial order allowing involuntary medical treatment. • Contact hospital superintendent, legal advisor, and/or ethics committee.
9. Not clear if (a) patient is competent, and/or (b) patient is in favor of or opposed to treatment.	• Reassessment of patient's capacity for decision-making and/or patient's preferences by primary physician. If possible, the source of the patient's ambivalence should be identified. • Psychiatric consultation if competence still unclear or if patient continues to express contradictory preferences. • If still unresolved, consult ethics committee.

(Reprinted with permission of *American Journal of Critical Care*, March 1994, 3[2].)

(Continued)

DISPLAY 8–1 *(Continued)*

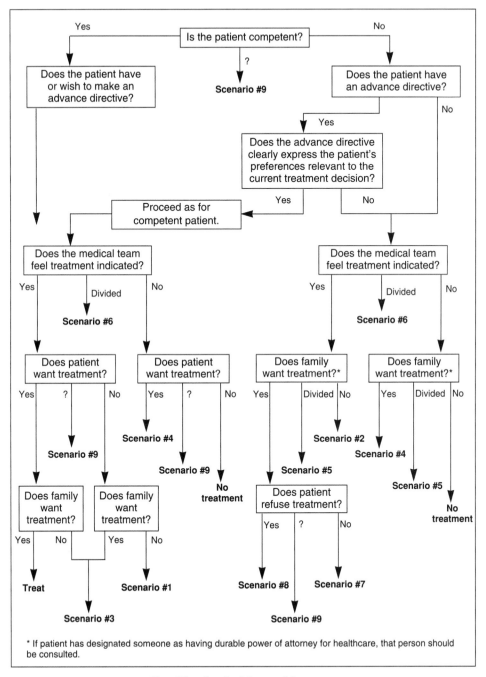

Algorithm for decision making.

The Guide for the Uncertain in Decision-Making Ethics (GUIDE), along with its companion algorithm, takes into consideration advance directives, proxy decision makers, and healthcare teams' preferences in their recommendations (Levenson & Pettrey, 1994). These guidelines contain nine scenarios, each defining key issues and conflicts between the patient-family and medical team. The recommendations use logically sequenced questions about the patient's competency, advance directives, treatment options, benefits and burdens of the treatment options, patient and family preferences, and patient prognosis (1994).The NCM should be cautioned that this GUIDE and algorithm are not intended to take the place of legal or risk management advisement. However, it is consistent with applicable law and good risk management (1994). It should also be noted that it was written in Virginia with that legislation in mind; as stated in Chapter 7: Legal Issues for Case Managers, know the statutory regulations pertinent to healthcare in your state. Last, the GUIDE is essentially for adult patients and perhaps for legally emancipated adolescents (1994).

Ethical Public Opinion: Polls and Studies

Ethical questions about life-sustaining treatments and about healthcare reform in the 90s have been in the news almost daily. In the spring of 1992, St. Joseph's Hospital and Medical Center in Phoenix, Arizona, conducted a nationwide Delphi study on ethics and healthcare. Both consumers and experts were polled with some interesting results:

- Both consumers and experts felt it was appropriate for people who engage in unhealthy lifestyles to pay more for healthcare.
- On administering or withholding medical treatment:
  1. Both groups felt it was appropriate to base the decisions on the chance for survival.
  2. Both groups were not as eager to base decisions on patient age, cost of treatment, or a patient's expected contribution to society.
- Fifty-three percent of the consumers placed individual rights over societal rights; 53% of the experts place higher priority on the good of society as a whole.

The following percentages are taken from "expert" polls. These experts include ethicists, hospital administrators, doctors, and insurance administrators.

- 76% feel rationing of healthcare to the poor is not ethical.
- 74% feel that healthcare should not be treated as a commodity.
- 72% agreed that setting a monetary capitation ceiling is ethical.
- 55% were concerned that, in healthcare reform, individuals are not encouraged to take personal responsibility for their health.
- 34% felt concerned that healthcare reform would lead to more rationing based on sets of criteria.

As an adjunct to opinion polls, research studies have been done in an attempt to clarify how much America would save in healthcare dollars if policies were written disallowing futile care (other than comfort care) to terminally ill people.

In a landmark $28 million (that's a lot of bone marrow transplants!) study, the following was discovered (Knox, 1994):

- Only $1 out of every $8 spent for medical care could be saved by a strict policy that ruled out life-prolonging care. The study found that this is because most dying patients or their families decide against being coded in advance. But most of that $1 savings would come from withholding care from relatively young, critically ill patients. (Consider the major diagnoses for this category of patient.)

- Only 14% of the 2150 critically ill patients who died during the study had an attempted resuscitation. Therefore, it was estimated that reducing aggressive life-sustaining treatment would save "at most" 3.3% of the total US healthcare expenditures. (Note that 3.3% of the over $900 billion spent in 1993 is over $30 billion.)

- Past projects to identify guidelines for withholding or withdrawing treatment based on objective criteria have not been very accurate. Newer prognostic criteria with very narrow criteria margins—in this case less than 1% chance of survival for 60 days—were more accurate. In this study, 75% of the patients died in 5 days, 98% had died within 1 month, and one patient survived 10 months with a good quality of life.

The study concluded that their prognostic criteria would be acceptable to most people and "would sacrifice very few patients who might have lived" (Knox, 1994, p. A26).

Ethical Dilemmas Specific to NCMs: Balancing Roles and Rationing

For all the cost and effort of this study, dilemmas that are a consequence of our contemporary healthcare climate continue to haunt us. The issues are not static, and more will be revealed as healthcare reform unfolds. As NCMs, we may be subject to ethical "discomforts" from the very roles we must perform: as gatekeepers of resources versus patient advocates and as coordinators–facilitators of the multidisciplinary teams. One common thread that appears over and over, sometimes in subtle disguises, is the issue of healthcare rationing.

The very idea of "rationing" healthcare is extremely distasteful to many Americans. But like any budget the healthcare budget is finite—and it is spiraling out of control. A few years ago when I read that Americans spend about $7.5 billion *per day* on healthcare (Doughery, Kizer, & O'Brien, 1990), I thought it was a typographical error. It was not. Since then, the price tag has gone up. The estimated cost of healthcare in the United States in 1993 was $903 billion. Other sobering statistical estimates state that between 5% and 6% of the population consumes 50% of the healthcare resources; 10% of the population consumes 80% of the resources.

And the average person consumes two thirds of his or her lifetime-accrued costs in the last 3 weeks of life (Boling, 1991).

When most people think of rationing healthcare, they have visions of cutting off life-saving, high cost procedures to a defined population. Perhaps people over 80 will not be allowed coronary bypasses; or anyone over 65 would not be allowed organ transplants or hemodialysis; or heroic measures would not be started on premature babies under 22 weeks gestational age.

The truth is that America already rations healthcare. The present discussions on newer, more stringent sets of criteria are for the purpose of rationing it further. Some feel that this is in order to serve a larger population (ie, the presently uninsured). Others believe it is for reasons of financial benefit to the payor agency.

The rationing fire is being fueled by the media. One newspaper article priced the cost of resuscitation of a cardiac arrest at $161,000, if the patient lives to be discharged (Wong, 1993). Another article estimated that very ill cancer patients "cost" $82,845 to $189,339 per year of life gained—not counting surgeries and post-surgical recoveries (Cancer Care, 1993).

Americans are grappling with the question of whether healthcare is a right or a commodity, which is another subtle way to evaluate whether healthcare should be rationed. The above articles are commodity-focused. But many of today's questions cross-examine whether healthcare is a right and how far should the rights of individuals go? Should noncompliant people who engage in unhealthy lifestyles be covered? Some question whether rationing, or limiting of healthcare, should be imposed on noncompliant persons.

Should ceilings be placed on their medical care dollars? Should those who can afford to pay have higher premiums? What is legal and what is ethical? Consider the Delphi study responses.

Even the definition of noncompliance does not consider all the ethical ramifications. Noncompliance is a failure of the patient to cooperate with the medical plan by not carrying out needed procedures or lifestyle changes. But the very concept of noncompliance betrays the professional's concern about patient autonomy; in other words, that patients are free to make life-directing decisions (Wright, 1987). And care must be taken not to label all those who don't follow a prescribed medical plan of treatment as "noncompliant." Cultural beliefs are highly ingrained in people's basic humanity. Food, health and religious ritual practices will not be changed simply because a western health practitioner dictated a prescription. Also, children and incapacitated adults who are in the care of noncompliant guardians may be penalized if society rations healthcare to "noncompliant" people. The kaleidoscope turns and the perspective changes.

NCMs deal with rationing on a daily basis. Two women have leukemia. Both could die. Both have families and young children. One is allowed a bone marrow transplant by her insurance carrier; one is not. Insurance companies "ration" their healthcare dollars through "allowed" benefits all the time: who is allowed "benefits" such as organ transplants, bone marrow transplants, home IV antibiotics, extended care benefits or "experimental" treatments. Subtle rationing of benefits takes many forms, and the NCM must be alert to a denial of benefits based on an interpretation of benefits that may be erroneous.

One case involved a cancer patient with stomach, esophageal, and intestinal tumor involvement. Surgically, there was little to be done for the patient and her prognosis was poor, although not imminent. She was alert and oriented and chose hospice care, as she was no longer trying to cure the cancer with medical treatment. She was on TPN as her only possible source of nutrition and was receiving radiation for palliative, not curative, purposes.

I was told that the TPN was disallowed because hospice does not cover services that are merely for prolonging life. Not feeling that basic nutrition falls under the "not prolonging life" umbrella in this case, any more than eating food would in a lung cancer hospice patient, I argued. She received hospice and TPN. The bottom line is that TPN is very expensive and is difficult to budget, so it is not routinely considered a covered service.

Some insurance companies cloak their rationing under terms such as "medical necessity" or "unnecessary" treatments. These vague terms must be treated with care, as they are arbitrary and prone to personal judgments when used as a measuring rod for insurance guidelines. "Clarifying the implications and usages of medical necessity requires semantic analysis, but it is not merely a semantic exercise. Confusion, conflict and refractory dilemmas inevitably emerge when the intertwined layers of meaning packed in the concept remain hidden" (Sabin, Forrow, & Daniels, 1991, p. 40). The authors of the above quote suggest that "choice would be a more applicable concept" and that the highly conflicted issues of medical coverage may soon be in the political and public arena (1991).

The NCM—as a patient advocate—must be alert to vague interpretations of benefits. In addition, "a payor inappropriately interpreting benefit language to cut its losses to the detriment of the claimant is courting malpractice" (Boling, 1993, p. 6).

In a positive sense NCMs help to ration healthcare. Through astute case planning and attention to detail NCMs avoid duplication and overutilization of finite resources. This is done through our "gatekeeper" role. As a gatekeeper, the NCM's job responsibilities may include monitoring of resources, allocating and authorizing resources, and introducing incentives to improve the quality of care providers (Kane, 1988). In essence, the gatekeeper controls and rations limited resources in a world where there appears to be unlimited need.

But when the NCM superimposes the role of patient advocate on that of a gatekeeper, role conflict and ethical dilemmas may result. Many feel that the combined patient advocate-gatekeeper role of a NCM is an impossible marriage. A gatekeeper controls entry to services and uses them economically; an advocate strives to gain all the services the client needs for a safe, efficient, and effective case plan.

Is it possible for one person to be both a patient advocate and a gatekeeper of healthcare resources? Can the NCM maintain quality while cutting costs? It is a challenge. There are factors that play into how effectively this merger can be accomplished.

The type and definition of the individual case management position may weigh one role heavier than another. A case manager for a Medicaid plan may feel that allocation of resources for her population of many thousands of clients (the whole) supersedes the needs of the individual (the part); therefore, her gatekeeping role may be stressed. A case manager in an oncology unit may feel that her client's needs are the most important factor, and this NCM may practice 75% patient advocacy and 25% gatekeeper. Potentially serious conflict of interests are possible when the agencies that provide services send their case managers to do the assessment of need and make the case plans (Kane, 1988). If the company's objective is to increase business, overutilization may be practiced; if the company's objective is to control utilization of services, underutilization may be the result. The NCM may be placed in the unfavorable position of asking, "How can I really advocate for this patient when it means fighting with this person paying my salary?" (Boling, 1991, p. 81).

Perhaps the most important factor in how effectively the merger is accomplished is your own personal style and ability to balance the two roles so that everyone wins. Although this is not always possible, it should be strived for. Whenever it is not possible, err on the side of patient advocacy: "A case manager misinterpreting his or her role to be primarily that of a provider or payor *employee* and secondarily that of a *patient advocate* is truly creating cause for divisiveness regarding case management" (Boling, 1993, p. 6).

Another NCM role that at times is the cause of ethical discomfort is that of a coordinator facilitator. NCMs are often asked to facilitate consensus of a large multidisciplinary team when a case is soaring out of control. This case conference may include any or all of the following: the patient, the family, the attending physician, physician specialists, residents or interns, respiratory therapists, speech therapists, occupational therapists, physical therapists, staff nurses, hospital administrators, risk management specialists, social workers, insurance company liaisons, insurance utilization review nurses or case managers, nutritionists, finance officers, or anyone else essential to that individual case. NCMs deal with so many people making decisions on each case, it's dizzying. Ethicist John Banja likens this facilitator role to an air traffic controller, who must coordinate flight patterns so that everyone is not crashing into one another (Boling, 1991).

At times, it feels as though some team members are on a collision course. Most NCMs have been in situations in which the payor (insurance company) was found to have a different agenda from the physician. The payor felt that the patient could be safely provided for at a lesser level of care. The physician felt that the patient was not stable enough for a step-down change. The payor felt that they must make wise and strict use of resources, since they have a very large population to manage and must ration the funds carefully. The physician was focused on the best care for this patient at this time.

Sometimes the biases come from opposing viewpoints about the best treatment for a particular case. One physician feels that a patient needs a lower extremity amputation; another physician feels that care should be "comfort only" at this point. The physical therapist feels the patient is unsafe to go home alone; the patient insists that he will go home. A patient refuses care for a gangrenous foot; the family is threatening to sue if this patient dies from a gangrenous foot. As the air traffic controller-NCM gathers a meeting and allows each dissenting opinion time on the runway—one at a time—to air their views on the best way to handle this situation—don't forget to state *your* agenda—that of patient advocate.

There are no answers at the back of a book on ethics. There are no assurances that the choice made is the best choice. But for decisions "to be truly ethical ones, they must be uncontaminated by personal gain, fear of reprisal, or other ulterior motives" (Boling, 1991, p. 81 [interview with John Banja]).

Although not all NCMs have the comfort of an ethics committee to call on when needed, more institutions are forming these important links to quality healthcare. All NCMs have their pet list of ethical doubts and difficulties. The names and faces change, as do some of the medical and psychosocial details, but often the dilemmas have common roots. As NCMs identify common ethical problems, it also becomes apparent that clear *ethical standards* are needed for the nurse case management profession. It is hoped that at some time in the near future NCMs will have a panel of ethical experts to turn to when dealing with these trying circumstances.

CASE STUDY

As a case manager for a large Medicaid plan, you feel ethically imbalanced as you perform your gatekeeper role in the following two cases.

Case Study 1: Mrs. Varo is a 46-year-old with advanced metastatic breast cancer. She finished a course of chemotherapy that left her with intractable nausea and vomiting. She has not vomited for 24 hours but is very weak and nauseated. She lives alone with little social support. She has no intensity of service with which to authorize any further hospital days. The physician advisor of the insurance plan felt that she could be managed at home.

Later the same day, you perform an initial review on the following case:

Case Study 2: Mr. Ciro's admitting diagnosis was "suicide attempt." He was placed in an ICU bed for close observation. Mr. Ciro had called 911, saying he had just swallowed most of a bottle of diazepam (Valium) and had drunk a fifth of whiskey. His toxic screen showed very little drugs or alcohol. However, it did test positive for cocaine. Later that day, Mr. Ciro told a social worker that he had spent his last dollar on cocaine and that he considered it too hot (Phoenix in August) to sleep outside, so he feigned suicide. On physical examination, the physician finds cellulitis on both of his legs from cocaine injections. His hospitalization is authorized for initiation of intravenous antibiotics for bilateral cellulitis.

CASE STUDY QUESTIONS

1. How would your ethical "equity meter" register?
2. If private insurance, rather than federal/state insurance, was covering the patients, what might have happened?
3. What conflicting personal and social values do you feel you are compromising, if any?
4. What rights does patient "A" have? Patient "B"?

5. Identify values and ethical principles that affect this situation.
6. Is there an actual ethical dilemma here? If so, what is it?
7. Discuss rationing of healthcare resources as it applies to these cases.
8. Discuss "patient advocacy" as it applies to these cases.
9. If you were the social worker, what would you have done with the information given about the deceptive suicide attempt? What are the confidentiality issues involved?
10. Discuss "medical necessity" as it applies to case A, case B.

Study Questions

1. What are ethics? What constitutes an ethical dilemma?
2. Would Nancy Cruzan's case be resolved differently today than in the 80s? Why?
3. Recall and discuss an ethical dilemma that occurred with one of your cases.
4. In each of the nine scenarios in the Guide for the Uncertain in Decision-Making Ethics:

    • Discuss a real case that matches each scenario.
    • Discuss the recommendations given for each case scenario.

5. If an ethics committee has ever been consulted on one of your cases, discuss the case, the ethical dilemma, and the committee's recommendations.
6. Is there an ethical difference between withholding and withdrawing life-sustaining treatment?
7. Under what circumstances can life-sustaining treatment be withheld? Withdrawn?
8. When does ordinary treatment become extraordinary?
9. Is withholding or withdrawing nutritional support from a person ethically justifiable? When, if ever? What criteria could be used? What about hydration?
10. Are nutritional support and hydration different from other forms of life support? If so, how are they different?
11. Is discontinuing nutritional support "active" euthanasia? Is it "passive" euthanasia?
12. What does the 1983 President's Commission for the Study of Ethical Problems in Medicine and Biomedical Behavioral Research say about withholding and withdrawing treatment?
13. Give case examples for each of the four positions about the contemporary consensus regarding withholding or withdrawing of artificial food or hydration.
14. Discuss differences between a patient who is "terminally ill" and one who is "imminently dying." Would the case plans differ?

15. Discuss your views on the points mentioned in the Delphi Poll.
16. Discuss a case that you felt had an ethical twist to it concerning rationing healthcare.
17. Discuss a case in which you felt your "patient advocate" role was compromised by your "gatekeeper" role.
18. Discuss a case in which your gatekeeper role was influenced by your patient advocate role.
19. Discuss a case in which you felt "medical necessity" was misused.

References

Boling, J. (1991, July). Profile—John Banja. *The Case Manager*, 76–81.

Boling, J. (1993, Aug/Sept). Conflict with case management...The ethical agenda. *The Case Manager*, 6.

Cancer care may cost more than it's worth, study says. (1993, February 11). *The Phoenix Gazette*, B8.

Curtin, L. (1992). On writing a column on ethics. *Nursing Management, 23*(7), 18–20.

Curtin, L. (1994). Ethical concerns of nutritional life support. *Nursing Management, 25*(1), 14–16.

Doughery, C., Kizer, W., & O'Brien, R. (1990). Covering America's uninsured: Who has the answer to rising health care costs. *Creighton University Window, 6*(3), 16–21.

Fiesta, J. (1992). Refusal of treatment. *Nursing Management, 23*(11), 14–18.

Issues in Law and Medicine (Vol. 6, No. 1, Summer 1990, p. 92)—A Publication of the National Legal Center for the Medically Dependent and Disabled, Inc.

Kane, R. (1988). Case management: Ethical pitfalls on the road to high-quality managed care. *Quality Review Bulletin*, 161–166.

Knox, R. (1994, May 27). Noted deaths reflect attitude shift: Most patients and families oppose resuscitation efforts, study finds. *The Phoenix Gazette*, A26.

Kolodner, D. (1992). Advance medical directives after Cruzan. *MEDSURG Nursing, 1*(1), 56–59.

Levenson, J., & Pettrey, L. (1994). Controversial decisions regarding treatment and DNR: An algorithmic guide for the uncertain in decision-making ethics (GUIDE). *American Journal of Critical Care, 3*(2), 87–91.

President's Commission for the Study of Ethical Problems in Medicine and Biomedical and Behavioral Research. (1983). "*Deciding to forego life-sustaining treatment.*" Washington, DC: US Government Printing Office.

Sabin, J., Forrow, L., & Daniels, N. (1991, December). Clarifying the concept of medical necessity. *Medical Interface*, 35–42.

Wong, S. (1993, March 17). Hospital resuscitation brings cost "avalanche": Price of reviving patients put at $161,000. *The Phoenix Gazette*.

Wright, R. A. (1987). *Human Values in health care: The practice of ethics*. New York: McGraw-Hill.

CHAPTER 9

Quality Improvement and Risk Management

IMPORTANT TERMS AND CONCEPTS

Adverse Patient Outcome (APO)
Continuous Quality Improvement (CQI)
important aspects of care
incident
incident report
Indicators
Occurrence Report
outcomes
Performance Improvement (PI)

Potentially Compensable Event
Quality Assurance (QA)
Quality Improvement (QI)
Quality Management (QM)
quality of care
Risk Management (RM)
Total Quality Management (TQM)
variances

The present healthcare climate contains elements that leave it open to accusations of compromised quality of care: utilization review criteria that is becoming more strict each year and demands prompt discharges to lower levels of care; scrutinized resource use and stricter allocation of healthcare resources; capitation and risk contracts in acute hospital settings placing hospitals at increased fiscal risk; and "downsizing," which changes the professional staff-to-patient ratio.

Quality Improvement (QI)—also referred to as Quality Management (QM) or Quality Assurance (QA)—has long been a function mandated by the Joint Commission for the Accreditation of Health Care Organizations (JCAHO). Some JCAHO requirements that improve various aspects of quality care include the creation of hospital policies and procedures, job descriptions, personnel evaluations, the provision of educational programs to ensure that knowledge and clinical skills are up to date, and continual monitoring activities.

Rather than merely emphasizing QA, which is often episodic in its assessments, JCAHO is now emphasizing the concept of CQI—Continuous Quality Improvement (Fanucci et al., 1993). Gleaned from the industrial sector that is typical of the Japanese automotive management philosophies since World War II, CQI attempts to meet or exceed the customer's needs. The "customer" is no longer just the patient but includes everyone associated with the healthcare industry, both externally and internally (1993).

The CQI concept is gaining strength in the healthcare industry as TQM—Total Quality Management. TQM, also taken from the industrial sector, has been customized for healthcare and incorporates Risk Management (RM), QA, and patient satisfaction as objectives. Customer-patient expectations may focus on provider attitudes, convenience, access, or costs. A provider's focus may differ; here TQM roles and commitments include employee motivation, enhancement of technical quality, excellence in structural and process aspects of care, and reduction in mistakes related to both clinical and administrative treatment of patients (Williams & Torrens, 1993). TQM and CQI emphasize a proactive rather than a reactive approach.

> Effective quality management is both a continuous and a systematic endeavor. Instead of centering on crisis, wrongdoing by individuals, and conformity to correct processes established by experts, quality management should engage everyone in the organization in continuous efforts to raise the organization's level of performance (Kongstvedt, 1993, p. 167).

This ideal of high level of performance is the goal of quality improvement and risk management programs. Unfortunately, at this time in the healthcare evolution, we must also continue to focus on crises when they occur and to monitor potential or actual problems. This troubleshooting is done through safety checks, infection control, incident reports, risk management activities, nursing care evaluations, and, most recently, through case management assessments and use of tools such as clinical pathways. Quality assurance cannot "assure" that risks and maloccurrences will not happen, but through the previously mentioned activities and prompt identification of problems, the risk manager can initiate the appropriate intervention to minimize "crescendo-ing" consequences.

Risk management and quality improvement are closely related programs with similar goals. The scope of this chapter will be to clarify the similarities and differences of traditional QI–RM programs, illustrate the importance of the NCM role to QI–RM activities, and describe circumstances and indicators that warrant close attention. An extensive body of literature has already been written about what the QA Ten-Step Process is and how it works; on traditional QA programs utilizing the three dimensions of structure, process, and outcome; and on the legal aspects of risk management. If interested, carry out further investigation.

It should also be noted that more organizations are using terminology for the newest generation of quality improvement functions—Performance Improvement (PI). Here the three dimensions of structure, process and outcomes have evolved into the following processes: design, measurement, assessment, and improvement. The *design process* is responsible for designing new functions, processes, and services based on the mission and vision of the organization, the expectations and needs of the customers, and the most up-to-date information regarding the focus of improvement. The *measurement process* evaluates the effectiveness of the previously mentioned redesigned processes, thus identifying opportunities for further improvement. The focus of the measurement process includes areas of care that are high volume, high risk, and problem-prone. The *assessment process* provides a systematic approach to determine whether the goals and priorities for the redesigned process were met and how further improvement could be made. The *improvement process* uses the Total Quality Management (TQM) process called FADE (Focus, Analyze, Develop, Execute) and team collaboration to improve outcomes and performance.

This performance improvement process translates into *quality of care*, one of the cornerstones of case management, and is essentially the degree of excellence concerning all aspects of patient care, including strict adherence to medical and nursing standards. Payors, such as insurance plans, also expect quality of care for their members. Quality of care is the measuring rod that determines the value of the commodity purchased (Williams & Torrens, 1993).

Traditional Quality Improvement— Risk Management Programs

Traditional *quality improvement* is a process that determines whether the care provided meets medical standards (Sederer, 1987). Quality improvement activities are designed to monitor, prevent, and correct quality deficiencies. In that sense, quality improvement is a proactive model. It is a continuous effort to raise the organization's quality level. This is accomplished through: *quality assessment*, which is the process by which quality of care is evaluated, and *quality assurance*, which includes the QA activities performed on an ongoing basis with the goal of *quality improvement* (Williams & Torrens, 1993).

Traditional *risk management* is the "art and science of how not to be successfully sued" (Sederer, 1987, p. 214). Ideally, the major emphasis is on identifying potential risk areas and on interventions that will enhance patient safety and prevent losses before they occur. In reality, in many organizations the risk management department is called in after the undesirable event has occurred. Its function then is to control and minimize losses through legal methods and public relations. Because of the latter situations, "risk management sometimes has been characterized as damage control: an attempt to remedy the effects of internal failures before they can become external embarrassments" (Kongstvedt, 1993, p. 166).

In this sense, risk management is a *reactive* model. But risk cannot always be prevented. Some adverse events do not become apparent until after the fact. Consider a case in which a patient received standard treatment for a disease and in which patient care was of high quality during the treatment phase: good quality management. Unfortunately, the disease was misdiagnosed: poor risk management potential. This case is not likely to get reported through routine quality improvement channels at the time of misdiagnosis.

Quality Improvement–Risk Management Language

Some terms frequently used during quality improvement and risk management activities are self-explanatory: mishap, patient safety problem, maloccurrence. Others require further definition.

Outcomes. Outcomes describe the results and consequences from the care received; outcomes also result from care that was *not* received. Outcome studies look for trends and potentially adverse events. Poor outcomes revealed through outcome studies often lead to policy and procedural changes in an effort to improve the problem.

Adverse Patient Outcome (APO). An APO is defined as any adverse patient occurrence which, under optimal conditions, is not a natural consequence of the patient's disease process, or the end result of a procedure (Northrop, 1987).

Potentially Compensable Event. A potentially compensable event is one in which the end result could be litigation (1987).

Incident. An incident is an accident or the discovery of a hazardous condition that is inconsistent with standards of care (1987).

Incident Report (Also Known as Occurrence Report). An incident report is a communication tool to record adverse events or unusual occurrences. Incident reports assess potential liabilities, are used for discovering existing problems, and assess the need for revising current policies or procedures. State law determines whether they are confidential or "discoverable," in court. It is not advisable to document in the medical record that an incident report has been filled out, although the events of the incident may be recorded in the patient's chart if they are important to future care and treatment. Be objective, factual, clear, and complete, since incident reports *may* be discoverable in court (Feutz-Harter, 1991).

Variances. Variances are deviations from expected care. Three types of variances are practitioner, system/institutional, and patient/family (see Lag Days and Variances in Chapter 6: Utilization Management for a more complete discussion).

Important Aspects of Care. These are aspects of care that occur frequently, affect large numbers of patients, or place patients at risk for serious consequences if not provided for optimally. These aspects of care are often the target of performance improvement activities.

How Quality Improvement & Risk Management Contrast & Compare

Like case management, the new direction in quality improvement emphasizes looking at the big picture and efficiently coordinating the whole system. But classic quality improvement, with its inherent limitations and flaws, is still necessary and required by regulatory agencies (Kongstvedt, 1993). Therefore, an understanding of how quality improvement and risk management differ, and how they work together, is important.

Quality improvement and risk management differ in the following ways:

- Their focus is different (Northrop, 1987). Risk management is concerned with acceptable care from a legal and financial perspective; risk management attempts to minimize the costs of liability insurance and liability of claims. Quality improvement emphasizes patient care issues rather than financial concerns.
- Risk management looks at all hospital exposures: environmental, patient safety, visitor safety, and so on. Quality improvement emphasizes patient-focused issues, which includes all services involved in patient care: optimal quality of

care, adherence to professional standards, reasonable and prudent delivery of care, and so on (1987).
- Risk management focuses on loss prevention activities. Quality improvement facilitates quality of care issues (1987).
- Overall, risk management wants to decrease the probability of adverse patient outcomes (1987). Quality improvement wants to increase the probability of quality patient outcomes.

The following are *areas of common concern in risk management and quality improvement:*

- Both are concerned with anything that may cause risk of injury to the patient. Both attempt to identify and avoid adverse patient outcomes (Northrop, 1987).
- Both stress monitoring of trends to identify risk patterns or problems in patient care (1987).
- Both require and emphasize the need for complete and clear documentation (1987).
- Both require cooperation and information from the medical staff, nursing staff, and hospital administration to assess trends and resolve problematic issues.
- Many of the "tools" used are effective for both quality improvement and risk management purposes (1987).
- Both attempt to correct identified problems by educational methods, changes in policies and procedures, or disciplinary action.

Importance of Nurse Case Management to QI–RM Activities

Nurse case managers are constantly overseeing all aspects of patient care: evaluating, monitoring, and reevaluating. For this reason, case managers are a critical team member in the QI–RM process. Consider these six high-risk areas for nurses: after reviews of occurrences and actual claims against nurses, these deficits have been deemed areas of practice that can become major sources of liability (Northrop, 1987). Many of these "failures" can be spotted through astute chart reviews and hopefully can prevent an adverse patient outcome.

1. Failure to take or properly assess a patient's history (1987)
2. Failure to perform a nursing procedure according to nursing standards (1987)
3. Failure to follow a doctor's order promptly; failure to follow a doctor's order correctly (1987)
4. Failure to report deviations from accepted practice (1987)
5. Failure to properly supervise the patient (1987). These cases can result in patient falls, intravenous line failures or infiltrates, patient extubation, all from inadequate monitoring.
6. Failure to summon the medical attending physician appropriately (1987)

Keeping these high-risk areas of concern in mind, consider how important an NCM's skills and responsibilities are from a QI–RM perspective. As a patient advocate who is involved in all areas of patient care, NCMs are always alert for hindrances to optimal outcomes.

In addition, a skilled and experienced NCM is adept at identifying problems in a timely manner, such as recognizing risk management issues, optimally before they have done maximum damage. Also, a skilled and experienced NCM can anticipate potential problems before they happen. NCMs identify traits in a patient that could make them vulnerable to high-risk incidents and adjust the case plan for maximum safety. Furthermore, NCMs function in a capacity in which they hear many patient and family complaints. One possible intervention is a wake-up call to the risk management department. Finally, NCMs may act as a liaison between the patient, the facility he or she is in, and the insurance company. In this capacity, NCMs assist in developing treatment and discharge plans. The NCM ascertains the best plan to meet the individual needs of the client—all within the constraints of the payor (insurance company). This often takes thought, creativity, and negotiation skills in today's resource-conscious atmosphere. At times, it is necessary to do some bargaining in order to meet the basic needs of the patient. Perhaps without the NCM's assessment of the need for these services—and the negotiation skills—this patient would be a future risk liability; many insurance companies realize this concept and are willing to cooperate by authorizing plans that have been negotiated by the NCM to enhance the patient's safety. The authorization may include more discharge supports than are normally covered or a "noncovered" service or piece of equipment.

Risk Management Recommendations and Prevention Skills

Consult a Risk Manager. When in doubt about *anything* that may preclude a risk management event, call a risk manager in your organization for clarification and evaluation.

Warn the Risk Management Department. A goal of risk management is *never* to be served with a lawsuit that the facility agency was previously not aware of! Through warnings by the NCM, the risk management department would have time to flag the chart, review the medical records, and possibly review court records.

Avoid Angry Clients. When a patient or family has complaints, **listen** and **be responsive**. This may not avert all lawsuits, but it is true that people get angrier if they feel no one is listening.

Notify Risk Manager of Potential Suits. If a patient or family member mentions a lawsuit or attorney, a call to the risk manager may be appropriate. Although unreasonable expectations may be the cause of the threat, it is still better to notify the RM department for their assessment.

Be Inclusive. Include the patient–family unit in the decision-making process about various aspects of care. Those inside the boat are less likely to rock it!

Carefully Consider Readmissions. Readmissions soon after a discharge from the hospital need careful consideration, especially if the previous admission had the possibility of suboptimal treatment or an inappropriate discharge, either a premature discharge or the result of poor discharge planning.

Pay Special Attention to High-Risk Neonates. Adverse outcomes in neonates need attention. All mothers reasonably expect a positive outcome—a healthy newborn; events that deviate from this expectation could benefit from a risk management evaluation.

Practice Quality Documentation. Documentation is a vital aspect of risk management. See following section for a detailed discussion.

Documentation

The theme surfaces often throughout this book. Its importance cannot be overstated and is especially critical in the courtroom when proving whether malpractice has occurred. The old adage, "if it's not documented, it did not occur" is important; what *is* documented versus what *is not* documented can determine the win–loss outcome of a case. Documentation in a medical record may be the only evidence available to indicate whether a standard of care was met. And since years usually have gone by between the care and the court date, important details may be lost without thorough documentation. The risk management department also depends on quality documentation for determining how to handle a particular case. What the old adage does not do for nurses is give specific guidelines that may be helpful if a case does go to litigation. Some further recommendations follow:

- Ask yourself whether you would mind if your charting was read aloud in a court of law. If the answer is "yes" on any case, assess why you feel the discomfort. For example, did judgment or frustration show up in your notes? Were your notes incomplete? Use the assessment for personal growth and improvement.
- Document communications between yourself and physicians. Include dates and times calls were initiated, response time, doctor's response to the reason for the call, and your intervention. Number 6 in the previous list of high-risk areas for nurses was a failure to summon medical attention. Perhaps, in some cases the physician was summoned, but, without documented proof, the nurse had to assume the responsibility for a poor outcome. Also note that if the physician paged does not answer within a reasonable amount of time and with a reasonable number of attempts, go through the chain of command until a doctor can be reached who will address the problem. Document all efforts.
- Falls are a major cause of litigation. They also fall under number 5 of high-risk areas for nurses: failure to properly supervise a patient. Document use of restraints, use of siderails, and visits to a patient's room for treatment and monitoring purposes. This is especially important for NCMs who also are direct care nurses.
- It is essential to follow some basic record-keeping rules. To begin, remember to date and time all entries. This is especially true in emergency situations. Furthermore, state all information clearly, factually, objectively, and completely. This should ensure that standards of care are met. Any measures used to prevent complications should be noted, since they may show good faith in the future. Avoid ambiguity. "Feels warm," "high blood pressure," "lower tempera-

ture" are too nonspecific. Chart the facts. Use words that are not susceptible to multiple meanings.

- In a court of law, the appearance of the chart is often equally as important as the content. Use JCAHO-approved abbreviations and recommendations. Using a white-out agent to delete for errors is not permissible in court and leaves room for suspicion of falsifying information. The chart for one case involving white-out had to be x-rayed to determine what was underneath (Northrop, 1984). Use a single line to cross out an error. Write "error" over the single line, and initial it. Sign all completed entries. Also, make sure all blanks and boxes are filled in or checked. Always, write legibly and with permanent black ink.
- Good follow-through should be evident from the chart. If a critical lab value or patient condition is noted, as stated above, keep track of who you reported it to and what the response was. Note all patient responses to any treatments or medications given (again, this is especially important for NCMs with direct patient care responsibilities). If a doctor's order is *not* carried out, explain reasons for the omission (1987).
- When documenting complications or mishaps, be factual, thorough, and objective. Do not assign blame or fault.
- Threats and complaints can be documented, but it is best to quote, if possible. Document follow-up actions to the threat or complaint.
- Patient or family concerns or worries can also be documented. Identify who is expressing concern; what was said (quote, if possible); your verbal responses; and any interventions that were done in response to the concern.
- Patient noncompliance needs to be documented, including what the patient is or is not doing. A diabetic eating candy bars or a patient allowed nothing by mouth (NPO) found munching on crackers is not an uncommon occurrence. But it can delay surgical procedures and extend length of stay. In many cases, noncompliance can harm a patient and interfere with optimal patient care.
- Document informed consent about medical procedures (more on this subject is discussed under Informed Consent in Chapter 7: Legal Issues for Case Managers).
- Document information about transferring patients to other facilities. Record on the chart who was spoken to and what was agreed on. This may include conversations or phone calls to the patient's family, the ECF, and the attending physician. Note who made the decision to transfer, when the transfer took place, and who approved the transfer. If there is a suboptimal outcome during or after a transfer, and there is no documentation that the family supported the transfer decision, repercussions can occur.

Reviewing the Chart

Many times a careful review of the medical record will reveal issues or situations that warrant a call to the quality improvement or risk management departments.

Any condition that may indicate poor or incomplete patient care, either inside a facility or outpatient, requires quality improvement or risk management notification. Outpatient management is an important consideration; many insurance plan NCMs use this information to trend patient treatment practiced by their primary care physicians, thereby ensuring quality care in all settings. Review the charts for the following clues to possible delayed diagnoses and suspicious admissions.

Delayed Diagnoses

Be aware that reasons other than missed early clues—such as patient noncompliance—can cause some of these delayed diagnoses:

- First admission for advanced disease processes including advanced metastatic cancer, perforated ulcer, advanced tuberculosis
- Diagnosis such as a perforated appendix when a chart review reveals an emergency room visit 3 days prior to admission for abdominal pain
- Severe diabetic ketoacidosis (note: watch for noncompliance or "brittle" diabetes)
- Shock (various types) or septicemia
- Possible poor monitoring for a patient's condition. Examples include pregnancy-induced hypertension (preeclampsia, eclampsia, and toxemia) and diabetic ketoacidosis.

Admissions Concerns

- Admissions for diseases in which immunizations are available. Did the pediatrician or primary care physician offer the immunizations? Did the parent refuse them or not take the child to the primary care physician for them?
- Admissions from complications following an outpatient or emergency room procedure. Examples include poorly set fractures, neurologic defects, wound infections.
- Admissions for side effects of outpatient drug therapy. Did the patient take more, or less, than was ordered? Did the physician or nurse improperly or incompletely educate the patient about the medication? Were the patient's blood levels adequately monitored for the medication? Examples include gastrointestinal bleeding, resulting from the patient taking aspirin while on coumadin, or hypokalemia while the patient is taking a potassium-depleting diuretic.
- Readmission for the same condition within 2 weeks. This can happen with any condition or diagnosis. The causes may range from patient noncompliance (a woman with congestive heart failure who goes home and eats pretzels) to poor outpatient monitoring or premature discharge.

Other Instances for Chart Review

Sometimes critical thinking and investigative work must precede the discovery of poor management or adverse events. For example:

- During a gastrectomy, the spleen is removed. Since this is not standard protocol for a gastrectomy, the curious NCM would investigate. No explanation is found in the progress notes. The pathology report states that the splenic artery had been injured, necessitating the removal of the spleen.
- Perhaps a hysterectomy patient returns postoperatively with bloody urine. A further review shows the ureter was inadvertently transected and repaired.
- A 6-week-old infant is admitted for seizures. A review of his birth chart reveals that labor was prolonged and difficult, and necessitated midforceps delivery.
- An infant with congenital heart disease develops severe bradycardia and arrhythmia and dies. An autopsy report shows his digoxin level was 10 times above the normal range.
- An infant with an Apgar score of 3 requires resuscitation. A review of the maternal predelivery record shows that the mother had been given excessive doses of narcotics.

Indicators

Quality improvement indicators are measurable, specific, and clear guides to monitor and evaluate important aspects of patient care. Indicators may be written for any area that enhances patient care, from ambulatory services and social services to nuclear medicine. Each medical service has its own specific indicators to monitor potential problems or opportunities to improve patient care. Ongoing monitoring should reveal trends. Several years ago, one study revealed a high trend in pneumothorax after central line insertions. Astute detective work disclosed a problem with a discrepancy between the insertion site and the use of an appropriate length of catheter. As nursing case management grows, NCM standards and NCM indicators may be a part of our future guidelines.

Following in the chapter appendix are several sample indicators from various services. A visit to the facility's quality improvement department is likely to reveal several books on screens and monitors. A review is recommended, especially in your specific service line; they often "red flag" situations that need a review and an alert to the quality improvement or risk management departments.

Also in the chapter appendix are sample clinical indicators of Generic Quality Screens (Display 9–1) put out by the Health Care Financing Administration (HCFA). A review of the HCFA Generic Screens demonstrates some circumstances that may signal inadequate quality of care. The chapter appendix also includes a compilation of 10 types of claims categories (Table 9–1) gleaned from the National Practitioner's Data Bank. These categories are used by risk management departments as a possible indication of suboptimal quality of care. A review of the indicators, the HCFA Generic Screens and the claims categories should arm the NCM with enough cues so that an "off" case will signal further investigation and monitoring and possibly a call to the risk management or quality management departments.

CASE STUDY

Twelve-year-old Jimmy was normal and healthy until 3 years ago. At that time, Jimmy developed a severe, unsubsiding headache. Magnetic resonance imaging (MRI) scanning performed 3 months later showed carotid and basilar aneurysms. Several months after that, Jimmy suffered a brain-stem stroke. A basilar aneurysm clipping was performed, but the basilar artery remained thrombosed postoperatively.

A long and stormy course followed surgery, with vocal cord paralysis and pneumonia manifesting as complicating factors. Jimmy worked tirelessly in an inpatient rehabilitation unit and was eventually able to return to school, where he was a well-liked "A" student.

Nearly 2 years later, Jimmy suddenly developed seizure activity. A residual right-sided weakness in this right-handed adolescent was disconcerting. A computed tomography (CT) scan again revealed the carotid aneurysm. A carotid repair and bypass were performed. According to records, Jimmy did well postoperatively and was discharged home.

The day after discharge, a fever and recurrent seizure occurred. An electroencephalogram (EEG) and MRI were both abnormal. Herpes viral titers proved to be high; Jimmy was treated with the appropriate medication, acyclovir, and restarted on dexamethasone for presumed herpes encephalitis. Urinary tract infections and gastrointestinal problems were also identified.

Inpatient rehabilitation was again provided, and soon Jimmy "graduated" to a day rehab unit. Because of constant gastrointestinal (GI) upsets and frequency of urination, the day hospital couldn't continue to provide care.

Multiple urinalysis cultures, with occasional exceptions, were negative. Jimmy responded well to an oral antibiotic prescribed for the presumed urinary tract infection.

Jimmy's GI symptoms persisted. GI workups were performed several times, with few conclusive returns. An esophagogastroduodenoscopy (EGD) showed mild gastroparesis. Jimmy showed a low iron on lab tests, but his mother stopped his iron at home because of GI complaints.

Jimmy is now readmitted 3 months after his last cranial surgery. The mother's stated concerns for her son are his persistent nausea, abdominal pain and vomiting, fevers to 102°F, urinary frequency every 3 minutes, constant seizures (low voltage), blackouts, head deviation, and facial twitching.

Another thorough workup is performed. Jimmy's dilantin level is low and IV dilantin is started. On hospital day 4, his potassium drops to 2.9 (normal levels, 3.5 to 5.5) requiring IV boluses. He is afebrile much of the time, with low-grade fevers to 101°F noted. Occasional small emesis (75 mL) is charted, although Jimmy is frequently complaining of nausea. Urinary frequency every 3 minutes has not been noted. His iron level remains low at 14 (normal level, 36 to 150).

Neurologic findings are nystagmus, perhaps a little more than Jimmy's chronic state, which is consistent with his old brain-stem stroke. Cognitively, Jimmy remains stable, according to neurologists. He does have a significant short-term memory loss.

Following are the hospital tests and their results for this admission:

- MRI—No acute changes; some atrophy that may be from the recent herpes infection.
- Twenty-four-hour Holter EEG—No acute changes; essentially negative for anything new
- Urinalysis—one of four was positive for leuk esterase
- UGI-SBFT (upper GI, small bowel follow-through)—negative
- Barium enema—negative
- CT of abdomen and pelvis—normal
- Lumbar puncture—negative, no growth of cultures

There are many unresolved issues between Jimmy's mother and the physicians. According to the physicians, these range from unreasonable demands by the mother to nonpayment of medical bills. Doctors claim that insurance reimbursement checks sent to the mother were never paid to physicians. The nursing staff states that they are under attack from Jimmy's mother for not charting mental status changes that she deems are occurring (and for not noticing them) and for not knowing all details about Jimmy when she asks.

Jimmy's mother is angry because she feels that no one is in charge. Her request for one doctor to give her overviews has been granted; however, she is displeased with him. The same day she requested two more specialists: a hematologist and an endocrinologist The request is carried out, although it is explained to the mother that this type of consultation can be provided on an outpatient basis, since the patient is stable.

The mother now demands a multidisciplinary team meeting immediately, and the social worker sets it up quickly—with only 2 hours' lead time. The mother has announced that she will be tape recording the session and clearly states, "This is not just a threat but a promise that everyone involved in this case will be going to court."

During the 1½-hour meeting that follows, "Mom" demands a diagnosis for all of Jimmy's problems before discharge or she will refuse to pick up her son and take him home. She also wants to know why her son was like his "old self" after a lumbar puncture.

CASE STUDY QUESTIONS

1. Who should attend the meeting called by Jimmy's mother?
2. What happens if an important person cannot attend on such short notice?
3. What is the legality of the mother taping the session?
4. What can be/should be done if the mother refuses to pick up her son when he is discharged?
5. Discuss the quality improvement issues involved in this case.
6. Discuss the risk management issues involved in this case.
7. Discuss the utilization management issues of this case.

References

Fanucci, D., Hammil, M., Johannson, P., Leggett, J., & Smith, M. J. (1993). Quantum leap into continuous quality improvement. *Nursing Management, 24* (6), 28–30.

Feutz-Harter, S. A. (1991). *Nursing and the law.* Wisconsin: Professional Education Systems.
Kongstvedt, P. R. (1993). *The managed health care handbook.* Gaithersburg: Aspen Publishers.
Northrop, C. E., & Kelly, M. E. (1987). *Legal issues in nursing.* St. Louis: C. V. Mosby.
Sederer, L. I. (1987). Utilization review and quality assurance: Staying in the black and working with the blues. *Gen Hosp Psychiatry, 9,* 210–19.
Williams, S. J., & Torrens, P. R. (1993). *Introduction to health services.* New York: Delmar.

Appendix: Clinical Indicators

Note: Some of these indicators are "undeveloped" and lacking specific criteria. Your institution's indicators will probably contain objective criteria to match the needs of the organization.

Cardiology and Cardiovascular Indicators

- Readmission within 30 days of discharge
- Congestive heart failure—not present on admission
- Pericarditis—not present on admission
- Pulmonary embolus—not present on admission
- Cardiac/respiratory arrest following cardiovascular procedure
- Complication of thrombolytic therapy
    Gingival bleeding
    Hematemesis
    Hematomas at puncture sites
- Unplanned transfer to special care unit
- Neurodeficit not present on admission
- Injury to organ/structure during cardiovascular procedure
- Return to operating room for postoperative thoracic bleeding
- Return for percutaneous transurethral coronary angioplasty (PTCA) of some lesion within 72 hours
- Post-PTCA complications such as hematoma at insertion site requiring evacuation
- Patients undergoing nonemergent PTCA with subsequent occurrence of either an acute myocardial infarction (MI) or coronary artery bypass graft (CABG) surgery needed within the same hospitalization
- Patient undergoing attempted or completed PTCA during which any lesion attempted is not dilated

Pediatric Cardiovascular Indicators

- Return to surgery for exploration of bleeding or other complication
- Complication of device or graft such as occlusion or malfunction

- Infection of device or graft
- Sepsis with positive blood cultures
- Postoperative neurologic deficits
- Wound infection or dehiscence
- Pulmonary emboli not present on admission
- Cardiac or respiratory arrest

- New-onset renal failure requiring dialysis
- Readmission for complication of surgical procedure within 30 days of discharge
- All deaths related to surgical procedure

Pediatric Indicators

- Apgar scores of less than 6 at 1 minute and less than 8 at 5 minutes
- Newborn injuries
- Transfer to neonatal intensive care unit after 24 hours of age
- Readmission to hospital within 72 hours of discharge
- Physically or sexually abused children

- Fever of unknown origin
- Errors in diagnosis and management
- Inpatient mortality including perioperative mortality
- Unscheduled admissions following ambulatory procedure
- Unscheduled return to ICU within 48 hours of transfer out

Neurology and Neurosurgical Indicators

- Unplanned readmission within 15 days of discharge
- Unplanned transfer to a special care unit
- Injury to an organ or structure during a procedure or treatment
- Pulmonary emboli or DVT (deep vein thrombosis) not present on admission
- Greater than five consultations
- Complication of anticoagulation therapy
- Complication of neurodiagnostics procedure
- Neurologic deficits not present on admission
- Organ failure not present on admission
- Cardiac or respiratory arrest

- Discharges against medical advice (AMA) or patient–family dissatisfaction
- Deaths
- Unplanned return to operating room
- Unplanned removal, injury, or repair to an organ or structure during an operative procedure
- Acute MI during or within 48 hours of an operative procedure
- Wound infection or dehiscence
- Pulmonary edema not present on admission
- Unplanned transfusion of greater than 2 units
- Acute hemorrhage or wound hematoma postoperatively

Internal Medicine Indicators

- Complications from invasive, diagnostic, or monitoring procedures
- Management errors including errors of omission or commission
- Death
- Delays or inadequacies in diagnosis increasing length of stay
- Adverse reactions to medications
- Unplanned admission to special care unit
- Pneumothorax following central line insertion
- Unplanned readmission
- Unplanned transfer to special care unit
- Cardiac–respiratory arrest
- Patient–family dissatisfaction or AMA discharge
- Pulmonary emboli or DVT not present on admission
- Complications of anticoagulation therapy
- Organ failure not present on admission

Utilization Indicators

- Admission not meeting acute criteria
- Readmission within 30 days for incomplete management of problems of previous hospitalization
- Peer review organization issue needs attention
- Readmission within 15 days for same diagnosis
- Receipt of Medicare denial
- Delays in diagnosis increasing length of stay

Anesthesia Indicators

- Malintubation or reintubation
- Morbidity or mortality for complications such as hose disconnection, incorrect gas flow, or too much or too little medication
- Patient's developing postural headache within 4 postprocedure days following use of spinal or epidural anesthesia administration
- Dental injury following procedure involving anesthesia care
- Ocular injury during procedures involving anesthesia care
- Unplanned admission within 2 postprocedure days following outpatient procedures involving anesthesia
- Vocal cord paralysis after intubation that was not present preintubation

Social Work Indicators

- Recognition of psychosocial needs
- Timeliness of interventions
- Quality of counseling/interventions
- Interdisciplinary collaboration
- Appropriateness of discharge or referrals

Ambulatory Indicators

- Unscheduled returns to the emergency room within 72 hours
- Cancellation of ambulatory procedure on day of procedure
- Unplanned admission to acute care related to surgery or complication

- Patient not accompanied home by a designated person
- Morbidity: vascular, neurologic, pulmonary, cardiac, drug reactions, or infections
- Local anesthesia supplemented with general anesthesia

Emergency Services Indicators

- Registered patients in emergency room more than 6 hours or delayed evaluations or treatment
- Registered patients who leave emergency room prior to completion of treatment or AMA emergency room discharges
- Transfers to another acute care facility

- Return visit for similar or same complaint
- Misadministration or adverse drug reaction
- Mortality after arrival and within 48 hours of admission
- Consultant responds within reasonable time
- Complications related to caseload

Dietary Services Indicators

- Appropriateness of diet order versus diagnosis
- Adequacy of dietary counseling/teaching
- Adequacy of parenteral nutrition

- Duration of NPO without nutritional support
- Adequacy of nutritional values of diets
- Diet orders—errors or ambiguous or improper dietary order

Pathology Indicators

- Monitoring of unnecessary tests
- Evaluation of appropriate sequencing and frequency of tests

- Evaluation of inadequate or improper specimens

Nuclear Medicine Indicators

- Turnaround time for studies acceptable to medical staff
- Comparison between nuclear medicine and pathologic diagnosis for inconsistencies

- Appropriateness of study requested to the diagnosis
- Misadministration of, or adverse reaction to, radionuclide agents

Radiology Indicators

- Turnaround time is acceptable to medical staff
- Number of "repeat" films
- Compare radiologic and pathologic diagnosis for any inconsistency
- Consistent reading by radiologist and nonradiologist (attending physician or others)

- Appropriateness of radiologic study to symptom

   CT scan when headache is isolated symptom

   Upper GI series in asymptomatic duodenal ulcer patient

   Routine chest x-rays

Obstetric Clinical Indicators

- Any maternal death
- Fetal mortality in pregnancy over 20 weeks (stillborns)
- Hemorrhage related to delivery requiring transfusion
- Any Apgar score of less than 6 at 1 minute and less than 8 at 5 minutes
- Third or fourth degree birth canal laceration
- Malposition accidents and/or extractions
- Anesthesia-related problems

- Intrahospital neonatal deaths of infants with birth weight of 750 g to 1000 g that were born in a hospital with an NICU
- Readmissions of the mother within 2 weeks of delivery
- Infants delivered in a hospital without an NICU weighing less than 1800 g
- Unattended delivery
- Unplanned return to obstetric or surgery unit
- Newborn injuries

Intensive Care Unit Indicators

- Mortality
- Medication errors
- Appropriate admission and discharge criteria
- Patient returned to ICU

- ICU psychosis
- Physician response time to calls
- Response time to code blue alerts
- Complications of immobility

Respiratory Care Indicators

- Hypoxemia is documented for oxygen therapy (exception: MI)
- Arterial blood gases (ABGs) criteria

   Patient's clinical condition changes (exception: continuous ventilation therapy)

   For home oxygen authorization (room air ABGs)

- No PRN oxygen
- Mechanical ventilation is based on established criteria

Rehabilitation Indicators

- Timeliness of referral into rehab unit
- Appropriateness and adequacy of treatment plan and goals
- Quality of treatment techniques
- Number and types of readmissions
- Adequacy of interdisciplinary collaboration
- Patient's understanding of instructions
- Availability of inpatient and outpatient services
- Therapy sessions missed versus reasons

Pharmaceutical Indicators

- Time response to medications orders
- Accuracy of medication, dosage; dispensing errors
- Appropriateness of medication ordered
- Identification of interaction, compatibilities
- Preparation of all mixtures
- Food or drug interactions or compatibilities

Death Indicators—Criteria Guidelines

- Unexpected death criteria

  1. Death within 24 hours of hospitalization, which does not meet the expected death criteria (three out of first four).*
  2. Death within 24 hours of a DNR order, which does not meet three out of first four expected death criteria.*
  3. Death that occurs after a steady downhill course with multiple interventions, which does not meet three out of first four expected death criteria.*

- *Expected death criteria—Must have three out of the first four criteria (any combination)

  1. Clearly documented prognosis that death is expected
  2. Patient/family/next of kin are aware of and in agreement with medical plan
  3. Interventions—comfort care only
  4. DNR status—documented in orders and progress notes

*Not otherwise classified.

DISPLAY 9–1
HCFA Generic Quality Screens: Some Circumstances That May Signal Inadequate Quality of Care

Adequacy of Discharge Planning
- No documented plan for appropriate follow-up care or discharge planning as necessary, with consideration of physical, emotional, and mental status needs at the time of discharge.

Medical Stability of the Patient at Discharge
- Blood pressure on day before or day of discharge: systolic, <85 mmHg or >180 mmHg; diastolic, <50 mmHg or >110 mmHg
- Oral temperature on day before or day of discharge >101°F or rectal, >102°F (38.3°C oral/38.9°C rectal).
- Pulse <50 beat/min (or <45 beat/min if patient is on a beta blocker) or >120 beat/min within 24 hours of discharge
- Abnormal results of diagnostic services not addressed or explained in the medical record
- Intravenous fluids or drugs on the day of discharge (excludes the ones that keep veins open [KVOs], antibiotics, chemotherapy, or total parenteral nutrition)
- Purulent or bloody drainage of postoperative wound within 24 hours before discharge

Deaths
- During or after elective surgery
- After return to intensive care unit, coronary care, or special care unit within 24 hours of being transferred out
- Other unexpected death

Nosocomial infections
- Temperature increase of more than 2°F more than 72 hours from admission
- Indication of infection after an invasive procedure (eg, suctioning, catheter insertion, tube feedings, surgery)

Unscheduled return to surgery within same admission for same condition as previous surgery or to correct operative problem (excludes staged procedures)
Trauma suffered in the hospital
- Unplanned removal or repair of a normal organ (ie, removal or repair not addressed in operative consent)
- Fall with injury or untoward effect (including but not limited to fracture, dislocation, concussion, laceration)
- Life-threatening complications of anesthesia
- Life-threatening transfusion error or reaction
- Hospital-acquired decubitus ulcer
- Care resulting in serious or life-threatening complications not related to admitting signs and symptoms, including but not limited to neurologic, endocrine, cardiovascular, renal, or respiratory body systems (eg, resulting in dialysis, unplanned transfer to special care unit, lengthened hospital stay)
- Major adverse drug reaction or medication error with serious potential for harm or resulting in special measures to correct (eg, intubation, cardiopulmonary resuscitation, gastric lavage), including but not limited to the following:
  1. Incorrect antibiotic ordered by physician (eg, inconsistent with diagnostic studies or patient's history of drug allergy)
  2. No diagnostic studies to confirm which drug is correct to administer (eg, culture and sensitivity)
  3. Serum drug levels not measured as needed
  4. Diagnostic studies or other measures for side effects not performed as needed (eg, blood urea nitrogen, creatinine, intake and output)

Source: Healthcare Financing Administration, 1986.

Table 9-1. Claims Categories Used by Risk Management Departments

Diagnosis-related

- Failure to diagnose (ie, concluding that patient has no disease or condition worthy of further follow-up or observation)
- Wrong diagnosis (misdiagnosis, ie, original diagnosis is incorrect)
- Improper performance of test
- Unnecessary diagnostic test
- Delay in diagnosis
- Failure to obtain consent or lack of informed consent
- Diagnosis-related (NOC)*

Anesthesia-related

- Failure to complete patient assessment
- Failure to monitor
- Failure to test equipment
- Improper choice of anesthesia agent or equipment
- Improper technique or induction
- Improper equipment use
- Improper intubation
- Improper positioning
- Failure to obtain consent or lack of informed consent
- Anesthesia-related (NOC)*

Surgery-related

- Failure to perform surgery
- Improper positioning
- Retained foreign body
- Wrong body part
- Improper performance of surgery
- Unnecessary surgery
- Delay in surgery
- Improper management of surgical patient
- Failure to obtain consent for surgery or lack of informed consent
- Surgery-related (NOC)*

Medication-related

- Failure to order appropriate medication
- Wrong medication ordered
- Wrong dosage ordered of correct medication
- Failure to instruct on medication
- Improper management of medication regimen
- Failure to obtain consent for medication or lack of informed consent
- Medication error (NOC)*
- Failure to medicate
- Wrong dosage administered
- Wrong patient
- Wrong route
- Improper technique
- Medication administration related (NOC)*

Intravenous- and blood products-related

- Failure to monitor
- Wrong solution
- Improper performance
- IV-related (NOC)*
- Failure to ensure contamination-free
- Wrong type
- Improper administration
- Failure to obtain consent or lack of informed consent
- Blood product related (NOC)*

(Continued)

Table 9-1. Continued

Obstetrics-related

- Failure to manage pregnancy
- Improper choice of delivery method
- Improperly performed vaginal delivery
- Improperly performed cesarean section
- Delay in delivery (induction or surgery)
- Failure to obtain consent or lack of informed consent
- Improperly managed labor (NOC)*
- Failure to identify or meet fetal distress

- Delay in treatment of fetal distress (ie, identified but treated in untimely manner)
- Retained foreign body—vaginal or uterine
- Abandonment
- Wrongful life or birth
- Obstetrics-related (NOC)*

Treatment-related

- Failure to treat
- Wrong treatment or procedure performed (also improper choice)
- Failure to instruct patient on self-care
- Improper performance of a treatment or procedure
- Improper management of course of treatment
- Unnecessary treatment

- Delay in treatment
- Premature end of treatment (also abandonment)
- Failure to supervise treatment or procedure
- Failure to obtain consent for treatment or lack of informed consent
- Failure to refer or seek consultation
- Treatment-related (NOC)*

Monitoring

- Failure to monitor
- Failure to respond to patient

- Failure to report on patient condition
- Monitoring related (NOC)*

Biomedical equipment/product-related

- Failure to inspect/monitor
- Improper maintenance
- Improper use
- Failure to respond to warning
- Failure to instruct patient on use of equipment/product

- Malfunction or failure
- Biomedical equipment or product-related (NOC)*

Miscellaneous

- Inappropriate behavior of clinician (ie, sexual misconduct allegation, assault)
- Failure to protect third parties (ie, failure to warn or protect from violent patient behavior)
- Breach of confidentiality or privacy
- Failure to maintain appropriate infection control

- Failure to follow institutional policy or procedure
- Other (provide detailed written description)
- Failure to review provider performance

*Not otherwise classified.

CHAPTER 10

Discharge Planning: Understanding the Levels of Care and Transfers

IMPORTANT TERMS AND CONCEPTS

air ambulance
ALS ambulance
BLS ambulance
custodial care
extended care facility (ECF)
grievance process
home healthcare services
hospice

intermediate care
long-term care (LTC)
nonskilled nursing services
notice of noncoverage
rehabilitation services
skilled nursing
subacute care
transitional hospitals

Safe transfers to alternative levels of care are a major nursing case management responsibility. The Joint Commission for the Accreditation of Health Care Organizations (JCAHO) requires hospital policies and procedures on discharge planning (InterQual & Tennant, 1993). As utilization management criteria tighten in this decade, patients are being moved to lower levels of care with more physiologic needs than ever before. The sooner the nurse case manager (NCM) can start the assessment process on a case, the more time can be spent matching appropriate services to the client's needs.

When considering discharge planning, all levels of care options should be explored. Discharging home with family support is preferable in most cases. If family is unavailable, friends, neighbors, religious affiliation volunteers or community referrals can sometimes provide the needed link between the client's independence and his or her having to go to a supervisory or foster care setting. Social services can be an invaluable asset in case planning with this type of client.

If more skilled care is required than can be provided by family or volunteers, perhaps the client is safe to go home with the addition of home nursing services. Consider the use of home RN visits for care, teaching, or assessments, home physical therapy, occupational therapy and speech therapy, home aides (restrictions apply), home psychiatric nursing, or home social services. Most insurance plans

Powell: Nursing Case Management. © 1996 Lippincott–Raven Publishers

provide home health services only if the patient is homebound; this is an important point to assess. Also, determine just what the client's insurance plan provides; many plans allow only a few intermittent visits, which do not always meet the client's total needs.

If a patient is not homebound or can easily be transported by family or volunteers, consider the use of outpatient services such as outpatient rehabilitation departments, which provide physical, speech, and occupational therapies. Freestanding clinics may provide a wide range of services from wound care to the administration of intravenous antibiotics or chemotherapy.

Outpatient pharmaceutical benefits need to be assessed when sending patients home at discharge. Recent studies have revealed that one of the primary causes for readmission to the acute care hospital setting is improper medication administration. Educational deficits may contribute to this problem; assessing knowledge deficits relating to medications is an important NCM responsibility. Another underlying contributor to the problem may be financial; not all insurance plans have adequate prescription coverage and some people cannot afford the prescriptions. For example, patients with traditional Medicare have few pharmaceutical benefits, and even most Medicare supplements do not supply them; some detective work may be needed in order to see whether the supplement plan covers medications.

Until recently no home intravenous antibiotics were supplied by Medicare (see Chapter 5: Insurance under Medicare for 1993 medication exceptions that are supplied on a home basis). Sending a Medicare patient home with intravenous antibiotics was nearly impossible unless the patient could personally finance the drug. This is changing. Again, detective work is needed. If the Medicare plan is one of the new "risk" contracts that pays for hospitalizations on a per-diem or capitated basis (instead of diagnostic-related groups [DRG]), it is financially beneficial to the plan to send the patient home with intravenous medications; therefore, the insurance company often works with the NCM on this discharge plan. Note that under the traditional Medicare DRG reimbursement, only the hospital is financially penalized for keeping a patient in-house for a long time for antibiotic administration, which is why the traditional Medicare plans have little incentive to change this benefit.

If the insurance company does not pay for home intravenous antibiotics and the patient is otherwise stable for discharge, assess whether the patient can receive the antibiotics at a free-standing clinic or at the doctor's office. It may be necessary to set up an observation admission or an outpatient admission on weekends for the dosage. Sometimes emergency rooms can be used, although this should be a last resort and done with the facility's approval. Traditional Medicare *will* pay for the nurse to administer the medication, so if the patient can afford the drug, this plan sometimes works.

Medicaid plans generally pay for most prescriptive needs. They often have a "negative formulary" disallowing certain prescriptions. Some newer, expensive medications may need prior approval. No over-the-counter medications are covered (applies to most insurance plans).

Managed care pharmacy benefits may vary from the member paying 100% to the insurance company paying 100% (rare). Some members must purchase prescription riders on their policies to receive the benefit. Usually, the benefits require a copayment of $3 to $20 per prescription, an annual deductible, or a 20% coinsurance fee. The client may also be reimbursed only at a generic rate if a generic equivalent is available (Kongstvedt, 1993).

Many insurance plans with pharmaceutical benefits require the member to fill the prescription at designated contracted pharmacies. The NCM may need to find out where these pharmacies are if the client doesn't know.

Discharging clients home is often the best plan of care for the patient and is also the least resource-intensive plan for the insurance company. But this is not always safe or possible. Discussions about the alternatives—nursing home, rehabilitation, long-term care, hospice—along with more details on home coverage follow. In all discharge plans, insurance verification of coverage is essential. Occasionally nonbenefit options can be negotiated, but in all cases prior authorization should be obtained.

Early discharge planning, even in the preadmission phase, has been emphasized several times. But even with a good plan and prior authorization, the discharge plan may fall through. The patient's medical stability may change, family members may change their minds 30 minutes before transfer time, various other surprises may pop up! Sometimes the NCM has already had a nagging feeling that something was going to delay the discharge and therefore had an alternative plan in mind. NCM intuition is a useful skill, and it prepares us for sudden stops and detours.

If a mentally competent patient decides to go home refusing all available services, documentation may be all that is needed. If there is a question of mental incompetency and the patient would be unsafe with his or her chosen discharge plan, a psychiatric consultant may be necessary to assess the patient's mental capacity.

Sometimes patients who are deemed medically stable refuse to be discharged. Federal law mandates that all Medicare-certified facilities provide patients with a written statement about their rights to discharge planning and their right to pursue a *grievance process* if they feel that they are being discharged too soon or without adequate posthospital arrangements. These papers are usually on the front section of the hospital chart. Essentially, the grievance process starts when the attending physician and utilization review department feel the patient no longer meets medical criteria for the acute hospital level of care. If the patient or family disagrees with the "Denial for Continued Stay," also called "Notice of Non-Coverage," they can appeal it with a prompt phone call to the Peer Review Organization (PRO) by noon of the first day. A written notice may also be recommended. This call or written notice starts the grievance process. Without the phone call or written notice to the PRO the patient or family may be liable for hospital charges, starting on the third day after receiving the Notice of Non-Coverage.

From the NCM perspective, careful documentation of the patient's medical status and adequate discharge planning are needed. This documentation should show good faith and evidence that the patient is medically stable and that the discharge is based solely on medical status and not related to a DRG payment.

Grievance proceedings initiated by patients or families are not common. But often, after the grievance procedure is initiated, the patient/family is satisfied with the discharge plan during the 3-day grievance process and the discharge goes as originally planned! Occasionally the patient's medical status does deteriorate, and the denial notice is rescinded or a revised discharge plan is needed.

If the PRO agrees with the original notice of noncoverage, the patient may be billed for all charges beginning on the day after he or she received the PRO's final decision. If the patient/family continues to disagree with the discharge provisions, a request for reconsideration can be made.

This chapter discusses several issues pertaining to discharges and safe transferring of patients. Note that within federal guidelines each insurance plan has its own interpretation of these guidelines. Some coverage is disappointing, whereas other coverage may be surprisingly generous. The NCM can often get optimal coverage by reflecting clinical needs and backing up the request for services with good critical reasoning. Interpretations about what constitutes skilled, subacute, intermediate, or custodial levels of care also vary in extended care facilities (ECFs); a definition of skilled care in one may constitute the subacute level in another facility. Hospice benefits are interpreted differently among hospice companies. What follows is a solid foundation about levels of care and coverage; learn the individual idiosyncrasies of the plans and facilities for insurance "assurance."

Evaluating the Client's Level of Care Requirements

The following definitions and criteria demonstrate various degrees of care that a client may require. Appropriate assessment of a client's needs is essential and may provide clues to the NCM as to whether or not insurance will pay for the planned level of care. These definitions and criteria may vary from facility to facility, so clarification may be needed. Note that some of these patient care levels do not require an ECF and can be safely carried out in a more home-like environment. Figure 10–1 helps to summarize the levels of care from the most to the least complex care needs among the acute and subacute phases.

Long-Term Care (LTC)

The expression LTC used to be synonymous with nursing home placement. This is no longer always the case; chronically impaired people who are dependent on others to care for them can be found in homes, foster homes, day care centers, and a variety of other institutional and noninstitutional settings.

There is no single regulatory definition of LTC, but most emphasize the dependence and chronicity of the client (Williams & Torrens, 1993). In general, LTC is targeted at persons with functional disabilities that may present as a physical or mental problem. The goal of LTC is to promote or maintain as much independence and quality of life as possible. If the client is terminally ill, the goal is to

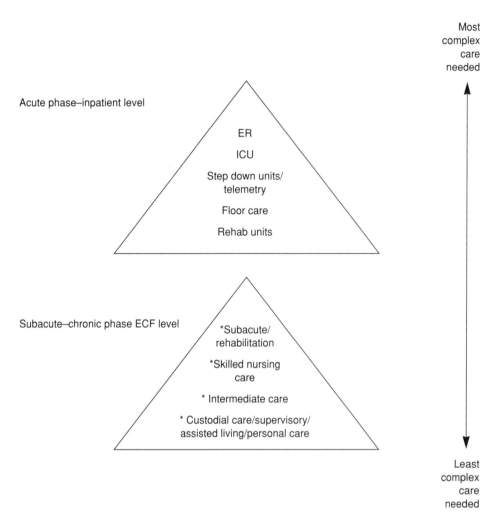

Figure 10-1. Levels of care.

* ECF terms and definitions for levels of care may vary among different facilities.

maintain comfort and dignity. A broad spectrum of services is provided, depending on the unique needs of the individual and family.

Limited LTC coverage is available, although the number of individual LTC policies grew from 815,000 in 1987 to almost 2 million in 1990. It is rarely financed with company insurance policies, and the consumer must usually pay for the entire, somewhat expensive premium (Kongtvedt, 1993). State coffers provide LTC to persons who can pass the strict medical and financial requirements.

Candidates qualifying under the definition of LTC fall into one of two groups: (1) those requiring complex care and extensive convalescence such as a major trauma victim and (2) those with chronic and multiple medical, mental health, and social problems, who are unable to care for themselves (Williams & Torrens,

1993). Some clients with diagnoses such as severe mental retardation, cerebral palsy, or spastic quadriplegia fall into the chronic category. They live in group homes where all of their needs are taken care of. If these clients need hospitalization, insurance authorization is not usually required to return them to that facility. In many cases, LTC clients have fairly stable discharge dispositions.

There is no inherent limit to the number of medical or custodial resources that a LTC client can consume. Consider the changing demographics of the United States: chronically ill patients are living longer; the number of elderly people and younger people with chronic diseases such as AIDS or ESRD (end-stage renal disease) is increasing, and they are making a significant impact on the LTC budget.

Many clients have acute medical insurance and short-term extended care benefits. But the NCM needs to see beyond these benefits and assess the need for LTC. Even if the patient meets the strict state requirements, the process to qualify for state LTC coverage can take up to 90 days; again early assessment and planning can avoid future problems.

Custodial Care

Custodial care may also be referred to as personal care, supervisory care or assisted living. Group homes and foster homes may also be included at this level of care. The Health Care Finance Administration (HCFA) definition of custodial care is care that is primarily for the purpose of helping clients with their personal care needs such as activities of daily living (ADLs); this care could safely and reasonably be supplied by persons without professional skills or training.

Custodial care requires the least skilled personnel of all the levels of extended care. I have never had an insurance company pay for a client who needed only custodial care (LTC clients may be an exception). The rule of thumb for Medicare and most insurance companies is as follows (HCFA, 1994):

- If custodial care is the only kind of care needed, Medicare will not pay.
- If skilled care is required, custodial care can be included in the services.

This level of care is generally characterized by clients who can:

- Ambulate independently with or without assistive devices such as walkers, wheelchairs, or canes
- Transfer from the bed to a chair or toilet with standby assistance
- Accomplish ADLs such as eating, dressing, grooming. or bathing with only minimal assistance. Food preparation may be needed.
- Be considered continent of bowel and bladder although may require minimal assist in caring for indwelling urinary catheters or colostomy appliances
- Take their own medications with general staff monitoring; no sliding scale or adjusted dosages
- Socially interact. These patients may have intermittent episodes of confusion, impaired judgment or agitation but do not require restraints to control behavior.

Note: Sometimes home health nursing and an assisted living arrangement can be provided if, for example, an otherwise custodial care client needs help only with sliding scale insulin or physical therapy. Call the home's main caretaker or owner. Many of these clients are considered family in their group homes, and they will work with the NCM in discharge planning.

Intermediate Care

The client needing intermediate care requires a moderate assistance with ADLs and often restorative nursing supervision for some activities. These persons are not as independent as those classified under custodial care, and in some facilities the distinction between the two levels of care is blurred. Insurance companies usually do not pay for this level of care unless skilled care is also required. The intermediate level of care is generally characterized by a client who:

- Needs no more than one staff person for transferring from a bed to a chair or toilet
- Needs assistance with ambulation but can self-propel a wheelchair
- Requires a moderate amount of assistance in bathing, grooming, eating, and dressing
- May need restraints
- Has routine medications and treatments that can be provided for with general staff monitoring
- May be intermittently incontinent of bowel or bladder and may need help with an indwelling Foley catheter or colostomy
- Is socially acceptable but may have periods of confusion, agitation, or emotional outbursts that can be controlled with moderate staff intervention

Skilled Nursing—Subacute Care

In some ECFs, the delineation between skilled nursing care and subacute care is one of progressing complexity of the client's medical and functional needs. This level of care is considered the most intensive in the ECF system. The clients may require a maximum assistance with ADLs, may be totally incontinent of bowel and bladder, and may be disoriented, confused, combative, or even obtunded. Yet these characteristics alone will not qualify a client for insurance coverage. For an insurance company to pay for care at an ECF level, a need from a skilled licensed professional provided on a daily basis *and* the assessment that this care must take place at the ECF level for reasons of patient safety and economy are also required. The skilled services below represent some services covered under many insurance plans. A patient with injections, more frequent or complex dressing changes, or more invasive tubes to care for may be considered subacute, rather than skilled.

Note: Even if a client is medically stable, if the care is too complex, ECFs may not be able to provide the level of care needed owing to staffing restraints. Consider a transitional hospital in these complex cases.

Skilled nursing services may include (but are not limited to):

- Daily injections: intravenous fluid, intravenous medications, intramuscular injections, subcutaneous injections (such as sliding scale insulin)
- Daily wound care requiring aseptic technique
- Tube feedings or tube care: nasogastric tube, duotube, gastrostomy tube, jejunostomy tube, tracheostomy care (initial teaching and care)
- Frequent observation and assessment by licensed personnel in order to prevent deterioration of the patient's condition or complications; this change would require prompt nursing response.
- Treatment of decubitus ulcers (severity of grade 3 or worse) or severe skin conditions
- Initial phases of a regimen involving administration of medical gases such as bronchodilator therapy
- Early postoperative care and teaching for colostomies, ileostomies, Hickman catheters, and other tubes
- Physical therapy and possibly adjunctive speech or occupational therapies
- Newly diagnosed diabetic teaching of diet, sliding scale insulin injections, and foot care (for further comparisons, see Table 10–1)

Levels of Care

The following represent various levels of care that a client may qualify for, based on his or her assessment level of medical or custodial need. These levels may vary from total care of a client to home-based services, which may only entail an intravenous medication administration. These levels of care are often very costly, so that insurance verification should be obtained.

Extended Care Facilities (ECFs)

Extended care facilities offer a *level of care below acute hospitalization*, in which the client still requires ongoing skilled care from licensed personnel on a daily basis. The following types of ECFs all subscribe to this definition:

Nursing home—NH
Nursing home placement—NHP
Intermediate care facility—ICF
Extended care facility—ECF
Skilled nursing facility—SNF

The use of acronyms is fine for medical personnel, but it is best to use the entire term when talking to patients or their families. I usually use the term "extended care facility" and explain that this is an extension of the hospital care they are now receiving, but at a less intense pace. I don't like using the term "nursing home" or "convalescent center." These terms often bring up unfavorable images or frightening memories of neglect or of loved ones dying.

Table 10-1. Subacute Levels of Care

Levels of Care	Subacute & Rehabilitation	Skilled Nursing	Intermediate Care	Assisted Living/ Custodial Care
Medical stability	Can be complex and unstable; requires ongoing monitoring by RNs; complex care for multimedical problems may be provided	Can be complex and generally stable; requires skilled nursing observation and modification of care plan to prevent further deterioration	Client medically stable; intermittent nursing and medical services needed to maintain medical stability	Client medically stable
Injections	Complex IV therapy regimen; multiple IV meds requiring infusion pumps	IV push therapy; simple IV therapy; central line care	IM and SC injections	No IV, IM, SC injections; may retain home health nurses to provide these services
Medication regimen	Complex medication regimen due to unstable conditions; at least five medication changes per week by the attending physician may be required to meet this level of care	Medication regimen requiring some adjustments in dosages or frequency of medication; done through observation and assessment of vital signs or laboratory data	Administration of routine medication; RN or LPN monitoring may be necessary with occasional dose or frequency changes when ordered by attending physician	Stable regimen of oral medications; home health nurses may be hired to monitor more complex medications such as sliding scale insulin
Respiratory treatments	Some facilities care for patients on respirators, including frequent suction and SVN PRN treatments	May have oxygen, SVN treatments, inhaler therapies	Routine oxygen administration and a stable respiratory therapy regimen	May have home oxygen, simple inhalers
Suctioning	Frequent (more than every four hours) tracheal suctioning allowed; new tracheostomy care	Nonsterile suctioning or intermittent sterile suctioning	Simple, routine nonsterile suctioning	No suctioning

(Continued)

Table 10-1. Subacute Levels of Care (Continued)

Levels of Care	Subacute & Rehabilitation	Skilled Nursing	Intermediate Care	Assisted Living/ Custodial Care
Invasive tube care	Can handle complex tube care including trach tube, G tubes, J tubes, ileostomies, colostomies, indwelling tubes, T tubes, catheters; may include irrigation, monitoring, replacement PRN, site care and self-care instructions	Same as subacute, but patient and care must be fairly stable; patients at this level with several types of tubes not accepted at some facilities	Routine maintenance and care of uncomplicated catheters, tubes, ostomies; may do intermittent irrigations.	Empty drainage tubes and do simple, routine care (more complex care may require intermittent home health nursing visits)
Wound care/ dressings	Complex treatments and wound care; Criteria: treatment over 20 minutes, performed by RN level nurse, two or more times per 8 hour shift	Will perform complex, sterile, and frequent dressing changes or wound cases needing close monitoring (wounds can be infected and acute)	Will perform routine care for non-infected, chronic wounds and skin conditions	May perform simple care such as salves and simple dry dressing; may call in a home health RN for further care
Rehabilitation	Usually require minimum of two therapies (physical, occupational, or speech) and patient's ability to tolerate at least 3 hours of therapy daily	Rehab therapy needed on a daily basis and performed by a licensed therapist	May be supervised by a licensed therapist (restorative nursing); may include assistance with ambulation, range of motion, positioning, and so on	Not a safe level of care if patient requires rehabilitation, unless home health is involved in non-complex case
Mobility	Requires complex assistance from licensed personnel	Usually requires assistance of more than one person in mobility, transfers to chair, bed, toilet, or bath; unable to help very much in these activities; assistive devices may be used	Patient possibly able to participate in mobility and transfers to chair, bed, toilet, or bath; assistive devices may or may not be needed	Often allows wheelchair-bound clients, but must be independent in getting to and from bathroom and eating areas and independent in getting in and out of bed

(Continued)

Table 10-1. Subacute Levels of Care (Continued)

Levels of Care	Subacute & Rehabilitation	Skilled Nursing	Intermediate Care	Assisted Living/ Custodial Care
Patient education	Teaching needs identified and taught by licensed professional staff; administration of medications, self-care of tubes, wounds, use of equipment are taught on ongoing basis in preparation for discharge to a lesser level of care	Teaching needs identified and taught by licensed professional staff; administration of medications, self-care of tubes, wounds, use of equipment, and other needs taught on an ongoing basis in preparation for discharge to a lesser level of care	Simple teaching done by non-licensed professionals but under the supervision of licensed staff; may teach basic ADL support, feeding techniques, use of assistive devices, and so on	No teaching skills at this level of care; home health nurses may be retained if needed
Nutrition	Can accommodate TPN, IV fluids, use of infusion pumps, tube feedings with residual checks	TPN and IV fluids accommodated at some facilities; tube feeding with or without infusion pump and maximum assistance with oral feeding accommodated	Requires some assistance with self-feeding	Most require client to be able to get to dining room and feed self
Personal hygiene and toileting	Can accommodate total care of personal hygiene and toileting including disimpaction when needed and perineal care	Can accommodate total care of personal hygiene and toileting, including disimpaction when needed and perineal care	Assists with toileting, perineal care, bathing and grooming	Most require client to be continent; some accept indwelling catheters and assist with dressing and grooming efforts
Behavioral /Mental		May be confused, disoriented, combative; may need physical or chemical restraints for safety of patient or others; patients with active, serious psychological disorders are not legally allowed at this level of care in many states	May be intermittently confused or disoriented requiring staff intervention and possibly restraints for protective purposes; patients with active, serious psychological disorders not legally allowed at this level of care in many states	May be slightly forgetful; not a safe level of care for confused, disoriented clients

ADL, activities of daily living; IM, intramuscular; PRN, as needed; SC, subcutaneous; SVN, small-volume nebulizer; TPN, total parenteral nutrition.

Most communities have books listing their ECFs, along with names, addresses, and telephone numbers. Other information such as ratings, level of care offered and Medicare certification is usually provided. Not all facilities provide the same levels of care or even quality of care. It is worth a visit to these sites for a thorough understanding of the level of skilled care each one can provide. These visits can be real eye openers. I visited an ECF in which one licensed nurse was on duty from 6 o'clock in the morning until 10 o'clock at night. I could not send anyone to that facility with even a TKO (to keep open) intravenous line, in case it needed attention at 2:00 AM, for example. This ECF had a good physical therapy department, and if that was the client's sole need, this facility would be a good match.

Keep the following factors in mind when choosing an ECF:

- Does the facility's skill level meet the assessed needs of the client?
- Will the patient/family agree to this facility? Is it an acceptable location for visiting purposes?
- Does the patient's primary physician go to this facility? If not, would the doctor prefer another ECF that is also acceptable to the patient/family? Or, perhaps the physician, family, and patient would agree to have another doctor follow up at the ECF of choice.
- Is the chosen ECF a contracted facility with the payor?
- Will the services that the patient needs be covered at the ECF level of care by the payor?

Insurance Criteria

Traditional Medicare patients (those reimbursed under the DRG system) may enter an ECF level of care when certain criteria have been met:

- The patient must be in the hospital for 3 consecutive days. *Note:* This criterion may not be needed for the newer-risk Medicare plans.
- The 3-day stay must have been medically necessary.
- The ECF reason for admission must also be congruent with the reason the client was in the hospital (InterQual & Tennant, 1993)

or

- Posthospital ECF placement may take place within 30 days of hospital discharge. The 3-day rule applies (1993).

Note: The 3-day hospital stay is for an *inpatient* status only; patients admitted under *observation* status do not qualify. If it appears that the client will need ECF placement *and* meets acute inpatient medical criteria, ask the physician for an order to change the patient to inpatient status.

In addition, Medicare and other insurance plans also mandate the following criteria before a client can be admitted into an ECF:

- The medical condition requires daily, skilled services of a licensed professional.
- Those services cannot be provided at a lesser level of care or it would be impractical, uneconomical, or inefficient to do so.

- The care provided must be based on physician orders (HCFA, 1994).

The following ECF coverage options are specifically for Medicare-reimbursed clients, but many insurance companies have the same or similar provisions. Major ECF services covered under Medicare Parts A & B include (HCFA, 1994):

- A semiprivate room
- Meals, which may include special diets
- Nursing services
- Physical, occupational, and speech therapies
- Blood transfusions (non replacement fees may be required)
- All medications furnished by the ECF during the admission and prescribed by the attending physician
- Medical supplies such as splints, casts, and dressings
- Use of durable medical equipment such as walkers or wheelchairs

Some ECF services not covered by Medicare include (HCFA, 1994):

- Personal convenience items such as televisions and telephones (not all ECFs provide them unless the client requests them and rents them)
- Private duty nurses
- The extra charge necessary for a private room, unless the private room is deemed to be medically necessary

Rehabilitation Services

Rehabilitation services, physical therapy (PT), occupational therapy (OT), and speech therapy (ST) can be provided at various levels of care depending on the client's functional ability and support system. Home PT/OT/ST can be provided on an intermittent basis. For daily rehabilitation needs, an ECF level may be required. Inpatient rehabilitation facilities generally require that the client can tolerate 3 hours of combined rehabilitative services daily and follow, at least one- to two-step commands. Transitional hospitals can take patients at any level of rehabilitation needed and can generally move them within the hospital structure to the appropriate therapies.

Often a trauma or stroke patient in an acute hospital requires an inpatient rehabilitation consultant. If the patient is said to be "too high a level" for inpatient rehab, this means that he or she does not require the intense focus of this level of care. An ECF level may be more appropriate, or even home may be appropriate with home therapy services. If the patient is said to be "too low a level" for inpatient rehabilitation, this may mean that the patient cannot follow commands or cannot yet tolerate 3 hours of intense rehab. Again, an ECF level may be more appropriate, with the hope and intention of the client improving enough to graduate to an inpatient facility.

Again, insurance coverage is the key in most cases, since some companies cover their members at varying degrees of dysfunction in the different rehabilitative levels.

Note: Medicare exception to the 3 hours of rehab daily. If the client has a complicating condition that prevents him or her from participating for 3 hours, but inpatient rehab is the only reasonable means by which even a low-intensity rehab program can be safely carried out, it may be authorized. Documentation must support the claim (InterQual & Tennant, 1993).

Inpatient Rehabilitation Centers

Inpatient rehabilitation care is covered under many major insurance plans but strict criteria must be met because this is a cost-intensive setting. The criteria listed below follow reimbursement guidelines under Medicare. As in any discharge plan, consult the client's insurance coverage or request that the rehabilitation hospital/unit of the client's choice look into coverage. Most admission departments can let the NCM know about coverage within 24 hours. Some insurance plans use stricter guidelines than the Medicare criteria. If the NCM and rehab physician feel strongly that the client is an excellent rehab candidate but the insurance company is reluctant to cover services, try negotiation. Sometimes a short stay can be agreed on, with frequent monitoring of the patient's progress toward self-care.

Insurance Criteria

Four main categories of criteria reflect Medicare requirements for authorization in an inpatient rehab facility. Other insurance companies may use the same general criteria.

1. Admitting diagnosis must include at least one of the following conditions:

    - Amputation
    - Arthritis
    - Cardiac conditions
    - Chronic pain
    - Congenital disorder
    - CVA (cerebral vascular accident)
    - Diabetes mellitus
    - Fracture
    - Head trauma/brain injury
    - Multiple trauma
    - Musculoskeletal disorder
    - Neurologic disorder
    - Orthopedic condition
    - Pulmonary condition
    - Spinal cord injury

2. The primary problem must include a *recent* functional loss, whereas prior to the illness or accident, the client was independent in that function. There also must be *dependence* on the assistance of another person to carry out that function. Some functional categories include the following:

- Bladder dysfunction—incontinence, external catheter
- Bowel dysfunction—incontinence, maintenance of an excretory pattern
- Communication—major receptive or expressive aphasia
- Cognitive dysfunction—change in client's attention span, memory, or intelligence
- Medical monitoring—patient's medical status requires intensive medical monitoring or nursing attention at least once daily because of a cardiovascular, gastrointestinal, urologic, endocrine, or neurologic disorder. This is in addition to the primary diagnosis as stated in #1.
- Medical safety—client either exhibits or is at risk for, secondary complications such as decubitus ulcers, contractures, urinary tract infections, or major spasticity.
- Mobility dysfunction—must learn safe transfers to chair/bed/toilet/shower, walking (usually with appliances), negotiating stairs, wheelchairs, and so on.
- Pain control—pain severely prohibits active motion or functional use.
- Personal safety—the patient is physically unsafe alone.
- Self-care activities—ADLs (activities of daily living) must be renegotiated, such as feeding, drinking, dressing, grooming, brace and prosthesis care, bathing, toileting, and perineal care.

3. The physician must document the expectation of *significant* improvement in functional ability within a reasonable time frame.
4. If a patient was previously in a rehabilitative program with an unsuccessful outcome, this patient *must* have some change in condition or circumstances that would indicate that progress is now possible.

Other important criteria for admission to an inpatient rehabilitation unit include medical stability, mental ability to follow one- to two-step commands, and ability to withstand at least 3 hours of therapies daily, five times per week. The 3 hours can consist of any time frame combination of physical therapy, occupational therapy, and speech therapy.

A patient may be discharged from a rehab unit for several reasons including:

- The stated goals of rehab have all been met.
- There has been no progress toward stated goals after an adequate trial (usually a period of 1 week without any appreciable headway).
- A severe complication develops necessitating a transfer to acute care.
- A complication develops, which inhibits the multidisciplinary approach for over 1 week. In this case, it is sometimes necessary and reasonable to transfer care to an ECF level until the modalities can be reinstated.

Transitional Hospitals

Transitional hospitals are acute care hospitals for medically stable patients with long rehabilitative needs and care that is too complex for ECFs. These hospitals are DRG-exempt (at this time) and are paid on a cost basis (Anonymous, 1991).

These hospitals have a lower price structure than traditional acute hospitals mainly because fewer specialists are on staff and they contain only basic diagnostic or surgical equipment. They usually do not have expensive computed tomography (CT) scanners or magnetic resonance imaging (MRI) equipment but do have x-ray capabilities. Major surgeries are not done on site, but surgical procedures such as surgical feeding tube placement or tracheostomies can be performed. RN staffing is reported to be the same as other acute hospitals.

These hospitals can handle patients just below the ICU level with multiple complex medication regimens and treatments, which may include:

- Ventilator-dependent patients including weaning patients
- Use of TPN (total parental nutrition) or hyperalimentation
- Extensive wound care
- Infectious disease management
- Intravenous medication therapies
- Burn care
- All rehabilitative modalities (OT/PT/ST)
- Hemodialysis clients
- Prehospice clients–pain control therapies
- Coma recovery, cognitive rehabilitations, neurobehavioral rehabilitation
- Most other treatments that can be done at other acute hospitals or levels of care

Several years ago, one of my clients with AIDS also developed Guillain-Barré syndrome and became ventilator-dependent for many months. It took almost 1 month to obtain placement in an ECF that handles ventilators because of their long waiting periods. A Gallup poll in 1991 revealed that there was an average waiting period of 35 days between the time that a chronic ventilator-dependent patient could be discharged and the availability of an appropriate bed (Anonymous, 1991). It now takes an average of 24 to 48 hours to place a complex patient, pending availability of these beds and authorization from the payor source.

If a client's condition is very complex but "too low a level" for inpatient rehab, these facilities should be considered. One client came in for a coronary catheterization. During the procedure, she suffered a stroke and a cardiac arrest, requiring a tracheostomy. Eventually, this patient was weaned from the ventilator. She was alert and oriented, but too weak to tolerate intensive rehabilitation modalities. She also required more frequent tracheal suctioning than ECFs can usually handle. The transitional hospital further stabilized the respiratory function and strengthened her. Later this woman was placed in an inpatient rehab unit, where she did very well.

Home Care Services

Most clients who were living independently before the present episode of illness prefer to return to their own homes. Perhaps they are not completely independent or back to their baseline, but have family support for basic needs. Sometimes home care services provide the vital link to a client's independence. A thorough social and medical assessment can evaluate the safety of a home health plan. For example, if the patient is a debilitated 94-year-old who lives with her daughter, the daughter also needs to be assessed to see if she can still safely care for her mother. (The daughter will likely be in her 70s.)

Home health agencies are public or private organizations that specialize in providing both skilled and nonskilled services in a client's home. This line of service is not new, and several agencies have already celebrated their centennial. They are, however, the fastest-growing component of healthcare in the 90s. Changes in the way that America is delivering healthcare is having a significant impact on the home healthcare industry. There is an increase in patients being sent home, necessitating more nurses. Patients have more medical needs than ever before, requiring clinically and technically astute nurses with developed critical thinking skills and advanced practice degrees (Gookin, 1994). And more patients are being sent home on weekends and late in the day, necessitating staff that is available and flexible (1994).

Perhaps the most far-reaching change is occurring because of the new Medicare risk contracts. Although this chapter discusses the criteria requirements of the traditional Medicare model, these risk contracts are touching all areas of healthcare, including home health agencies. As more members choose the Medicare health maintenance organizations (HMOs), more hospitals, physician groups and home health agencies are agreeing to capitation as a means of reimbursement (Gookin, 1994). (See Chapter 5: Insurance, for further discussion on capitation.) Although this puts home health agencies at some risk, it has some advantages over the traditional, and some feel archaic, Medicare model.

Insurance Criteria

In the traditional Medicare model, both Part A and Part B cover home health services. Home health visits are authorized only if all four of the following criteria are met (HCFA, 1994):

1. The client is homebound, which means that he or she is confined to the home or that it would be a great hardship to come to an outpatient facility for treatments.
2. The care required includes intermittent (not necessarily *daily*, as in the ECF criteria) skilled nursing services and possibly physical, occupational, and speech therapies.
3. The client is under the care of a licensed physician who has set up a home health plan and oversees it. The plan is reasonable and necessary and is reviewed at least every 60 days.
4. The home health agency is Medicare-certified, which means that the strictest federal standards are met.

It is doubtful whether this basic criteria set will change. But consider the following covered and noncovered services. Under the traditional Medicare model home services covered by Medicare, if the above criteria are met, include the following (HCFA, 1994).

Part-Time or Intermittent Skilled Nursing Care. This may include up to 8 hours of reasonable and necessary care per day for up to 21 consecutive days (more, under some circumstances). Few cases are allotted 8 hours per day, and the key phrase is "reasonable and necessary." Most clients who need 8 hours of skilled nursing care are not in the home environment. Occasionally, this does happen. But for the most part stress to your clients that an average home visit from an RN lasts 45 minutes to 1 hour, not 8 hours, and that the services must be skilled.

Physical Therapy or Speech Therapy. PT and ST may be added if skilled nursing services have been assessed and they are deemed reasonable and necessary. This also opens the gate for occupational therapy and home health aide services.

Home Health Aide Services. If skilled nursing services have been assessed as necessary and physical or speech therapies have also been deemed necessary, the client may qualify for intermittent home health aide services. Aide visits occur two to three times per week to help with personal care such as bathing, grooming, and changing linen.

Home Social Services. If skilled nursing services have been assessed, the client may qualify for home social services. This is at times more effective than a social worker seeing the client in an acute or subacute facility. The client is seen and assessed in his or her own environment, and this often elicits a more realistic appraisal of the social situation.

Medical Supplies. Supplies, such as dressings, will be made available if needed by the RN for the client's care.

Durable Medical Equipment. This equipment must be approved, since not all equipment is covered. There is also a 20% coinsurance for most equipment. Some durable medical equipment such as oxygen has strict criteria that must be met. The *home oxygen criteria* are added here because so many clients such as those with chronic obstructive pulmonary disease (COPD), diffuse interstitial lung disease, cystic fibrosis, bronchiectasis, or widespread lung cancer need it for comfort and survival. (*Note:* if the client is admitted into hospice, the oxygen guidelines are not as strict).

To qualify for home oxygen:

1. First, arterial blood gases must be drawn *on room air.*
   a. The PO_2 must be 55 or below or with an arterial saturation of 88% or below, *or*
   b. If the PO_2 is between 56 and 59 or the arterial saturation is 89% or below, there must also be evidence of one of the following: dependent edema suggesting congestive heart failure; or P pulmonale on electrocardiogram (ECG) (P wave above 3 mm); or erthrocythemia with a hematocrit over 56%.
2. If the PO_2 is between 56 and 59 or the arterial saturation is 89%, the client must be retested between the 61st and 90th day of oxygen therapy. A renewal prescription with the qualifying test result will be required in the fourth month for further home oxygen coverage.

Home Medications. Some intravenous antibiotics and selected medications are now offered by Medicare in the home setting (see Chapter 5: Insurance, under Medicare for further discussion).

Psychological Nurse Assistance Under Specific Criteria.

Services that are *not* covered under traditional Medicare in the home setting include the following (HCFA, 1994):

- General homemaker services such as shopping, cleaning, laundry, and meal preparation
- Standby services such as 24-hour per day nurse or nurse aide care at home so the patient will not be left alone
- Blood transfusions
- Medications—except when specifically authorized

These strict criteria have been somewhat lifted with the newer Medicare HMOs. They provide more freedom to choose and use whatever services best meet the client's healthcare needs and the plan's financial needs. The newer Medicare plans now act more like independent HMOs or even some Medicaid plans; criteria such as a 3-day hospitalization being required before a patient can be placed in an ECF or intravenous antibiotics not being provided for in the home setting no longer makes any fiscal sense.

The previous regulations and limitations on Medicare patients are being lifted with these new plans. The contracts allow "in lieu of" services. This means, for example, that if a patient could be discharged sooner from the hospital if he or she had, in addition to skilled nursing services, some personal care and provisions for meals, the home health agency has flexibility to do this. The hospital (who may also be capitated on these plans) may choose to reimburse the home health agency for these services in lieu of an extended hospitalization (Gookin, 1994).

Occasionally, the distinction between skilled services and nonskilled services becomes blurred. Essentially a skilled service is one that is performed by a licensed professional such as an RN, physical therapist, respiratory therapist, occupational therapist, or speech therapist. The care given must be for the purpose of patient safety or medical stability. Table 10–2 shows some examples of *skilled care* and *nonskilled care*; these may be appropriately applied in any level of care.

Home health agencies are becoming more sophisticated every year, and many furnish almost any service that can be provided at the acute care level as long as the client is medically stable. Even if the client needs blood products (RBCs, fresh frozen plasma [FFP]), many agencies can accommodate with a 24-hour advance notice. However, emergency transfusions must be handled at a higher level of care. It is helpful to know which agencies can provide specified services. Like ECFs, home health agencies differ in their level of acuity. It is important to secure insurance authorization before calling an agency. Many insurance companies use only specific contracted agencies; calling the correct one at the onset can save a hospital day and a dose of aggravation.

Table 10-2. Comparison of Skilled and Nonskilled Services

Service Provided	Skilled Care	Unskilled Care
Vital signs	Takes vital signs; may record and report worrisome vital signs to physician; observes cardiopulmonary stability; teaches caregiver how to take and record vital signs and when to call physician	Takes vital signs; may record and report to appropriate person
Medications	Administration of medications, injections, sliding scale insulin, suppositories, eyedrops; teaches families about medication, side effects, what to do for side effects, observation of client's ability to comply with medication prescriptions, perhaps teach to give injections; assesses for negative side effects such as toxic levels	May assist in giving medications by reminding client of times to take them or helping open the lid
Skin care	Teaches diabetic skin and foot care; assesses skin for breakdown; aseptic wound care that may include packing, wet to dry dressings, dry dressing with sterile technique, irrigations; teaches family wound care; takes wound cultures, reports negative assessment to the physician or any negative change in skin condition; care of grade 3 or worse decubitus ulcers	Baths, applying lotions, ointments, creams, powders; application of nonsterile dressings; may reinforce dressings; treatment of chronic, noninfected surgical wounds and minor skin problems
Diet and nutrition	Instructs in special diets such as a low sodium, diabetic, renal, administer TPN, or tube feedings; instructs in administration of TPN or tube feedings; assesses nutritional status, monitors and teaches fluid restriction or fluid status; teaches and assesses fluid intake and output; replaces some indwelling tubes	Helps prepare meals; assists with feeding
Elimination	Insertion of straight catheter or Foley; teaches straight catheterizing procedure; observes and teaches signs of urinary tract infection; bowel or bladder training; provides care, observation, and teaching of new ostomy; assesses and reports skin breakdown	Cleansing of perineal area; empties drainage bags such as colostomies, indwelling Foley; measures urine; tests urine for sugar and acetone; assists client on and off commode; treats incontinence with diapers or rubber sheets; provides general care of colostomies or ileostomies including assisting in appliance changes in stable ostomy

(Continued)

Table 10-2. Comparison of Skilled and Nonskilled Services (Continued)

Service Provided	Skilled Care	Unskilled Care
Respiratory	Teaches and administers medical gases in the initial stages; in tracheostomy clients, suctioning and tracheostomy care; instructs client/family in trach self-care; observes and reports signs of respiratory distress or infection; administers oxygen; respiratory therapists may make ventilator changes per doctor's orders; small-volume nebulizer and chest physiotherapy treatments and instruction	Administers medical gases after initial stages; small-volume nebulizer and chest physiotherapy treatments after initial phase; assists in tracheostomy care of stable tracheostomy patient
Rehabilitation	Assesses and instructs use of assist devices, range of motion exercises, gait training, transfers; administers hot packs, ultrasound treatments, TENS units, whirlpools in compliance with doctor's prescriptions; speech therapist assesses and helps with communication problems and swallowing difficulties	Supervises exercises taught to client; performs passive and active range of motion in conjunction with physical therapist; assists in applying and removing prosthesis; assists with use of canes, walkers, wheelchairs, and Hoyer lifts
Miscellanous	Assesses any complex set of unskilled needs that requires putting together an overall picture of the patient for that patient's medical safety	

TENS, transcutaneous electrical nerve stimulation.

Hospice

Hospice programs began in Great Britain several decades ago. The concept reached the United States in the 1970s and has recently gained much respect and popularity. The philosophy of hospice is that terminally ill patients should be allowed to maintain their final days of life comfortably and with dignity. Ideally, these last days take place at home with family and loved ones present, if desired. When nothing further can be done medically for the patient, the family and patient agree that death is imminent, and the family and patient want only palliative and comfort measures taken, not aggressive curative measures, then hospice may be the plan of care of choice. Hospice does not hasten or postpone death but allows nature to take its course.

Often families and medical staff are confused about the difference in services between home health and hospice. Although hospice is similar to home health services in many ways, it differs in some important aspects. Following are some differences between Medicare home health coverage and Medicare hospice coverage services as the standard guideline. Be aware that insurance companies other than Medicare may or may not include hospice benefits; and if they do have the hospice benefit, it may include different covered services.

Comparison Between Hospice Coverage and Home Health Coverage

Skilled Nursing Services Provided on an Intermittent Basis. Both home health and hospice provide this, but hospice covers these services on a 24-hour, 7-day-a-week, on-call basis.

Unskilled Services. Most home health agencies do not provide unskilled nursing services because they are rarely covered under insurance agreements. Nurse aides may be covered under Medicare for two to three 1-hour visits per week for personal care, but only under strict criteria. Hospice can provide 12 to 16 hours of personal aides per week if needed, including some homemaker services.

Physician Services. Both home health and hospice care must be under the guidance of an ordering physician.

Bereavement Services and Counseling (Including Spiritual Counseling). This is perhaps the most important distinction between home health services and hospice services. Bereavement and counseling services are often offered to the family for several months after the death of the patient. But more important, if hospice is called in early enough, these trained persons help to prepare the family for the impending death, often averting shock and crisis situations.

Social Services and Volunteers. With hospice, social service personnel and volunteers are part of the multidisciplinary staff. Home health agencies are allowed very limited social service attention at home.

Homebound Requirement. Under home health criteria, the client must be homebound or must need to undergo an unusual hardship to get care through outpatient facilities. Although terminal hospice patients are often homebound, this is not a mandatory requirement for hospice care.

Prescription Drugs for Symptom Management and Pain Control. Traditional Medicare rarely pays for prescription medications at home (exceptions are noted in Chapter 5: Insurance, under Medicare). Under the hospice benefit, prescription medications to manage symptoms and control pain are covered. There is a 5% or $5 charge toward each prescription, whichever is less.

Durable Medical Equipment and Home Oxygen. Medicare has strict criteria for many types of durable medical equipment including oxygen (see oxygen criteria under Home Health). Hospice guidelines for various types of durable medical equipment are more lax and can be provided for the comfort of the patient.

Respite Care. This is not a covered service under home health. With hospice, limited respite care in an ECF allows the family to take care of needed business or take a break so that they do not get overwhelmed with the extensive care that most terminal patients require. The respite is limited to 5 consecutive days per benefit quarter.

Physical, Occupational, and Speech–Language Therapy. These therapies are carried out for the purpose of symptom control or to allow the patient to maintain basic ADL function. Both home health and hospice benefits cover this service.

Continuous Care During Periods of Medical Crisis. Only hospice carries this benefit. For some families, continuous care during this period is the key benefit that allows the patient to die at home with dignity.

Deductibles. There are no deductibles under the hospice benefit.

Medicare Hospice Criteria

The hospice benefit may be used in a Medicare client if *all three* criteria are met (HCFA, 1994):

1. A physician certifies that the patient is terminally ill.
2. The patient (or family) chooses to use the hospice benefit.
3. The hospice agency is Medicare-certified.

If these three criteria are met and the client is in the hospital, a physician order for hospice will be needed. After a call is made to refer this patient to hospice, a representative will come to the hospital, meet the patient and family, and answer questions. A hospice referral can also be made while a client is at home, but also with the above criteria.

Although a client chooses to forego standard Medicare benefits in lieu of hospice benefits, standard benefits begin if treatment for a condition unrelated to the hospice condition is needed. For example, if a patient with terminal AIDS falls and breaks a leg, then the necessary care for this accident will be paid for by standard Medicare.

Hospice Benefit Periods

Special benefit periods apply to the hospice portion of Medicare. When a client opts for the hospice benefit, the benefit periods define the extent of his coverage. (See also Chapter 5: Insurance under Medicare for standard Medicare benefit periods.) Part A will pay for two 90-day benefit periods and a 30-day benefit period. Extension periods of indefinite duration protect the client in case of long terminal stages of illness (HCFA, 1994).

Patients can choose to cancel hospice and return to Medicare benefits or vice versa as long as there are remaining benefit periods; when someone cancels the hospice benefit, the remaining days in the benefit period are lost. If any benefit periods remain, they may still return to hospice and use those remaining periods (1994).

Perhaps the best way to explain the use of hospice benefit periods is through examples (HCFA, 1994):

Mr. Jones cancelled his hospice care at the end of 59 days during his first 90-day benefit period. He lost the 31 remaining days of the first 90-day period. If he wants to, he can choose hospice care again. He still has a 90-day and a 30-day period and the indefinite extension period. However, Ms. Smith cancelled hospice care during her final extension period. She cannot use the Medicare hospice benefit again.

Myths and Realities

Perhaps because hospice is so similar to home health or because it is simply misunderstood, myths about hospice abound. These are some myths that are commonly heard from patients and families.

Myth: Hospice is only for terminal cancer patients.

Reality: Hospice is for any terminal condition: COPD, AIDS, cystic fibrosis, and any end-stage disease (cardiac, liver, renal, Alzheimer's disease to name a few terminal conditions).

Myth: The patient must only have 6 months to live.

Reality: Although in general the prognosis for life expectancy should be in months rather than years, it is often difficult to say for certain how long a patient will live. Unfortunately, this misunderstanding has caused healthcare teams to wait until the "last minute" before calling in hospice, thereby losing valuable time in which patients and families could be receiving care and counseling that could improve the quality of the remaining time. Also, remember that Medicare allows 210 days (two benefit periods of 90 days and one benefit period of 30 days), which equals 7 months; add to that the indefinite extension. This is fact enough that demise is not "required" in 6 months.

Myth: A 24-hour caregiver is required.

Reality: This one requires careful assessment. I have admitted some patients to hospice who were still independent, although this is rare. Others do well with the 12 to 16 hours of assistance provided. If a patient is terminal, is dependent on others, and does not have a strong support system, then an ECF for terminal care (under Medicare Part A) may be a better choice.

Myth: Nursing home patients cannot receive hospice care.

Reality: Medicare does not pay for the room and board of an ECF under the hospice benefit. However, if the family can fund the room and board or the patient's private insurance policy covers this, as some do, then hospice can be used at the ECF level of care. The bereavement and counseling portion of hospice can then be used; it is an important part of terminal care.

Myth: To be accepted into hospice, all further medical treatment must be forfeited.

Reality: The important distinction here is whether the care is for aggressive, curative purposes or for palliative, comfort means. Radiation therapy has been used for palliation treatment. If someone may have several months to live and cannot tolerate food or tube feedings, total parenteral nutrition has been authorized. The main question to ask is *why* the care is being given. Hospice patients in distress are readmitted into the hospital; often they are stabilized and sent back home with hospice again. Conditions not related to the hospice condition are treated under Medicare Part A. But if a client wants to try chemotherapy with the hope of a cure, he or she will have to leave the hospice benefit period and opt for standard Medicare benefits.

Transferring Patients

The Transfer Packet

When a patient is transferred to another level of care or to another acute hospital, specific information must accompany the patient. The transfer packet includes the following:

- Physician transfer orders
- Chest x-ray (preferably within 30 days)
- History and physical
- Laboratory results
- ECG
- Urinalysis
- Preadmission screening (PAS), preadmission screening and annual resident review (PASAAR) forms
- Assessments from nursing, physical therapy, occupational therapy, speech therapy (as needed)
- Social service assessments
- DNR forms (if appropriate), Living Wills, Medical Power of Attorney
- Copies of important information such as results from CT scans, echocardiograms, Dopplers, MRIs, miscellaneous cardiodiagnostics, and so on.

A complete and thorough transfer packet is necessary for continuity of patient care, and it avoids a lot of trouble and problems. Patients have been returned to emergency rooms for not having a chest x-ray accompany them to the facility. ECFs must ensure that their residents are free from tuberculosis, and the chest x-ray is usually nonnegotiable. Patients with a positive Mantoux skin test may also need a signed and dated letter from the physician stating that the resident is free from pulmonary tuberculosis or that three consecutive sputum cultures have shown negative results for 3 days in a row.

Another required form in many states is the PAS document. It is also known as a PASAAR form. This program, started by Medicaid in the mid-80s, was originally designed as a technique to manage long-term care costs and utilization of services in nursing homes. It includes an on-site (or hospital) assessment of the client's needs (Kongstvedt, 1993). In some states, this assessment is extensive and includes an evaluation of physical and mental health, functional status, and formal and informal social supports (1993). Although the PAS program was not deemed successful as a utilization control measure, it was praised for its ability to help assess the level of care and type of facility that is best for the client (1993). Some PAS programs contain a level I and level II. Level I is essentially used to assess medical necessity for an ECF. Level II indicates whether a psychological referral is needed. This may hold up a transfer to an ECF for a week or more. State laws prohibit ECFs or supervisory homes from accepting clients with active mental illnesses that may cause them to be a danger to themselves or other residents in the ECF. If a client might need to pass a level II PAS, start the paperwork early in the admission.

One last detail: a patient must have an accepting physician at the ECF. If the patient's primary physician cannot follow up at the ECF, the facility often helps to find a doctor to follow up.

Transportation

Safe patient transportation between levels of care is an important consideration. Several levels of transportation are available for transferring patients to an outside destination, and the patient's needs must be matched to the appropriate mode of transportation. In many instances, the patient or family is responsible for the cost of transportation. Some rare insurance policies pay for expensive forms of transportation, so if the patient claims to have this policy rider, check it out. I had one patient air-ambulanced from Phoenix, Arizona, to Alaska with full payment from the insurance supplement. Some family members may request a more intensive level of transportation than the NCM has assessed, and they may be willing to pay for it. In one instance, I had assessed that this patient could safely be transported to another hospital using a stretcher van. The family wanted an ACLS ambulance plus an RN. Therefore, even when planning the mode of transportation, one must include the patient and family in the decision. There are several types of transportation:

Private Vehicles

Private vehicle is the most common mode of transportation. Usually, the patient is accompanied by family or friends, but occasionally the patient drives him- or herself to the hospital. Then arrangements must be made for the vehicle if the physician feels it is unsafe for the patient to drive. The simplest solution here is for a family member or neighbor to be dropped off at the facility to drive the vehicle and patient home. The facility's personnel can help get the patient into the vehicle. The NCM should assess whether there is enough help at the destination to safely get the patient inside. Assessment is also needed for any equipment needs for the trip. For example, many patients have their portable oxygen tanks at home and must make prior arrangements to retrieve them before they leave the facility. Also, assess the length of the trip and the possible need for more than one oxygen tank. Assess whether the patient can remain sitting for the trip: very ill patients and some orthopedic procedures make this mode of transportation unrealistic. Assess whether the patient has stairs to climb at the other end. If the patient cannot negotiate stairs, a car, taxi, or wheelchair van will not work and a stretcher van should be considered; the stretcher van personnel will take the client up the stairs and help him or her to get settled.

Taxicab

Ask some of the same questions as above for taxis, realizing that cab drivers are often less helpful at the other end than family members because of their legal constraints. Also, find out whether the client can afford a taxi. Many hospitals have funds or cab vouchers to help needy people. From a fiscal perspective, a cab ride is less expensive than a day in the hospital if a patient cannot get someone to take him home until tomorrow.

Wheelchair Van

Wheelchair vans are a good choice for several types of clients. If a person who is quadriplegic or who has cerebral palsy uses a wheelchair at home, he often has his own wheelchair at the hospital. Notify the van company whether they need to provide a wheelchair or whether the patient has one. If a patient can sit up for a designated length of time but may be slightly confused, he may need to be restrained. Careful assessment is imperative when sending a client needing restraints in a wheelchair van. For example, it would be safer to use a higher level of transportation if the patient is combative or requires maximum restraining. (Consider what the risk management issues would be if the patient is maximally restrained and the van catches fire or goes over the side of a road!) Orthopedic clients can often use wheelchair vans with adaptive equipment such as leg lifts. Specify what equipment is required when ordering the van. Again, assess the whole medical picture before deciding on this level of transportation.

Stretcher Vans

Stretcher vans allow a patient to lie down for the entire ride. The patient is transferred from the facility bed to the stretcher and taken to the destination, even transported up or down stairs, in the same position. Very ill, debilitated patients who cannot sit for any length of time are candidates for stretcher vans, as are some orthopedic patients or those who must stay on their abdomen or back because of medical considerations such as skin flaps or graft procedures. No form of cardiac monitoring is included in this mode of transportation.

Ambulances

There are two types of ambulances: Basic Life Support (BLS) and Advanced Life Support (ALS). BLS ambulances include a BLS paramedic and limited cardiac monitoring. Psychiatric patients or suicidal clients who are being transferred to a mental health unit require minimally this level of care; if the transfer is involuntary and the client is likely to become combative, extra help should be requested and restraints may be necessary. In general, assess patient's medical stability and decide whether it would be beneficial to have a BLS paramedic on board.

ALS ambulances include paramedics trained in advanced cardiac life support (ACLS) procedures. Cardiac monitoring and a drug box are available for use. Any patient who has a running intravenous line or who requires medications (including potassium) will require minimally this level of care.

Air Ambulance

Air transport is the most cost-intensive type of transportation available, often costing thousands of dollars for even short flights. But when an unstable patient is being transferred to another acute care facility and speed is of the essence, it may be the only safe mode of transfer. As in an ALS ambulance, the air ambulance has cardiac monitoring, a medication box, and ACLS-trained personnel, including an RN.

Almost any patient can be safely transferred, when necessary, with enough support provided. Some cases require careful consideration and advanced planning. More insurance companies are requiring their members to be transferred to contracted hospitals than ever before but are willing to pay the transportation costs. One member had a chest tube and needed an ALS ambulance with an RN on board. Since most ambulance companies retain only a few RNs, it took an extra day to provide the required services. Again, this is a case for early planning.

Considerations in Planning Transportation

Further important considerations to assess when planning a mode of transportation are as follows:.

Tubes and Lines. Most tubes can be capped off for shorter rides and require only a doctor's order to do so. This may include intravenous lines (peripheral or central), tube feedings, tubes to suction such as nasogastric tubes, or percutaneous endoscopic gastrostomy (PEG) tubes, gastrostomy tubes, or jejunostomy tubes. Most modes of transportation—even taxis—allow capped-off tubes, although that is not to say that a taxi is the safest vehicle assessed. If a tube cannot be capped off, an ambulance may be the lowest level of transportation allowed. If, for example, intravenous fluid containing potassium is running, then an ALS ambulance must be used. The transportation company can clear up any questions, since they carry on their business under legal guidelines.

Oxygen. Some state laws mandate that oxygen cannot be supplied by the transportation company for wheelchair or stretcher vans. The company can provide only oxygen in a BLS or ALS ambulance. However, if the client has his or her own portable oxygen tank, a wheelchair van or stretcher van may be provided in conjunction with the client's personal equipment. The van personnel are not allowed to adjust the oxygen, so that the client's ability to care for his or her own portable tank must be considered.

Prices of Transportation. Since the patient is responsible for the cost of transportation in many instances, the NCM may want to compare the prices of various companies for the best rate. Ambulance prices are essentially set by the government, but taxi, wheelchair van, and stretcher van prices may vary.

Transportation Reimbursement. Insurance companies often reimburse for transportation between two medically necessary levels of care; they usually do not reimburse for transportation to the client's home. Medicare reimbursement for transportation is very strict and includes only ground ambulance or air ambulance transport.

- Ground ambulance may be reimbursed under Medicare Part B for a medically necessary transfer if (HCFA, 1994):
  1. The ambulance, equipment, and personnel, meet Medicare requirements and approval.
  2. Any other mode of transportation could endanger the patient.
  3. The destination is to or from a hospital or skilled nursing facility. This does not include such destinations as hemodialysis facilities, doctor's offices, or ambulatory surgery centers.

4. Usually the transportation must be to a local facility. If the facility is outside the local area, Medicare will *help* pay for the transportation to the *nearest* appropriate facility.

- Air ambulance may be reimbursed by Medicare if (HCFA, 1994):
  1. The medical condition seriously endangers the member's life.
  2. Immediate medical attention is necessary for the person's survival or necessary to avoid severe health damage.
  3. Land ambulance is unavailable or would be so time-consuming that health or life would be further endangered.

Study Questions

1. Discuss various pharmaceutical benefits. Cite an example of how this benefit may influence the case plan.
2. Discuss differences between traditional Medicare and the newer-risk Medicare contracts and how discharge planning is affected. Do you see these changes positively or negatively?
3. Discuss the Medicare denial process. How would you handle a family/patient who disagrees with the hospital discharge date? What steps would you take?
4. Give an example of a patient who is appropriate for the custodial level of care; the intermediate level of care; the skilled and subacute levels of care? Discuss possible pay sources for each level of care.
5. What might constitute a client being too high a level for inpatient rehabilitation? Too low a level?
6. Cite an example of a good candidate for a transitional hospital.
7. Cite an example of a good home healthcare client? Give reasons that may be contrary to home health services.
8. Compare and contrast home health services with hospice care.
9. Cite examples matching clients needs to safe transportation.

References

Anonymous (1991). CMs find innovative options for clients between the ICU and the acute care bed. *Case Management Advisor, 2* (8), 113–117.

Gookin, L. (1994). Effects of capitation on home health care. *Geriatric Nursing, 15*(3), 167–168.

Health Care Financing Administration. (1994). *The Medicare 1994 Handbook.* DHHS Publication No. HCFA 10050, Baltimore, MD.

InterQual & Tennant, T. (Ed.). (1993). *Utilization review and management training manual.* North Hampton: Author.

Kongstvedt, P. R. (1993). *The managed health care handbook.* Gaithersburg, MD: Aspen Publishers.

Williams, S. J., & Torrens, P. R. (1993). *Introduction to health services.* New York: Delmar.

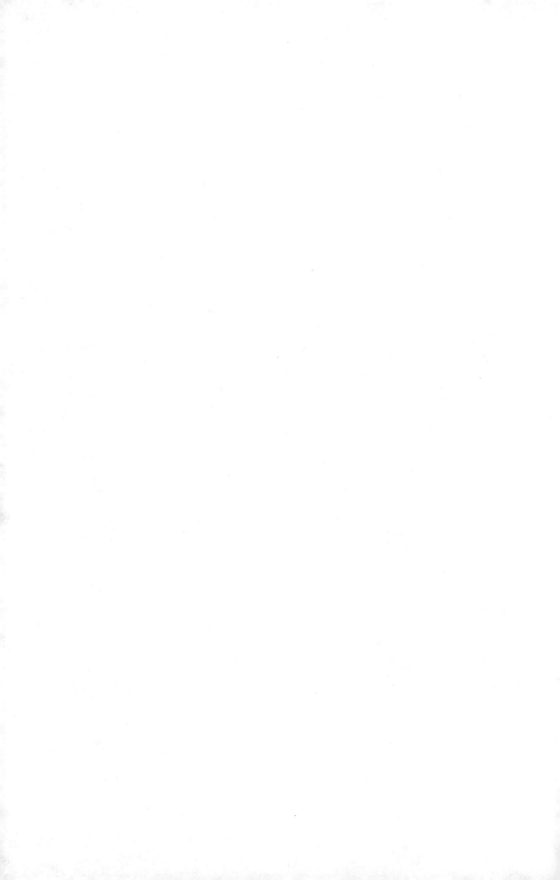

PART III

The Case Management Process

"You ought not attempt to cure the eyes without head, or head without body; so you should not treat body without soul."

SOCRATES

PART III
IMPORTANT TERMS AND CONCEPTS

assessment
case selection
continuous case management
coordination and development of the treatment/discharge plan
final evaluation and/or post discharge follow-up
implementation of the final plan

CHAPTER 11

Introduction to the Case Management Process

This section discusses the direction and activities needed to guide a client through the complex healthcare maze. Nurses will find the process familiar, because it uses some of the same components as the nursing process: assessment, planning, implementation, and evaluation. The focus, however, is much broader in case management. In the nursing process, the client is assessed for changing physical, medical, psychosocial, and safety needs on a shift-by-shift basis. The case manager must also assess the patient prior to this illness, determine whether his or her environment will continue to meet present needs, investigate how the needs will be met financially, and then plan posthospital care. Therefore, the steps may be slightly reordered with new ones added, and the emphasis and purposes may be altered.

This reordering and altering may also apply when considering different types of case management. *Case selection* for a hospital nurse case manager (NCM) may be filtered through the institution's admissions. An independent case manager may get referrals from a variety of sources such as physicians, insurance companies, and private citizens. Other case managers may select cases according to a predetermined specialty such as a specialty in spinal cord injuries, AIDS, or cerebral palsy. The *monitoring component* may be done less frequently for an NCM with clients in private homes or in sheltered care than a hospital NCM, who may have to monitor patients on a daily basis. Some hospital case managers are finished with a case at discharge. Others perform posthospital follow-up for a brief time frame. Hospice case managers may assess their clients in the home or hospital, but they do not actively take on the case until clients are admitted to hospice, which is usually when the patient arrives home or to a skilled facility after discharge. Hospice case managers may follow up the client until death. Still other case managers follow up their clients in whatever setting they need.

Each client is unique and case management styles are individual; therefore, the result is a very personalized process in each and every case. Considering this, the process discussed in this chapter should be used as a guideline: the skills and creativity of each NCM are still the essential ingredients.

Stages of the Case Management Process

In general, the case management process involves the following stages: (1) case selection; (2) assessment; (3) coordinating and developing the plan; (4) continuous monitoring, reassessing, and reevaluating; (5) implementation of the final plan; and (6) final evaluation and postdischarge follow-up. Independent case managers and NCMs who work outside institutional settings may require added steps, such as getting signed consents for case management services from the payors or for release of information or release of medical records. Insurance case managers may or may not perform all the steps. For example, Medicaid case managers rely on hospital personnel and other sources for much of the assessment, especially for medical and psychosocial aspects. They often work closely with hospital discharge planners and NCMs to fulfill a safe and timely discharge.

Stage I: Case Selection

Case selection is the "first cut" in the process. Basically, this step weeds out patients who probably will not need case management services. Occasionally, one of the patients put on the "probably not" list will actually need services. A patient's condition can deteriorate to the point of needing extended care facility (ECF) placement, or, more simply, a piece of durable medical equipment may be needed. Sometimes a quirky hitch arises such as a patient losing a lease or being evicted from an apartment by a roommate during the time of hospitalization. On the other hand, not all those who *are* put on the "probably" list (ie, needing case management) will need case management services; some may need only a bit of education or a walker for safety purposes. All patients who are selected need a basic assessment, at the minimum.

Stage II: Assessment

After the selection process has "red-flagged" a case, stage II—assessment—follows. Unless it is obvious that at this time the patient needs little or no case management services, a thorough and accurate assessment is done. Data collecting and analysis focus and direct the NCM to the treatment and discharge plans needed for that individual. Potential or actual problems are exposed; goals start taking shape. In this stage, the NCM finds out what gaps need filling, what services are needed, and what quality of life issues need focusing on. All anticipated needs are considered for a discharge plan that will allow the optimal quality of life for that client. A lengthy discourse on assessment is contained later in this section. The reason so much attention is given to it is because assessment is the critical pivot around which the NCM process revolves. If one misses an important enough condition, event, or circumstance, the whole discharge plan becomes unstable. At best, much confusion results and last-minute changes may be needed, sometimes delaying the discharge for 1 or 2 days. Remember the case discussed in Chapter 6 in which the NCM worked hard to set up a complex discharge, complete with "hi-tech" equipment, only to discover at the last minute that the patient's house had no electricity. This was a troublesome situation and was caused by misattention to details. At worst, an inaccurate or poor assessment can lead to an unsafe discharge plan— and a possible lawsuit. A complete and concise evaluation of all data is key to a holistic and individualized management of the patient.

Stage III: Coordinating & Developing the Treatment/Discharge Plan

If assessment aids the NCM in deciding where to go with a particular case, then stage III helps the NCM to choose the best way to get there. In this stage, the needs and services are matched into a seamless plan based on the assessment data. Creativity is the keynote at this point; often there is more than one "best" way to do something. Flexibility is very important; patient and family may desire changes, or patient conditions may change. Here is where the role of patient advocate becomes most evident. Creatively finding ways to meet the basic needs of your patient is reflected in quality treatment and discharge plans. The "gift" a patient advocate gives to the client is a plan that promotes the patient's optimal level of self-care and control over his or her own life.

Stage IV: Continuous Case Management

Case management continues until the case is officially closed and is, therefore, not really a "stage." Ongoing activities include monitoring and reassessment and reevaluation of the patient's status, treatment, and discharge plans. Rarely does the case management process proceed from stage I to stage VI, where the patient is miraculously being fully and perfectly cared for! More often, this continuous monitoring reveals changes in the patient's medical condition or hidden social circumstances hitherto unknown, necessitating changes in "the plan." This back-and-forth flow may occur several times before implementation of the final plan (stage V) becomes reality. The stability of the case determines the frequency of the monitoring and reevaluating. Some hospital cases need more than daily attention, whereas a "stable" spinal cord–injured patient residing in a rehabilitation center may need only weekly or monthly visits (of course, the patient would be monitored daily at the facility). Through the activities of this step, the service plan is revised, refined, and further fine-tuned.

Stage V: Implementation of the Final Plan

In the implementation of the final plan, the patient's assessed needs have been linked up with private and community services. The gaps are filled, there is no duplication of services, and the patient and support systems are in agreement with the plan. The goal of this stage is to maximize the safety and total well-being of the patient. A cost-effective setting for the discharge plan must match the client's capabilities, desires, and financial abilities. This is where the NCM shows a talent for coordinating and facilitation. The client is now discharged home, transferred to a supervised setting, or remains in the same setting but with a more appropriate service and treatment plan because of case management.

Stage VI: Final Evaluation and Postdischarge Follow-up

The activities of the final evaluation and postdischarge follow-up depend on the type of case management used. Some case managers do very little posthospital follow-up, with perhaps only a phone call being required. Other NCMs continue monitoring the case until it is closed (ie, the patient regains independence, no longer desires case management services, or dies). In general, episodic case management, as seen in many hospital settings, stops at discharge.

Information-Gathering Techniques

Good communication and interpersonal skills are required to do effective case management. Within the case management process is the need at times to conduct an interview for the purpose of gathering data. This activity has been elevated to the form of "art" and has made several talk show hosts a healthy living. Like any skill, it takes practice. Asking sensitive, personal, and sometimes disturbing questions cannot always be avoided in nursing case management, but there are some basic steps to take and some paths to follow to make it less intimidating and more productive:

Introduction. Introduce yourself and explain why you will be asking so many questions. Reasons may include helping the patient to regain independence and assisting him or her to provide a safe treatment and discharge plan. Ask permission to proceed.

Empowerment. Let the client do most of the talking. Be patient if he or she has a memory block or an inability for self-expression. Allow the patient to finish all sentences.

Trust. Establishing trust is not always easy in sensitive situations, especially if this is a first meeting. However, trust is essential to best help the client. Using layman's terminology avoids a language barrier and puts the patient more at ease. Self-disclosure (in small doses) often makes you appear more human. Reassurances that you are capable of managing this case and conveying commitment to it are necessary.

Respect. Maintain a level of respect and empathy. Being judgmental can be picked up in nonverbal body language.

Body Language. Observe the client for general appearance: nervousness, withdrawal, avoidance, congruence. Use all the senses.

Active Listening. Listening, in contrast to hearing, is an active cognitive process requiring sensitivity and focused attention. Hearing is what adolescents do with their parents; it does not require paying attention and not much sinks in. Active listening requires real participation and uses attending behaviors such as facial gestures, head nodding, and reflecting back what is said.

Data Collection. Use a pad and pencil as a tool to prevent omissions, but avoid taking too many written notes during the interview, because it is distracting and can promote suspicion about what you are writing.

Questioning. Ask about the major problem first (if appropriate). The more detailed, delicate questions may be answered without asking as the patient talks about other topics. Use open-ended questions whenever possible; these require more than a "yes" or "no" answer. Too many "why" questions may sound accusatory. Attempt to combine several questions into one, so that you're not "firing" short questions at the client. Example: Tell me about your family, employment, and what you do to relax and enjoy yourself.

Testing Discrepancies. Sometimes clients' words do not match their body language. In general, words are easier to change than the way they are expressed. If the words are positive but the expression is not, consider the message negative. If the words are negative but the expression is positive, consider the message positive.

Close the interviews with a verbal summary that captures the essence of the interview. This allows the client to add or correct the summary and also shows that you were listening.

Interviews are influenced by both internal factors such as anxiety and external factors such as noisy rooms. For some NCMs, the interview can take place in the client's home. This is often ideal, because the client usually feels less anxious. Some clients reside in an ECF or are temporarily in a hospital, making privacy more difficult. If the patient doesn't have a private room, interview him or her while the roommate is having a procedure done or is out of the room for some other reason. Attempt to have as few distractions as possible. Let the staff nurse know you'll be conducting an interview and time it for between medications or tests. Turn off the TV or radio and close the doors or curtains. Make sure the patient is as comfortable as possible.

CHAPTER 12

Stage 1: Case Screening and Selection

Universal case management is not necessary. Some cases neither require case management nor benefit from it. Previously healthy people who are admitted for uncomplicated procedures such as hysterectomies, cholecystectomies, transurethral resection of the prostate (TURPs), an occasional exacerbation of asthma or chronic obstructive pulmonary disease (COPD), and who have some social support, usually require little or no posthospital support. However, a simple ailment in combination with a poor social environment may signal further assessment.

Several indicators are commonly used to "red flag" situations that may require nursing case management services. Some indicators, although useful to trigger a case management investigation, warrant careful use. By their very nature, they are intrinsically flawed and may defeat some of the goals of case management, such as early intervention and cost containment. Consider the following common indicators:

- Length of stay over 5 (or another arbitrary number) days
- Charges over $50,000 (or another dollar amount)

Both indicators exclude the possibility of early case management. Perhaps with nursing case management, the client who is now on hospital Day 6 could have been discharged by hospital Day 4. In addition, if this client requires intensive needs postdischarge such as an extended care facility, it may take an extra day (or more) to plan and implement the discharge or transfer.

The second indicator, even if it was considerably less, such as $10,000, may still pose barriers to the case management process. Again, early case management is precluded. Chances to effect improved utilization of resources, to establish a relationship with the client and family early in the illness, and to steer any variances back on track are lost.

Other commonly used indicators are too general to be used on their own merit and warrant secondary screening for possible case management needs.

Lives Alone (or With Someone With a Disability). A psychosocial assessment would be useful. If the patient lives alone, is there an informal support system strong enough to match the client's needs? If the patient lives with a disabled or debilitated roommate or family member, can that roommate or family member meet the patient's needs at discharge. Often the patient has been the primary caregiver in the relationship. If so, who is caring for the person left at home?

Age Over 65 Years. People of all ages may need case management. (Some facilities use age indicators of 70 or 75 years.) Most nurse case managers (NCMs) have discharged spunky patients in their 90s. On the other hand, as the AIDS epidemic grows, more young men and women need supportive care.

Payor Source. Some types of insurance may be clues to possible medical or psychosocial needs such as Medicare disability. Also, clients without any insurance resources may need creative case management and discharge planning.

Readmission Within 15 Days. This may be a quality issue or a sign of an inadequate discharge plan during the previous admission. It could also signal patient noncompliance, such as a patient with congestive heart failure who loves pretzels and pizza or the diabetic who does not check his or her blood sugars, take insulin as directed, or follow a diabetic diet.

Physicians. Some physician practices such as those of trauma surgeons or geriatric specialists signal a possible need for case management. Other physicians request the services of nursing case management because of its efficacy and patient satisfaction. Another red flag indicator may be a chart with multiple physicians in consultation or with an extensive multidisciplinary team. Here, the NCM can serve as the conductor, ensuring that all the disciplines are in time and playing the same song.

Diagnosis or DRG. Not all people with a specific diagnosis require case management, especially in the early stages of a disease process; educational activities may be all that is needed. A chart review and possibly a client interview or assessment will show the level of independence and severity of illness. Some diagnoses and medical conditions do require further case screening. These are included in Display 12–1.

Certain mental health, behavioral, and substance abuse conditions warrant, at the very least, a psychosocial assessment. Often a psychiatric evaluation is also required. The specific case details will guide the NCM to the appropriate referrals. The following are some red flag indicators:

Overdose (Unintentional). Unintentional overdoses of prescription medications can result from lack of knowledge about correct dosages or inability to properly self-medicate, as a result of confusion or poor eyesight. Unintentional overdoses can also be of the illegal, polydrug variety.

Overdose (Intentional). Suicide gestures always need careful assessment and initiation of proper referrals.

Alcohol and Drug Abuse. This may present as a primary or secondary cause of admission.

Eating Disorders (Such as Bulimia, Anorexia Nervosa, and "Failure to Thrive"). Psychological causes may warrant psychiatric assessments. Conditions such as anorexia and failure to thrive may also have medical causes. Assessment will determine the extent of case management that may be needed.

Chronic Mental Illness. This may include various psychoses, schizophrenia, neurotic disorders, depression, bipolar disorder, and severe anxiety. Is the mental

DISPLAY 12–1
Diagnoses and Medical Conditions That Require Further Case Screening

AIDS/HIV	Intracerebral hemorrhage
Abdominal aortic aneurysm (ruptured)	Intestinal malabsorption (adult or child)
Amputations	Myocardial infarction
Arthritis (debilitating)	Multiple sclerosis
Autoimmune diseases	Muscular dystrophy
Burns (severe)	Neonatal high-risk infants
Back problems (severe)	Neurologic diseases
Birth trauma	Osteomyelitis
Chronic illness	Organ transplants
Cystic fibrosis	Pregnancy (high-risk)
COPD/emphysema	Pancreatitis
Congestive heart failure and other cardio-vascular conditions	Parkinson's disease
	Premature birth
Cancer (newly diagnosed to advanced cases may need NCM services)	Parenteral and enteral nutrition therapy
	Paraplegia
Cardiovascular accidents with paralysis	Postoperative wound infection
Cerebral palsy	Paralytic diseases
Congenital anomalies (if debilitating)	Pain (intractable)
Dehydration	Quadriplegia
Diabetes mellitus/DKA	Renal failure (chronic/acute)
Encephalitis	Respiratory distress syndrome
Failure to thrive (adults and children)	Subarachnoid hemorrhage
Fractures (multiple or major as in hip)	Spinal cord injuries
Gastrointestinal bleeding	Terminal illness
Head injuries	Traumas (multiple)
Hyperemesis gravidarum	Ventilator-dependent
Hemodialysis	

or emotional condition stable enough for the client to return to previous living arrangements or is the condition unstable and the client a danger to self or others?

Alzheimer's/Dementia. Any form of confusion or disorientation.

Noncompliance. Frequent readmissions may be an indicator.

Uncooperative/Manipulative/Aggressive Behaviors. The perpetrater may be the patient, a family member, a friend, or any combination of the above. Often these people create havoc in a case by refusing tests and procedures (delay of diagnosis), "firing" physicians, or making outrageous demands for unnecessary and costly tests (overutilization of resources). Early recognition of potential manipulative behavior and identification of ways to limit these behaviors are necessary.

Miscellaneous Conditions Such as Munchausen Syndrome or Munchhausen Syndrome by Proxy. The very definition of Munchausen syndrome lends itself to overutilization of resources because these people intentionally produce symptoms of illness in order to assume the sick roll. Munchausen syndrome by proxy is a form of child abuse where, for example, the parent (usually the mother) produces illness in the child. This, as in all forms of child abuse, is a reportable event. The extent to which one with Munchausen syndrome will go in order to receive medical care can be dramatic and often requires investigative work to make the diagnosis of Munchausen syndrome.

Socioeconomic Indicators

Some socioeconomic factors alert the NCM that further screening for case management is required. High-risk situations such as reportable events need immediate and close assessment. The occurrences may include:

- Suspected child abuse or neglect
- Suspected elder abuse or neglect
- Victims of violent crime

  Other socioeconomic red flags include:

- Homelessness
- Poor living environment such as inadequate housing, poor sanitary conditions, and lack of water or electricity
- No known social or familial support systems
- Admission from an extended care facility or other sheltered living arrangement
- Need for transitional care in an extended care facility or sheltered living arrangement
- Out-of-state or out-of-country residence
- Residence in rural community where services are poor or nonexistent, thus limiting posthospital follow-up
- Limited or no financial resources
- No health insurance of inadequate amount of health insurance
- Single parent (assessment of care of minors left at home)
- Dependent in activities of daily living (ADLs)
- Repeated admissions to acute care
- Frequent visits to the emergency room, family physician, or clinic
- Disruptive or obstructive family member or significant other

Some general clues found in a chart or found on assessment may reveal possible future problems. Appropriate case management, referrals, and support may make a tremendous difference in the client's quality of life. Be alert for situations such as:

- Any condition that will necessitate a major life change or a major quality of life change: Will the patient no longer be able to carry out his or her previous type of employment? Can the patient no longer live in his or her home of 40 years?
- Any condition that will negatively affect physical or sexual function or self-image.
- Unrealistic expectations about the prognosis, treatment, or ability to go back home.

With the exception of reportable events, no single condition or diagnosis is automatically a problem that necessitates full case management services. Certainly, those with obvious home health needs or hospitalizations that include any quality or risk management issues need careful attention. The lists that have been provided here serve as a guide, and many clients meeting these guidelines will need some discharge or transition services. The next step is a thorough assessment.

CHAPTER 13

Stage II: Assessment—The Critical Link Between the Patient and the Treatment Plan

Time spent performing a careful in-depth assessment may be time saved later on. Backtracking and changing plans can be confusing and frustrating for the patient, leaving him or her perhaps less than confident with the idea of case management.

There are several sources for assessment information. The patient is the primary contributor of social and functional data. If the patient is incapable of an interview, secondary sources can be used starting with the patient's closest support system: parents (especially if the patient is a child), spouse, significant other, adult children, other family members, close friends, neighbors, foster parents. It is important, when using surrogate sources for information, to ensure that the plan will incorporate what the *patient* might desire.

Sources for medical information include the family physician and related office records, hospital and ancillary medical staff and hospital records (both past and present), any supervisory care staff and those related medical records, and home health personnel and those related records. Dental, hearing, and vision records may also be helpful. Other types of important data can be gathered from physical, occupational, and speech therapists, social workers and discharge planners, and psychiatric nurses.

The patient's home environment is a crucial piece to evaluate for safe discharge planning. Sometimes the insurance company social worker or case manager has visited the patient's home for evaluation purposes and can be asked to share that review. Other important people who make home visits are therapists, home health nurses, social workers, and psychiatric nurses. They may contribute data needed for a safe discharge plan.

The client's employer can often be helpful in evaluating the patient's functional capacity prior to this illness or event. Care must be taken not to violate confidentialities.

Sometimes in the course of gathering information, conflicting stories are revealed. These contradictions can show up in medical records where several different doctors are charting medical, social, and functional data. Inconsistencies need further probing. The nature of the incongruity determines the route to clarification. Some contradictions clarify themselves; for example, a patient whose clinical picture is consistent with an alcohol problem may deny such a problem, then experience delirium tremens. In other cases, interviewing the sources of the conflicting data may be necessary. Care must be taken to avoid accusatory or confrontational tones, because it puts people on the defensive. The reason for the contradiction may be a seemingly insignificant typographic or dictating error. If resolution of the conflict is vital to the treatment plan (Grandma wants full resuscitation measures taken versus only comfort care given), a family or even multidisciplinary team conference may be required to sort it out.

A discussion of several assessment categories follows.

Client History

- Note all medical history. Most hospital charts contain a "History and Physical" section. This may or may not be comprehensive. A thorough medical history may include all previous diagnoses, diseases, childhood diseases, serious/chronic illness, accidents, injuries, hospitalizations, surgeries, obstetric procedures, and mental health.
- Look for complicating factors, chronicity, and comorbidities.
- Look at noncompliance issues. They can often be uncovered in the history. Reasons for noncompliance can be explored and hopefully altered. Noncompliance has many causes, some of which can be resolved such as lack of money for medications and lack of understanding or education about the disease process. Other reasons for noncompliance make behavioral changes more difficult. These reasons can range from burnout caused by the chronicity of a disease, to an "I don't care" attitude (sometimes so severe it appears to be a form of passive suicide).
- Note all medications the client is taking, including over-the-counter drugs, illicit drugs and alcohol, and herbal preparations.
- Be familiar with the use of nontraditional or "holistic" modalities. People are increasingly using alternative healing methods, especially patients with incurable diseases or chronic conditions for which traditional medicine did not help. It is estimated that in 1990 13.7 billion American dollars—mostly out of pocket—were spent for alternative healthcare. Although many give no credence to alternative healing methods, the National Institutes of Health (NIH) in Washington DC, has a $2 million budget for the study of "unconventional" methods of healing. Several medical schools, including Harvard University and the University of Arizona, are now offering courses on alterative medicine. The following are some of the many forms of alternative healing:

Homeopathy	Biomagnetics
Naturopathic/holistic healing	Imagery
Chiropractic	Vitamin–minerals
Acupuncture/acupressure	Reiki
Shiatsu	Tai chi

Ayurvedic medicine	Reflexology
Prayer	Massage
Herbalogy	Rolfing
Medicine wheel	Crystal healing
Meditation	Energy healing/laying on of hands
Bio-acoustics	Myotherapy
Sound therapy/toning	Feldenkrais
Biofeedback	Bach flower remedies

Some of these therapies are thousands of years old, and new forms and variations of them are cropping up. It is recommended that nurse case managers (NCMs) have knowledge of some of these modalities, since more clients are using them.

- Look at family histories for possible diabetes, cancer, Alzheimer's disease, heart disease, hypertension, epilepsy, sickle cell disease, renal disease, alcoholism, mental illness, and others.
- Be aware of allergies: food, drug, and environmental.
- Evaluate how your client uses care facilities. Is he or she inconsistent in the use of medical resources? For example, does your client rush to the emergency room when the clinical condition could be taken care of at a lesser level, such as in the physician's office?

Current Medical Status

- If the patient is at home, interviewing home health professionals can be useful: physical, occupational, speech therapists (PT/OT/ST), and home health nurses and social workers. The family physician and insurance company may also be able to provide helpful information. If part of your job responsibilities includes a physical appraisal, a head-to-toe assessment can be done.
- If the patient is in the hospital or an extended care facility (ECF), all available data can be used: medical charts including lab results, special tests, x-rays, MRI and CT scans, vital signs, progress notes, nurses notes, PT/OT/ST notes, consultations, respiratory therapist notes, surgical reports, allergies, and your own personal observations.
- Utilization review modalities. Use of intensity of service/severity of illness criteria, Milliman & Robertson or critical pathways, should be reviewed. This alerts the NCM to possible needs for changing the level of care, and it may also be necessary for insurance authorization of resources.
- Find out the patient's health goals and major health concerns.
- Check assessments of direct care nurses.
- Evaluate diets. Does the client follow a special diet for health conditions, religious purposes, or personal preference? Is the diet adequate or is a dietary consultation needed?
- Evaluate all skin conditions.

- Determine what tubes and equipment will continue at discharge. Are urinary catheters, tracheostomies and suction machines and supplies, J-tube and G-tube care, drains, feeding tubes, intravenous or feeding tube pumps, oxygen, miscellaneous ostomies, and supplies required? Is any wound care needed?
- Review medicine. Is the medicine regimen complicated enough to require a visiting nurse to help coordinate proper intake? Do medications such as anti-coagulants and isoniazid require laboratory studies? Assess any over-the-counter drugs for possible problems. Assess patient compliance in the use of medications. Can the patient afford the medications? Is there a problem getting transportation to the pharmacy?
- Assess bowel and bladder incontinence.
- Analyze client understanding of conditions and educational needs pertaining to diagnosis/illness.

Demographics

The client's name, age, ethnic group, address, marital status, children (with ages), employment, languages spoken, educational level, and religion should be noted.

Financial Assessment

- Does the client have inadequate insurance coverage or no coverage?
- Look for any governmental entitlements (Medicare, Medicaid, SSI, SSD [see Glossary]).
- Can the client/family meet copayments and deductibles?
- Can the client/family pay for necessary supplies, medications, and miscellaneous not covered by their insurance?
- If necessary, can the family contribute toward an ECF placement or supplemental home help?
- Can the patient meet basic financial obligations during this illness—rent, utilities, food?
- If the patient must be discharged with "hi-tech" equipment, can he or she afford the additional utilities? For example, some air-flow beds may increase the electric bill up to $200 per month. Clients on fixed incomes cannot usually afford this monthly increase.

Functional Assessment: Environmental Factors

It is very important to assess for patient safety in discharge planning. Was the patient safe and at an adequate level of care *prior* to this event? Many elderly patients fall in the home and are admitted to hospitals. If hospitalization has been caused by an unsafe home environment, can it be modified for safety, or is a more supervised setting needed?

It is also vital to look at the patient's level of independence. How well did the patient perform functional tasks *prior to* this event? Was he independent in all activities of daily living and ambulatory, or was there a prior psychomotor deficit?

The Home Environment Assessment

The home environment assessment is a key activity for safe discharge planning. The following should be checked:

- Stairs. Can the patient get into and out of the house or apartment? Are there stairs inside that the client needs to negotiate?
- Telephone. Telephone communication is especially important to consider if the patient lives alone or is alone for several hours at a time. Can the patient see and hear adequately to use the telephone? If not, can adaptations be readily made?
- Utilities. Check electricity, heat, fans, and air conditioning to ensure that they are in working order. Many older people are admitted to hospitals with dehydration or heat stroke in the summer, and pneumonia in winter, both caused by poor environmental conditions. Often gas heaters and heat from gas stoves are major fire hazards. Is the electrical wiring safe for the durable medical equipment use?
- Sanitation. Are running water, working toilets, and clean conditions available? Are rodents or roaches a problem? I have seen more than one patient readmitted with maggots invading postsurgical wounds, caused by poor sanitary conditions.
- Equipment needs. Does the patient have a bed? Does he or she require a special hospital bed, other durable medical equipment, a Hoyer lift, or portable ramps?

Activities of Daily Living (ADLs) Assessment

Both prior and present self-care deficits and present learning capabilities are to be noted. If the patient is presently less independent in daily activities than at a prior time, discharge compensations may be needed. The discharge disposition must match and compensate for the client's deficits. The following questions about the client's capability for self-care must be addressed:

- Can the client dress and undress?
- Can the client put on vision and hearing aids and stump prosthesis?
- Does the client have the ability to perform the following hygiene tasks?

    Bathing
    Shaving
    Brushing teeth or dentures
    Testing temperature of bath or shower water
    Entering and exiting tub safely
    Lowering and raising self from toilet
    Cleaning self after elimination

- Can the client handle nutritional needs: shopping for and preparing food, using utensils, chewing, and swallowing? Is extra help needed such as for shopping and food prep or perhaps Meals on Wheels?
- Is the client able to do housekeeping and yard work?
- Can the client take prescription medications as ordered or is this too complicated, requiring home health RN supervision? Are wrong dose or expired medications still in the patient's possession?
- Can the client handle transportation needs to get to stores, pharmacy, or place of worship?
- Does the client have balance and coordination problems? Does he or she tend to fall or have difficulty with motor skills?
- What is the client's ability to see, hear, speak, read, and write? Is his or her native tongue English? Are translators or bilingual nurses needed?
- If client uses a wheelchair, is this a new development? Is the previous dwelling accessible to the wheelchair? If not, can modifications be made, or does the client need to change living arrangements? Is the wheelchair the correct size and type, with properly fitting cushions and trays?
- Does the client know how to phone for emergency services? This is especially important in areas without 911 capabilities. Does the client have phone numbers for utility companies and medical equipment supply companies in case of equipment malfunction or a need for medical supplies.
- The Big Question—Is safe home care a possibility for this patient? (The psychosocial assessment is the other major factor that affects the patient's ability to be discharged home safely.)

Psychosocial Assessment

In the psychosocial part of the assessment process, the NCM treats the whole family unit as the patient; the family or significant other is an extension of the patient, and all needs and desires should be heard. The family's effect on the patient is too important to overlook; in some social cultures, the extended family is a primary social unit. (*Note:* The word *family* will also include the client's significant other in this section.)

A relationship does not necessarily exist between the severity of the illness and psychological functioning; therefore, the patient's response to the illness or event must be assessed, along with the family's adjustment to it.

- What other stresses are taking a toll in the client's family life at the time of the illness? These possibilities include divorce, moving, a death in family, job change, or a new baby. What family dynamics are revealed? How does the patient and family usually cope with stress? These methods can include religious activities, meditation, sports, talking it over with friends or a professional counselor, anger, physical violence, and the use of alcohol and drugs. Even if the family dynamics were functional and safe prior to this event, will they continue to be so now?

- Who is at home? If the patient is a single mother, are the children safe? If the patient is a casualty of the "sandwich generation" and is responsible for caring for an ill parent, who is caring for that parent now? If the patient is elderly, is there a spouse (or other relative) at home who is unable to care for their own needs without the patient's assistance? Are there pets at home that need attention?
- Assess the family for exhaustion and burnout. Can respite be provided to help ease the burden?
- Ask about hobbies and recreational activities. I had one chronically ill patient who loved to sew as a diversion, but she lost an arm. With her primary form of entertainment made so much more difficult, we needed to find another way for her to relax. For this type of situation, it is necessary to explore other relaxation outlets.
- Assess the *formal* support system. Is it adequate, inadequate, or lacking or dysfunctional?
- Assess client's *informal* resources such as neighbors, church/synagogue groups, friends, and relatives. Can these be expanded if more help at home is needed?
- School or employment records may be assessed if job placement is part of your particular case management responsibilities. Patient-signed release forms may be required.
- Assess client's level of care prior to this illness. Can the patient return to the same environment, or is short-term ECF or long-term care needed? Do the people associated with the previous living arrangement agree to have the patient discharged back into their care? Sometimes even family members have reached their limit, but the decision to send the patient to a ECF is a difficult one, especially when the patient is fairly lucid and wants to go home. Early intervention with family or team conferences should begin.
- Secondary gains to illness often serve conscious or unconscious needs. Sometimes patients do not want to get well. They like the special attention from family and medical staff. Some feel it is a way to gain power over others. For others, dependency needs are met while ill. For still others, a hospital stay represents a warm or cool place to sleep and eat. Occasionally, the hospital is a refuge—a safe place—where a parent or spouse cannot abuse them. Patients such as these are often the "frequent fliers," who are admitted regularly for exacerbations of their basic problem (often rotating from hospital to hospital). A psychiatric consultation with possible referrals to outpatient support groups may assist this person. Depending on the problem, an adult protective/child protective service referral may be needed. If the patient is homeless, referrals to shelters may help, or preferably, a social service plan can provide a more permanent solution.
- Mental status or cognitive assessment may be needed. Not infrequently, a client at home or a patient in a hospital desires an unsafe or detrimental disposition (in the medical team's professional judgment). If that person is otherwise alert and oriented, ancillary assistance may be all you can provide. If the person's mental capacity is in question, the next step would be a psychiatric

referral to evaluate the patient's judgment, competency, and orientation. If the psychologist or psychiatrist feels this person is incompetent, court action must commence. Mental incompetence must be verified in a court of law.

- The brick wall syndrome; occasionally, a psychosocial situation occurs in which a very ill patient requires intensive care 24 hours a day. Family members insist that they can handle the patient at home. Your instincts are that it won't work, that the family will not be able to get enough rest or the patient may not be cared for adequately. Families have the right to try to care for their loved one, and all necessary equipment and available help can be provided. But many times after this plan has been implemented, the family "hits the brick wall" and requests ECF placement. If there is considerable chance that the home placement will not succeed, making necessary copies of the medical record for an ECF placement before the chart goes to the hospital records department may ease and speed a transfer request by the family. Suggestions for supervisory homes may also be given to the family "just in case."
- Be aware of language barriers. These can reach beyond simply not speaking the same language. Misunderstood basic language concepts can hinder the NCM relationship. Ruth Beebe Hill writes in her introduction to *Hanta Yo*:

Admit, assume, because, believe, could, doubt, end, effect, faith, forget, forgive, guilt, how, it, mercy, pest, promise, should, sorry, storm, them, us, waste, we, weed—neither these words nor the conceptions for which they stand appear in this book; they are the Whiteman's import to the New World, the newcomer's contribution to the vocabulary of the man he called Indian. Truly, the parent Indian families possessed neither these terms nor their equivalents.

The word "maybe" is another concept not readily understood by some Native American tribes, and use of this word may instill lack of trust in a relationship.

- Be aware of cultural traditions, differences, and taboos. For example, some people do not approve of eye contact, either feeling that it is impolite or believing that it robs them of their spirit. Some do not like casual touching. Silence is essential in some cultures and uncomfortable in others. In some societies, a smile and a nod "yes" may not indicate agreement, but rather the wish to be polite and respectful.

  Some ethnic groups are uncomfortable discussing topics that the medical profession and NCM may consider necessary. In some cultures, healthcare decisions are the responsibility of the elder family members (parents/grandparents) rather than of the patient. Expressions of pain, from stoic to expressive, vary among different cultures. Knowledge that the client may be acting stoically can help you to determine how to offer optimum comfort.
- For some, the spiritual belief system is a major source of strength. Assess the feasibility of pastoral/rabbinical visits, or tapes and reading material for spiritual nourishment. If daily prayer or meditation was previously an important part of the patient's life, an effort to include time alone without interruption could be arranged for this purpose.

Some religious practices may affect healthcare subtly, such as dietary practices or beliefs that illness is a punishment from God. Overt practices, such as the Jehovah's Witness's rejection of blood transfusions, can affect the treatment plan and have far-reaching consequences. Consideration should be given to all spiritual–cultural differences, because they can affect the patient–NCM relationship.

CHAPTER 14

Stage III: Coordination and Development of Treatment and Discharge Plans

The nurse case manager (NCM) and the social worker have just spent many hours amassing a thorough clinical and psychosocial assessment. The client's individual strengths, weaknesses, resources and lack of resources have been identified. Now the team, which can include several people such as the NCM, social worker, patient, family, physician, and others in the client's case, must decide the following:

- What needs to be done
- How to do it
- Who will provide necessary services
- When each need will be met
- Where the disposition will be

For this planning stage to be successful, the patient and family must actively participate in all decisions, including any changes in the plan. If the patient or family is not in agreement with the plan, it probably will not be successful. The family can add to a successful plan by identifying any informal resources that may be needed to fill in the gaps. These informal resources may be friends, neighbors, or volunteers from religious affiliations.

Establishing Goals

The first step in this stage of coordinating and developing treatment and discharge plans is *establishing goals*; what must be accomplished by when? For example, the family must pick out a skilled nursing facility for Grandmother, and all transfer details must be approved and completed within 72 hours, assuming that the patient is stable for transfer.

Most goals are composed of many smaller goals or tasks that must be met for successful completion of the main goal. Missed details can delay or hinder the smooth sequencing and progression of the plan. An objective such as home safety at discharge or the promotion of an optimal level of independence for the patient may require two, three or a dozen or more modifications in the home setting to make the goal of home safety a reality. Grandmother's transfer to the extended care facility (ECF) may consist of several tasks, such as finding an appropriate ECF, finding a physician who will follow her at the ECF, setting up appropriate transportation and durable medical equipment, copying all the necessary medical records, notifying the family of transfer time, obtaining doctor's orders for her care at the ECF, and obtaining reports from the multidisciplinary team. The ultimate goal of case management is *quality of care* and *efficient use of resources.* This entire book is dedicated to the smaller tasks needed to ensure that these two major goals will be met.

Establishing long-term goals and short-term goals may also be required. Consider short-term goals for a previously independent, elderly gentleman who recently had a total hip replacement surgery. These goals may include the removal of all tubes and drains, stable blood tests, transfers to a chair with assistance, and walking a few steps with assistance. This man's long-term goals—possibly in an ECF—may be walking 300 feet or more with a walker and independence in activities of daily living, which would allow the patient to return home safely.

Prioritizing Needs and Goals

The second step in the planning stage is to *prioritize the needs and goals* that were assessed. Again, the patient's and family's input is insightful here. What is their idea of the most pressing problem? Each person views life and adversity from his or her own perspective and value system. A "can't live without" for one person might be a minor irritation to someone else.

There may be times when the patient's or family's idea of a priority problem does not match the professional staff member's idea of a priority. I had a case that involved an elderly lady who was in the terminal stages of cancer. While the NCM, physicians, and social worker repeatedly tried to speak to the daughter about hospice, the daughter focused on her mother's dental cavity. The prospect of hospice was too much for this daughter, so she narrowed down the problem into something she could handle. Sometimes hard reality is just too overwhelming.

At other times, families or patients may adamantly disagree with the assessed priority needs. An alert and oriented elderly lady may insist on going home alone, when a short-term ECF placement is the obvious safe choice. Or, perhaps a patient is readmitted to the acute care level within 1 week of discharge. During the first admission, the family and patient refused services that the NCM deemed to be priority and in need of immediate attention. Through education and negotiation, a revised plan may be successful the second time around.

Often some limiting factors narrow down the choices, which may make prioritization easier but treatment and discharge plans less than optimal. Consider financial and insurance resource allocation and limitations. The limitation may be as simple as the fact that the insurance company will not pay for both a front-wheeled walker and a wheelchair, which both patient and NCM feel are needed. On the other hand, the limitation may be as critical as a need for a bone marrow transplantation with no payor source. Therefore, concentrating on conditions that can be improved is one way to prioritize. Since not all circumstances can be "fixed," focus on attaining the best quality of life possible.

Service Planning and Resource Allocation

After priority goals have been ascertained, the NCM compensates for assessed deficits, fills in healthcare gaps, and reduces duplication through coordination of services. This third step, *Service Planning and Resource Allocation*, requires knowledge of public and private organizations which may be helpful. Healthcare insurance is often the first place to try for funding needed services, and they usually consent to "medically necessary" requests. If your idea of medically necessary does not coincide with the insurance company's idea of medical necessity, you have the options of negotiation, speaking to the company's medical director for clarification, or finding other resources.

Resource allocation for a client with no insurance or inadequate insurance is a challenge and requires creative case management. The second place to look is at "informal" resources such as the patient's family, friends, neighbors, and religious affiliation groups. Matching the client with government entitlements such as Medicare, Social Security Disability (SSD), or Medicaid may be helpful, but may sometimes require long waiting periods. Geographically convenient resource books are a funnel of information for local social services. Make use of social service personnel, who sometimes can provide invaluable help. A partial list is in Display 14–1.

The unique features of each individual case will determine the service planning and coordination details. If a client can be independent with intensive education and a few follow-up home health visits for education and review of the skills taught, then education and home health are provided. If long-term placement is needed, a facility is matched with the client's skilled needs and available resources. If the family and multidisciplinary team agree that hospice and a duplication of the hospital room at home are required, the NCM will coordinate these services. Discharge plans can be simple or multifaceted and complex, but they are *always* personalized.

Even with the best intentions and the most careful planning, changes, stops, and detours are common. During busy winter seasons, many ECFs may be full, with waiting lists of several days to several weeks. If one ECF gives you a "definite maybe" for 2 days hence, it may be good insurance to place the patient on a second waiting list that also meets the family's approval.

An unexpected deterioration (or improvement) in the patient's medical status may necessitate an entire new service plan. Or, a change of heart/mind of the family members may cause an overthrow of the plan. Sometimes families, overcome by guilt, refuse ECF placement at the last minute or, overcome by exhaustion, they feel incapable of taking the patient home again. Family and team conferences should be convened as soon as possible to prevent additional hospital days. New goals and new plans may have to be evaluated.

DISPLAY 14–1

Organizations With Discharge Planning Resources

- United Way
- Easter Seals
- Ryan White Fund
- American Cancer Society
- Cystic Fibrosis Foundation
- American Lung Association
- Multiple Sclerosis Society
- Muscular Dystrophy Association
- National Hemophilia Association
- National Kidney Association
- Master Eye Foundation of America (guide dogs)
- American Association of Retired Persons (AARP)
- Helping Elder Adults Remain in Their Home (HEARTH)
- American Diabetes Association
- Food Stamp Program
- Women, Infants and Children (WIC) Program
- Adult Protective Services
- Child Protective Services
- Crisis nurseries
- SAIL program
- Meals-on-Wheels
- Adult foster care
- Shelters (homeless, medical, children, abused women)
- Family planning
- Medicare
- Medicaid
- Social Security categoricals (SSI, SSD)
- Adult day-care centers
- County mental health programs
- Senior citizen programs
- Jewish Community Foundation
- Knights of Columbus
- Miscellaneous: schools, churches, synagogues, women's clubs

With some clients who undergo planned, elective surgeries, discharge planning may be done prior to surgery. If complications occur and are serious enough, those plans may need reassessing. Anything can happen, so a Plan B or an alternate plan in the back pocket is a good idea.

Coordinating treatments and services during a hospitalization is another important function of the NCM. Efficiency not only saves valuable resources but can also save entire hospital days. This may be accomplished in several ways. "Clinical Pathways" have proved to be an effective tool in decreasing length of stays. Observation for correct sequencing of tests can also prevent unnecessary additional hospital days. Most NCMs have witnessed patients who have required barium clean-outs (sometimes requiring 2 days), when the barium tests could have been scheduled last.

Often several consultants on one chart are each making their own individual plans. The NCM can bring those plans into alignment in order to cause the least trauma to the patient. For example, if a patient needs major débridement for osteomyelitis and requires 6 weeks of intravenous antibiotics, the NCM can coordinate a long-term venous access placement to be done concurrently with the débridement. Or, perhaps a client needs a transurethral resection of the prostate (genitourinary surgeon) and a hernia repair (general surgeon). If the patient and physicians are in agreement, a single coordinated surgery saves the patient from two general anesthesias, saves operating room time, saves postoperative hospital time, and cuts down on use of lots of miscellaneous resources. However, good clinical judgment is necessary when suggesting a "better way"; poor or unsafe suggestions at the very least diminish NCM credibility.

Finalizing Stage III

The team has assessed the problems, ascertained what needs to be done, orchestrated a time frame (pending medical stability of the patient), and determined the contributions and limitations of the insurance company. Informal supports are verified and available. Referrals are in for skilled nursing facilities, rehabilitation facilities, mental health facilities, home health, Meals on Wheels, and whatever the client needs. Transportation needs are assessed. Durable medical equipment is approved. Educational factors—what needs to be taught to whom—have been evaluated. This stage culminates when assessed needs are linked with the chosen interventions.

CHAPTER 15

Stage IV: Continuous Case Management—Monitoring, Reassessing, Reevaluating

The process of case selection deletes clients who are essentially stable. The remaining cases, by their very nature of severity and instability, require continuous monitoring. Like a domino effect, a change in the patient's medical status could affect the entire continuum from the treatment plan to the final disposition. As the nurse case manager (NCM) monitors the medical and psychosocial stability of the patient, a moderate-to-severe change could necessitate the reassessment of the total balance of services planned for in stage III. The change may be minor, such as a new need for home oxygen, which would be added to any other home health needs that were previously evaluated. Or, a major reevaluation of the whole service, treatment and discharge plan may be needed. Most NCMs have at some time needed to upgrade a discharge disposition from home-based services to admission at a skilled nursing facility because of medical deterioration; the reverse may also take place. Following is an example of the importance of continuous case management.

Mrs. Bolton was a 97-year-old who lived with her 79-year-old daughter. Mrs. Bolton had a medical history, which included hypertension, osteoarthritis, congestive heart failure, and colon cancer necessitating J-tube feedings for nutrition. She was admitted into the hospital in a cachectic condition with hypotension, dehydration, acute renal failure (creatinine, 4.3), and pneumonia.

Within 48 hours of admission, Mrs. Bolton was unresponsive, with a temperature of 34°C. She was made DNR (do not resuscitate), and comfort care and gentle intravenous hydration were provided. It was also decided that intravenous antibiotics would be continued for the pneumonia. The next day her stools became grossly heme-positive and her hemoglobin and hematocrit dropped significantly. The daughter and physicians decided to transfuse 1 unit of red blood cells and monitor her hematocrit and hemoglobin daily. The family did not wish a colonoscope. By the week's end, the doctors assessed the prognosis as "grim."

The following Monday morning, I noted that Mrs. Bolton's name was still on the census board. I checked with the unit secretary and was told that she was indeed still with us. Imagine my surprise when, in the morning report, the night charge nurse mentioned that Mrs. Bolton was ambulating with assistance through the hallways! While the family and medical team were making "final disposition" plans, Mrs. Bolton had other ideas. She remained in the hospital for an additional 7 somewhat rocky days, during which time her pneumonia and gastrointestinal bleeding both cleared. Her creatinine decreased to a reasonable level, and physical therapy helped with strengthening. Once her J-tube feedings were tolerated at the prescribed rate, she was discharged home with her daughter.

It is said that the only constant thing is change; this is certainly true in case management. Constant change is the prime reason why this stage of continuous monitoring and reevaluation is so essential.

Each case has its unique features and important aspects that need monitoring. The following represent some basics that need to be monitored.

Changes in Medical Status (Improvement or Deterioration)

Change in medical status (improvement) is the desired outcome when a patient enters the hospital. When a patient comes in sick, it is hoped that the illness can be changed to a more homeostatic condition. If the lungs are wheezy, physicians try for clear lungs and to achieve acceptable arterial blood gases. If bowels are obstructed, the medical team attempts to clear the obstruction with conservative or surgical methods. A multisystem failure patient or a level I trauma victim may deteriorate further or may stabilize at a level of health that is less than the previous baseline. Each body system, lab results, and vital signs must be monitored. Patient changes may signal the need for change in the treatment plan. Anything that varies from the patient's baseline may indicate a need for compensations in the discharge plan.

Medical status changes must often be monitored for utilization and insurance authorization purposes. Clinical Pathways, Intensity of Service/Severity of Illness, and other utilization modalities may demonstrate a need for a change in the level of care. A patient who is not in an appropriate level of care may be at risk medically if a more acute level of care is needed; or he or she may be overutilizing resources if a less acute level of care is available to treat the medical condition.

Changes in the Social Stability of the Patient

Life changes that occur while a patient is in the hospital or in the convalescent phase of an illness can sometimes be more trying than the illness itself. A lost lease or apartment may leave a patient homeless and worried about his or her possessions. If pets or family members also live there, the emotional trauma is multiplied. During hospitalizations and convalescent periods, patients can lose roommates, significant others may depart, parents may die, spouses may also need to be hospitalized, pets are left uncared for, bills pile up, utilities are turned off, and employment is terminated—all of these may make a significant impact on the total psychosocial picture and often cause stress-related exacerbations of illnesses. Prompt attention from social services and modifications of the discharge plan may be needed.

Quality of Care

Acceptable standards of care and careful, ethical treatment of patients and their medical conditions are the minimal expected norms. Unfortunately, accidents and oversights take place. A clinically astute NCM can often prevent or impede an adverse outcome. Ideally, a maloccurrence can be averted. If that is not possible, quick action may minimize the negative consequences. If an undesirable outcome does take place, it may be wise to call the risk management department and follow the facility's protocol (see Chapter 9: Quality Improvement and Risk Management for further discussion).

Changes in Functional Capability and Mobility

Functional changes are especially important for older adults who were previously independent. Some conditions preclude early mobilization; new surgical patients (especially those with orthopedic conditions), profound weakness, deep vein thromboses, hemiparesis are examples. An aggressive approach to early mobilization is essential to prevent further weakness and decline. Patients often feel that illness and bed rest are a natural marriage, whereas nurses know that bed rest may lead to a host of possible comorbidities. Sometimes the physician's order for restorative nursing, physical therapy, or ambulation is missing and therefore not considered until late in the admission. Patients who may be restrained for safety purposes often are capable of walking with assistance. Guard against extra length of stay due to minimal mobilization until late in the hospitalization. It jeopardizes the independence of some patients and may cause insurance denials at the acute care level.

Evolving Educational Needs

As the client or family is ready, knowledge deficits about the disease process, its course, and treatment should be identified and educational sessions can be added. Opportunities for teaching seem endless. Education for staff nurses concerns the disease process, dressings, medical equipment, nutrition, rehabilitation activities, tube care, medication usage, interactions and side effects, suctioning, and many other techniques and informational aspects of care. As NCMs, the teaching aspect expands into areas such as explanations about the individual's insurance coverage, deductibles, copay plans, diagnostic-related groups, prescription costs, and location of contracted pharmacies and hospitals. Often patients are uncertain who their primary care physician is or how to access the medical system. Overuse of emergency rooms is often a clue to the latter knowledge deficit. Community resources and how to access these may be important to many individuals.

It is important to note that patients retain only about 10% of the information given to them in teaching sessions (Ferrell & Rhiner, 1994). Visual demonstrations, books and audiovisual handouts are helpful. As the patient's and/or family's readiness and receptivity increases they can review the material as needed.

Studies have shown that informational material is best understood when written at the sixth grade reading level, is in large print, and includes several illustrations (Ferrell & Rhiner, 1994). Tapes should be interesting but concise, since people who are ill often have short attention spans. If headphones are available, they can be used to block out distractions.

Education of patients and their families is not merely an option but a mandate by the Joint Commission on Accreditation of Health Care Organizations (JCAHO). According to JCAHO, the goal of educating the patient and family is to improve patient health outcomes by prompting recovery, speeding return to function, promoting healthy behavior, and appropriately involving patients in their care and care decisions. Patient and family education should:

- Facilitate the patient's/family's understanding of the patient's health status, healthcare options, and consequences of options selected
- Encourage participation in decision making about healthcare options
- Increase the patient's/family's potential to follow the therapeutic healthcare plan
- Maximize care skills
- Increase the patient's/family's ability to cope with the patient's health status/prognosis/outcome
- Enhance the patient's/family's role in continuing care; and
- Promote a healthy lifestyle (JCAHO, 1994).

Physical and psychosocial influences must be taken into consideration when assessing a patient's readiness to learn. Pain, weakness, nausea, and drowsiness from medications weigh heavily on a person's ability to learn. A person who is still in shock over a new diagnosis may be too depressed or in the denial stage and therefore unreceptive to learning. Body image is another powerful force. Occasionally, a previously independent client who lives alone may need to go to an extended care facility after a colostomy or tracheostomy because of refusal to accept—and subsequently care for—the tracheostomy or colostomy. Some people simply need more time. Learning cannot be forced; the information must be accepted and absorbed in cooperation with the free will of the client.

Pain Management

Pain management is one aspect of care that often brings out the "judge" in the medical staff. Perhaps it is because pain is a subjective experience that often does not correlate with objective criteria. It is further complicated by individual tolerance differences and psychological, sociologic, and cultural elements. Studies have shown that although pain is cited as the most common reason why people seek medical attention, the management of the pain is often inadequate (Henkelman, 1994).

The reasons for the inadequate relief of pain are many and include factors and misconceptions by the patient/family unit and by medical personnel. Patients and families may be concerned about becoming addicted and therefore ask for too little pain relief (McCaffery & Ferrell, 1994). They may also fear a tolerance ceiling of the pain medication and therefore may anticipate a time when further pain relief will not be possible (1994). Medical staff may feel there are ulterior motives when some types of patients with "drug-seeking behavior" ask for increased dosages. Medical staff may also be concerned about addiction or harm caused by higher doses, such as respiratory depression. Communication differences may also cause less than adequate pain relief. Some cultures are very stoic in their response to pain and won't ask for relief. Others may not look as if they are in pain while they are asking for pain medication, causing doubt among the medical personnel about the level of discomfort. Some patients may smile and use laughter as coping mechanisms while being in excruciating pain (*Acute Pain Management*, 1992).

Case managers may assess that much teaching is necessary for both patients and families and the medical staff. Misconceptions are common about this subject. However, relief of pain is essential. Pain-relieving strategies vary with different causes of pain. Postoperative pain medications are scheduled differently from that of a patient with terminal cancer who is readying to go home with hospice care. The postoperative patient will most likely be weaned off intravenous and intramuscular injections and be discharged on oral pain medication. The cancer patient may be admitted for intractable pain and may reach a comfort level only with a morphine PCA (patient-controlled analgesia) pump (see Figures 15–1 and 15–2 for surgical pain flow charts).

The bottom line is that early and adequate pain management is an obligation that we have in order to relieve suffering as much as possible. It also produces earlier mobilization of patients, shortened hospital stays, and reduced costs (Anonymous, 1994). Because home health agencies rarely send nurses out on a PRN (as needed) basis for a pain shot, a stable patient must stay in the hospital or transfer to an extended care facility for final management of pain when all systems are ready for discharge except for the pain management piece. Sometimes this is unavoidable; other times the medical attention has been focused on other parts of the treatment plan and has caused a delay in assessing this important aspect of care. Just like early mobility, early attention to pain management is essential when a discharge plan is being assessed. Constant monitoring and reevaluation of pain medications and the patient's response are essential.

Many excellent books and articles have been written on pain management (see references at the end of this chapter), and the NCM will need to be familiar with both pharmacologic and nonpharmacologic pain-relieving techniques (see Tables 15–1 through 15–3 for main types).

Patients should be made aware that total absence of pain may be unrealistic, although pain control is considered an important part of their treatment plan. Nonpharmacologic methods may be used successfully as an adjunct to pharmaco-

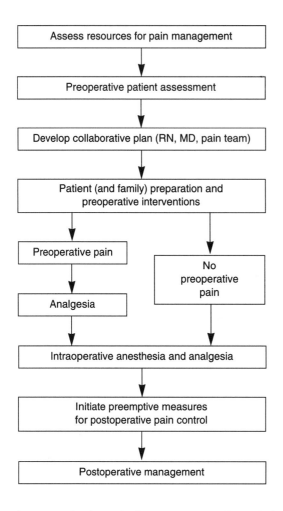

Figure 15–1. Pain treatment flow chart: pre- and intraoperative phases. (From Acute pain management guideline panel. Acute Pain Management: Operative or Medical Procedures and Trauma. *AHCPR Pub. No. 92-0032. Rockville, MD: Agency for Health Care Policy and Research, Public Health Service, US Department of Health and Human Services.)*

logic methods and often are especially helpful for chronic pain conditions. Some of these techniques include the use of heat, cold, massage, vibration, counterirritants, distraction, relaxation, acupuncture, imagery, music, biofeedback, patient education, and TENS (transcutaneous electrical nerve stimulation) units.

Important Pain Management Considerations

- Establish a positive relationship with the patient and family as early as possible and get them involved. Find out the pain management preferences of the patient. Some people prefer to avoid pain as much as possible, whereas others may opt for less obtundation while tolerating some level of discomfort.
- Whenever possible, discuss pain management options and elicit preferences preoperatively. Develop a plan for pain assessment and management. As in the doctrine of informed consent, the patient has a right to know what options are available to make informed choices about these options.

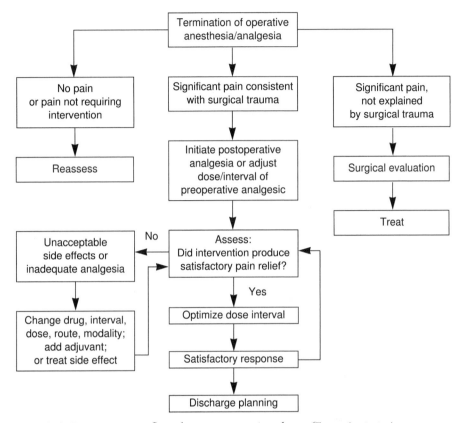

Figure 15–2. Pain treatment flow chart: postoperative phase. (From Acute pain management guideline panel. Acute Pain Management: Operative or Medical Procedures and Trauma. AHCPR Pub. No. 92-0032. Rockville, MD: Agency for Health Care Policy and Research, Public Health Service, US Department of Health and Human Services.)

- Fear and anxiety play a major role in the perception of pain. Often preoperative guidance helps dispel much anxiety. But only elective surgeries allow for this luxury. Many conditions other than surgery create pain. The NCM can help by being there to answer questions, dispel fears, and give appropriate information. Some patients respond well to active participation in their pain management. For those who would feel less anxious by actively participating in their pain management, a PCA device is often successful. Studies have shown that in the short term, postoperative patients who are able to self-medicate report less pain, are more satisfied with their pain relief, and tend to be discharged earlier than those who are given PRN drugs by the RN (*Acute Pain Management*, 1992).
- Teach the principle that pain is easier to control when it is prevented than when it gets out of control and must be brought back in line. This means that analgesics may be administered regularly instead of PRN. By taking the medication at regular intervals, a blood level is maintained, which relieves pain continuously (Ferrell & Rhiner, 1994).

Table 15-1. Pharmacologic Interventions

Intervention	Comments
NSAIDs	
Oral (alone)	Effective for mild-to-moderate pain; begin preoperatively; relatively contraindicated in patients with renal disease and risk of or actual coagulopathy; may mask fever.
Oral (adjunct to opioid)	Potentiating effect resulting in opioid sparing; begin preoperatively; use cautions as above
Parenteral (ketorolac)	Effective for moderate-to-severe pain; useful where opioids contraindicated, especially to avoid respiratory depression and sedation; advance to opioid; expensive
Opioids	
Oral	As effective as parenteral route in appropriate doses; use as soon as oral medication tolerated; route of choice
Intramuscular	Standard parenteral route, but injections painful and absorption unreliable; avoid this route, when possible
Subcutaneous	Preferable to intramuscular when a low-volume continuous infusion is needed and intravenous access is difficult to maintain; injections painful and absorption unreliable; avoid this route for long-term repetitive dosing
Intravenous	Parenteral route of choice after major surgery; suitable for titrated bolus or continuous administration (including PCA), but requires monitoring; significant risk of respiratory depression with inappropriate dosing

PCA, patient-controlled analgesia. (Adapted from Acute Pain Management Guideline Panel. *Acute Pain Management: Operative or Medical Procedures and Trauma*. AHCPR Pub. No. 92-0032. Rockville, MD: Agency for Health Care Policy and Research, Public Health Service, US Department of Health and Human Services.)

- Discuss the side effects of analgesics and the comfort measures to decrease them. These side effects may include dry mouth, constipation, drowsiness, and nausea. Teach that nausea often goes away in 3 to 5 days (Ferrell & Rhiner, 1994).
- If pain is poorly controlled, assess more frequently. Revise the pain management plan, if necessary. Teach the patient that factual reporting of pain is necessary to gain good control and to avoid either stoicism or exaggeration of symptoms.
- Pain assessment tools are often helpful. Visual tools such as those in Figures 15–3 and 15–4 are good guides; or, simply ask the client to describe the pain on a scale of 0 to 10, with zero expressing no pain and 10 being the worst possible pain. Make sure the pain assessment tools are developmentally appropriate. Children 4 to 12 years old often respond well to face scales, which show faces in different levels of distress. Vital signs and behavior as a sign of pain intensity should be used only if self-report (the most reliable indicator) by the patient is not possible (Anonymous, 1994).
- On discharge from the hospital or ambulatory setting, clients should be provided with a written pain management plan. Pertinent discharge instructions related to pain management include specific drugs to be taken; frequency of

Table 15-2. Pharmacologic Interventions

Intervention	Comments
Opioids	
PCA (systemic)	Intravenous or subcutaneous routes recommended; good steady level of analgesia; popular with patients but requires special infusion pumps and staff education; see cautions about opioids in Table 15–1
Epidural and intrathecal	When suitable, provides good analgesia; significant risk of respiratory depression, sometimes delayed in onset; requires careful monitoring; use of infusion pumps requires additional equipment and staff education; expensive if infusion pumps are used
Local Anesthetics	
Epidural and intrathecal	Limited indications; effective regional analgesia; opioid sparing; addition of opioid to local anesthetic may improve analgesia; risks of hypotension, weakness, numbness; requires careful monitoring; use of infusion pump requires additional equipment and staff education
Peripheral nerve block	Limited indications and duration of action; effective regional analgesia; opioid sparing

(Adapted from Acute Pain Management Guideline Panel. *Acute Pain Management: Operative or Medical Procedures and Trauma.* AHCPR Pub. No. 92-0032. Rockville, MD: Agency for Health Care Policy and Research, Public Health Service, US Department of Health and Human Services.)

drug administration; potential side effects of the medication; potential food and drug interactions; specific precautions to follow when taking the medication (eg, physical activity limitations, dietary restrictions; and name of person to notify about pain problems and other medical conditions).
• Document all discussions and teaching in the patient's chart.

These guidelines are in the public domain (ie, may be copied for clinical use) and contain charts and flowsheets that may be beneficial in clinical practice.

NOTE

For information about Clinical Guidelines, including the *Pain Management Guideline Manual,* call:
AHCPR Clearinghouse
(800) 358-9295
or
(301) 495-3453
or write:
Center for Research Dissemination and Liaison
AHCPR Clearinghouse
PO Box 8547
Silver Spring, MD 20907

Table 15-3. Nonpharmacologic Interventions

Intervention	Comments
Simple relaxation (begin preoperatively)	
Jaw relaxation Progressive muscle relaxation Simple imagery	Effective in reducing mild-to-moderate pain and as an adjunct to analgesic drugs for severe pain; use when patients express an interest in relaxation; requires 3–5 minutes of staff time for instructions
Music	Both patient-preferred and "easy listening" music effective in reducing mild-to-moderate pain
Complex relaxation (begin preoperatively)	
Biofeedback	Effective in reducing mild-to-moderate pain and operative site muscle tension; requires skilled personnel and special equipment
Imagery	Effective for reduction of mild-to-moderate pain; requires skilled personnel
Education/instruction (begin preoperatively)	
	Effective for reduction of pain; should include sensory and procedural information and instruction aimed at reducing activity related pain; requires 5–15 minutes of staff time
TENS	Effective in reducing pain and improving physical function; requires skilled personnel and special equipment; may be useful as an adjunct to drug therapy

TENS, transcutaneous electrical nerve stimulator. (Adapted from Acute Pain Management Guideline Panel. *Acute Pain Management: Operative or Medical Procedures and Trauma.* AHCPR Pub. No. 92-0032. Rockville, MD: Agency for Health Care Policy and Research, Public Health Service, US Department of Health and Human Services.)

Changes in Patient or Family Satisfaction

The patient or family may exhibit changes in satisfaction with the treatment or disposition plans. Ensure that the service plan continues to match the needs of the patient/family. Attitudes change and vacillate for a variety of different reasons. Sometimes the patient or family feels as if the attending physician is unresponsive to their questions or calls. Perhaps it is information that the NCM can provide, or a call to the doctor may be appropriate. Occasionally, families are so demanding that the doctor backs away and would appreciate any help from the NCM. Attitudes may shift because the patient/family gets frightened or feels guilt about the service plan. Should we have made Dad a DNR? Should we put him in a nursing home? A family conference may be needed to explore feelings and refocus back on the patient and on what is needed to ensure the best quality of care and quality of life. If revisions in the plan are needed, the NCM should keep the patient, family, physician, and other pertinent members of the multidisciplinary team informed and in full participation of the changes.

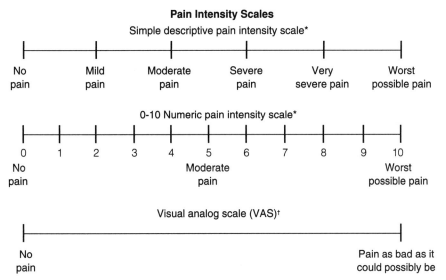

Pain Intensity Scales

Figure 15–3. Examples of pain intensity and pain distress scales. (Adapted from Acute pain management guideline panel. Acute Pain Management: Operative or Medical Procedures and Trauma. AHCPR Pub. No. 92-0032. Rockville, MD: Agency for Health Care Policy and Research, Public Health Service, US Department of Health and Human Services.)

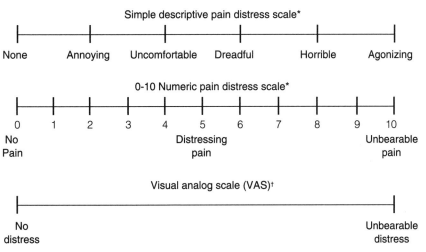

Figure 15–4. Pain distress scales. (Adapted from Acute pain management guideline panel. Acute Pain Management: Operative or Medical Procedures and Trauma. AHCPR Pub. No. 92-0032. Rockville, MD: Agency for Health Care Policy and Research, Public Health Service, US Department of Health and Human Services.)

Goals

Last, assess and reassess if all the goals determined to be essential to this case continue to be realistic and appropriate as the case evolves and unfolds.

References

Acute Pain Management Guideline Panel. *Acute Pain Management: Operative or Medical Procedures and Training.* AHCPR Pub. No. 92-0032. Rockville, MD: Agency for Health Care Policy and Research, Public Health Service, US Department of Health and Human Services.

Anonymous. (1994). Acute pain management in adults: Operative procedures—Quick reference guide for clinicians. *MEDSURG Nursing, 3*(2), 99–107.

Ferrell, B., & Rhiner, M. (1994). Managing cancer pain: A three-step approach. *Nursing 94, 24*(7), 57–59.

Henkelman, W. (1994). Inadequate pain management: Ethical considerations. *Nursing Management (Critical care edition), 25*(1), 48A, 48B, 48D.

Joint Commission on Accreditation of Health Care Organizations. (1994). *Accreditations Manual for Hospitals: Volume 1—Standards.* Oakbrock Terrace, IL: Author.

McCaffery, M., & Ferrell, B. (1994). How to use the new AHCPR cancer pain guidelines. *American Journal of Nursing, 94*(7), 42–46.

CHAPTER 16

Stage V: Implementation of the Final Plan

By this stage in the case management process, the nurse case manager (NCM) has accurately assessed the patient's and family's needs for a safe discharge. Weaknesses have been delineated and problems solved. The treatment plan may have made a few detours off the "clinical path," but variances were expediently identified and promptly brought back in line. The total case has been assessed, reassessed, negotiated, and coordinated. The treatment and discharge plans are realistic and workable and have been approved by the multidisciplinary team, the patient, family, and third party payor (insurance).

The NCM has the companies and facilities chosen and approved of by the team and the payor. All informal supports are in place. You are comfortable that this plan will work, but still, you are flexible and have a pretty good idea what "Plan B" might entail, if needed. The team and family are depending on you to have all the details taken care of and to get it right.

The Day Before Discharge

- Medical stability and discharge screens are monitored (see section on InterQual in Chapter 6: Utilization Management).
- Education continues and return demonstrations identify any misinformation or incomplete learning processes. Teaching is stepped up for discharge the following day. Home health is notified of learning weaknesses.
- Evaluate pain control and attempt to change to oral pain management, if possible.
- Anticipated tests (hemoglobin and hematocrit, room air, arterial blood gases for supplemental oxygen, prothrombin time/partial thromboplastin time, and so on) are ordered. Results are reported to attending physicians.
- Transportation needs are evaluated. If the patient is from out of state or county (or even out of country), transportation plans need clarification as early as possible. If the patient requires an ambulance or stretcher van, calls should be made 24 hours in advance; cancellation may sometimes be necessary but is preferable to holding up a discharge because an appropriate transport vehicle is not available. Wheelchair vans may also require 24-hour notice. Families can confirm approximate pick-up times on this day if they can transport the patient home.

- Find out when the attending physician and consultants need to see the patient after discharge and, if necessary, help the patient make follow-up appointments.
- Confirm outpatient physical therapy, occupational therapy, and speech therapy appointments, and give the patient the times, days, and a contact phone number.
- Any needed outpatient IV therapy (such as antibiotics, chemotherapy), wound care, and scheduled tests and procedures need orders and appointments. This is often needed for patients who are not homebound and therefore do not qualify for home health services.
- Coordinate the durable medical equipment (DME). All large equipment that must be brought to the home or apartment needs to be timed so that someone is there to accept it at the door. Smaller DME (eg, small volume nebulizer (SVN) machines, portable oxygen tanks) can be sent to the hospital. Often a patient cannot go home without continuous oxygen; a smaller E-tank must go to the hospital prior to discharge and the larger unit needs to be coordinated at the house. When assessing equipment needs, ask about room sizes and space availability. This should be done as soon as a DME need is assessed. Many patients require a hospital bed but must move out furniture to make it fit into the room. Even three-in-one toilets do not always fit if the patient lives in a small trailer. Shower equipment also needs to fit in the type of bathroom facilities the patient has (full-size bathtub, smaller trailer size tubs, or shower stall).
- Get all supplies ready for wound care, tracheostomy, ostomy, or other procedures. Some home health agencies want the patient to go home with a few days' worth of supplies for continuity purposes. This is especially important on weekends.
- Confirm hemodialysis days and times with the accepting facility.
- Call the home health agency and/or IV infusion company to confirm impending discharge, and update the company(s) on the social and medical status of the patient. Discuss any change of instructions.
- For transfers to an extended care facility (ECF), call for validation that the patient's bed is still available. Update the ECF on the social and medical status of the patient. Ask whether the ECF supplies transportation from the hospital to the facility, or set it up. Confirm that there is a doctor to follow up; if not, find one. If possible, get transfer orders written, get reports from the multidisciplinary staff, and copy pertinent parts of the medical record.
- Get confirmation from the patient, family, and attending physician that they still agree with the discharge plans (whether home or ECF transfer).
- Make a list of all pertinent agencies, companies, and community referrals and their phone numbers. Give this to the patient and family.
- Call the insurance company with up-to-date medical and discharge data; obtain authorization for the final hospital day (many insurance companies pay for the day of admission but not the day of discharge) and obtain authorization for any discharge disposition services.
- Gather any other details specific to a particular case.

The Day of Discharge

- Monitor medical stability and discharge screens.
- Give written discharge instructions. Work on fine-tuning any assessed educational insufficiencies.
- All test results have been reported to the physician. Those that are not normalizing have been discussed, and documentation verifies the physician's notification and permission to continue with discharge as planned.
- Transportation to home or another facility is set up. The patient/family/physician is notified of final times for pickup.
- The patient and family are given written instructions for follow-up with physician(s).
- The patient and family are given written dates, times, and addresses for any outpatient needs (physical therapy, occupational therapy, speech therapy, IV therapy, tests, hemodialysis, and so on).
- DME is delivered to the home or hospital.
- Supplies are delivered to the home or hospital.
- Home health agencies are called for medical updates and for confirmation of time and day when a first visit will commence. Often a home health agency will not begin servicing a client until the day after discharge if the care can be completed in the hospital on the day of discharge. If a patient needs a "BID" (twice daily) treatment or IV antibiotics, the home healthcare worker will come on the day of discharge.
- For ECF transfers, calls are placed with medical updates and to confirm transfer on that day. Final validation is obtained that physicians/family/patient all agree with the transfer, that transportation is set up, that the doctor will follow up, that the chart is copied, that orders are complete and correct, and that all reports are included.
- Gather any other details specific to a particular case.

CHAPTER 17

Stage VI: Final Evaluation— Postdischarge Follow-up and Case Closure

The stage of final evaluation, postdischarge follow-up, and case closure is an important one; it ensures case continuity and gives the patient and family a caring message. The job responsibilities of your particular type of case management determine what you do in stage VI and how you do it. Episodic case management is done for a specified episode in a client's life. Some hospital nurse case managers (NCMs) follow a client in the hospital during an illness episode with little follow-up after discharge. Other case managers start their responsibilities after the patient is discharged. Home health case managers follow up in the home; extended care facility case managers follow up clients while they reside in that facility; hospice case managers follow up their clients from admission into hospice until death (unless the patient or family opts otherwise); other NCMs manage their clients through all levels of care until independence, formal release of the case, or death.

Postdischarge follow-up from a setting such as a hospital, rehabilitation center, or extended care facility may be done by telephone or in person. The follow-up may be as minimal as one or two phone calls or visits or as significant as an extensive rehabilitation transitional period. This follow-up is usually appreciated, and often needed, by the patient and family. Many times after discharge unexpected events occur, questions surface, and ordered services fall through the cracks or do not meet expectations. Equipment does not arrive or is different from the type that the family was taught how to use in the facility. Perhaps the patient/family expected more hours of help or had a different idea of needed help from that of the home health agency. The patient may be more difficult to take care of than the family had anticipated; perhaps proper encouragement and a couple of added services would be all that are needed to turn the situation from one of panic to one of success. In addition, a family may be having a difficult time securing a medication. They may not know which pharmacy is contracted with their health plan, or the medication is not "covered" and they cannot afford the expense. Or, a patient may feel the physician is not responsive to their phone calls. Any number of unanticipated situations may surface.

This follow-up contact can be a vehicle to answer questions, discuss possible solutions, and often prevent complications and even readmissions or trips to the emergency room. One phone call or several phone calls may be needed before case closure. Phone calls to the physician, the home health agency, the durable medical equipment company, social service agencies, or any other part of the case plan within question may be required.

Familial Needs

Several research studies have been conducted about what families with ill family members need to help them cope with illness and hospitalization. The original landmark study was conducted by Molter in the late 1970s. The universal need identified as extremely important was the need for *hope* (Molter, 1979). Another study distilled the responses of 17 previous studies and revealed that 14 of the top 21 needs were concerned with obtaining information about the family member (Hickey, 1990; Kleinpell, 1990). NCMs are often the disseminators of the information that the family feels it needs in order to cope. Families are a total system in which a change in one member (eg, the ill patient) directly affects all other members (the family), often disrupting the equilibrium of the whole (Kupferschmid, 1987). By the NCM sharing accurate information, the family becomes empowered to make informed decisions; in this way, the NCM helps the family to gain understanding and a feeling of control over a difficult situation (Bouley, Van Hofe, & Blatt, 1994).

Fifteen of the most important family needs will be discussed in this chapter. The needs may have been ranked differently, depending on the study performed, and the year that a study was done has influenced its findings. Earlier studies show comfortable furniture in the waiting room, with the waiting and bathroom locations ranking higher in importance than in later studies. A reason for this may be that many hospitals have addressed these issues, and they no longer loom as major concerns.

It is interesting to note how often a NCM can make an impact on the 15 most important needs. When appraising the final evaluation of a case, assess the success and impact that case management had in meeting these needs.

1. To Feel There Is Hope. Hope helps people to cope with a present life crisis by helping them to believe that the future holds promise; it is the universal need expressed. There is a delicate balance that NCMs must achieve between giving too much or too little hope. Often we must talk about the gravity or difficulty of a situation. It is not always easy to do this without destroying hope. Assess how well this was done in some of your more difficult cases.

2. To Have Questions Answered Honestly. People respond to sincere honesty and expect it. In 10 studies, 100% of the respondents rated this need as extremely important (Hickey, 1990). Even grave news has the benefit of preparing family members for the worst. Less than honest answers—or false hope—can leave a family member in shock and disbelief if they were not told of the possibility of a poor outcome prior to its occurrence. This is especially difficult if the doctor or family member wants information kept from the patient or another family member. Assess how well this was done in a difficult situation.

3. To Be Assured That the Hospital Personnel Care About the Patient and That the Best Possible Care Is Being Given to the Patient. Families want to be *assured* that their ill relative is important to the staff and will be treated kindly. They also need to know that the care is appropriate for the illness. Clinical pathways, when shown to patients and families, have been noted to ease the worries of this point. If the patient is moving along the pathway fairly steadily, the family can see that the care is standard protocol and the family member is responding as expected.

4. To Know the Prognosis. Often after the family is told the prognosis by the attending physician, the family has many questions that do not always surface immediately. The NCM can act as a safety net, being there to allow the family to vent, grieve, or ask questions as they come up—perhaps to make one of the most difficult of decisions: whether or not to make the loved one a DNR (do not resuscitate).

5. To Know Specific Facts About the Patient's Progress on a Daily Basis. This knowledge was also an extremely important need to 100% of the respondents in 10 studies (Hickey, 1990). Some of the angriest family and patient complaints have resulted from their feeling that they were not updated regularly about the patient's progress and could not get the information they needed. Frequent visits by NCMs to answer questions and clarify any misconceptions can prevent unnecessary anger and anxiety. Assess the client's/family's satisfaction on this point.

6. To Have Explanations Given in Understandable Terms. There is an art to explaining complicated concepts in easy-to-understand language. Some physicians are excellent at this; other times it may be necessary for the NCM to assess for gaps and misunderstandings in the patient or family. When a patient is in pain or a family is in crisis from the acute, severe nature of the illness or injury, even clear and simple explanations may be more than a person can process. The explanations then must be concrete and clear, and only the most immediately necessary facts conveyed. Speaking slowly and calmly and making eye contact aid this process. Assess whether the family–patient unit received this kind of attention.

7. To See the Patient Frequently. This is more difficult in some areas of case management than in others, such as when the patient is in an intensive care unit. But the inability of a family to see, touch, and assess how their loved one is doing is a constant reminder of the threat of permanent loss of that person from the family unit (Mathis, 1984). This is especially true in sudden, acute situations such as traumas. I remember when, as a fairly new bride in the late 1970s, I was called at work with information that my husband was involved in a motorcycle accident. I arrived at the scene and stayed with him for 45 minutes until the ambulance came. During that time, he was in and out of consciousness, his pupils were dilated, and it was obvious that several bones were broken, including his clavicle, which was protruding through the skin. In the 7 hours that followed—during which he was in the emergency room—the only information volunteered to me was the name of the ward that he was being transferred to. The only time I saw him was when I sneaked into his room in the ER, and then I was promptly ushered out. The anxiety felt was intense; it could have been eased greatly by regular updates and closer physical proximity.

Perhaps because of that experience my unit uses more cots—and we've been known to run out of them!—than most other units. But both patients and families usually respond with decreased anxiety when they can be near each other. NCMs who work in ICUs or emergency rooms can plan times that are acceptable to the area and the family for visitation. Assess family satisfaction on this point as part of the final evaluation.

8. To Know Exactly What Is Being Done for the Patient and Why It Is Being Done. This is important in order for patients and families to make informed decisions. The NCM aids the family by sharing accurate and consistent information. This is a shared responsibility with the physician and has legal ramifications when this information is used for the purpose of signing an informed consent. As in all the informational needs, assess how well this was covered in the case plan.

9. To Talk to the Doctor Every Day. Usually a patient, if alert and oriented, speaks daily to his doctor. Issues arrive when family members and significant others are unable to make contact with busy physicians. After a couple of days pass with no word from the patient's doctors, family members are likely to become upset, displaying attitudes that lead the staff to label them as "difficult," "manipulative," or "interfering." Again, anxiety is often the cause of this behavior, and it can be diminished with a physician phone call to the family, sometimes supplemented with information offered by the NCM.

One communication disaster paired a doctor with a less-than-empathetic bedside manner with an angry man whose grandfather—his only living relative—was in the hospital. As the patient's hospitalization stretched longer and longer, the worried grandson threatened lawsuit after lawsuit, fired multiple physicians, and became tangential in his conversations. The doctor withdrew, doing his best to avoid communication. The situation was reaching a danger point, since staff nurses were becoming frightened of the grandson. When the case was transferred to my unit, I made a deal with the physician that if he would speak daily—at least briefly—to the grandson, I would fill in the gaps. The grandson agreed to this arrangement, after I assured him I was available for further informational needs. Working on the tangential nature of his personality was a little more challenging; however, I limited the number of main points for each conversation (frequent reorientations back to those main points were necessary), and the main points were written down for him to hold onto. At first, the grandson asked the same questions over and over without seeming to hear the answers. But within 3 days, he was much less hostile and the frequency of repeated questions was dramatically reduced. Finally, the patient was transferred to an extended care facility with the same physician following up, and the grandson was in agreement with the plan.

In the final evaluation, assess whether the family and patient were comfortable with the one-on-one attention from the attending physician.

10. To Be Called at Home When the Patient's Condition Changes. Since NCMs are not present 24 hours a day, calling to update families may fall on the staff nurses or physicians to fulfill. Many nurses are very conscientious about this. If the family is upset over poor communication, staff teaching and support may be needed.

11. To Have a Specific Person to Call If the Family Cannot Make It to the Facility. The three-shift structure of facilities that give 24-hour care translates into many caregivers for the client. Families often feel more peace of mind if they have a single contact person whom they can ask for by name. The NCM is a reasonable choice and beneficial for both parties. The family has a knowledgeable contact, and the NCM often picks up important information about discharge planning from these conversations. Information appears to be a vital need for families, and the NCM can be a primary link between that information and the family. If too many people are calling from one family unit, it helps to have the family appoint a spokesperson to call the NCM. The other family members can then call this designated person. In the final case evaluation, assess your role in this pivotal communication position.

12. To Be Told About Transfer Plans. When a patient is being transferred to another unit in the hospital, let the family know. It frightens family members when they visit and find an empty bed, especially if the patient is very ill. When the transfer is to another facility, the plans should be agreed to by the family and coordinated with them. One uncomfortable type of situation occurs when a family approves of the hospital that the patient is in, but the insurance company wants the patient transferred to one of their contracted hospitals. The present hospital could suffer financially if the transfer is not made, and few families can afford to pay for a hospitalization. In the final evaluation, assess transfer coordination with the family.

13. To Feel Accepted by the Hospital Staff. Family members often feel to be "strangers in a strange land" and need to feel supported if they are to be a support for the ill family member. I remember one very difficult case involving a husband and wife. The wife was a large woman who was essentially a quadriplegic caused by multiple sclerosis. She had many chronic conditions, including infections that frequently necessitated intravenous antibiotics. Although she required 24-hour care, the husband adamantly refused nursing home placement. He was a difficult person himself, and many home health agencies no longer could deal with his demands. Therefore, my challenge became finding a home health agency that would accept the wife each time she was discharged. The staff always groaned when this patient was admitted; although she was extremely pleasant, the husband could not be satisfied. One afternoon, while making rounds with the nurse manager of the unit, the husband went into his usual tirade of complaints and demands. The nurse manager approached him in a way no one else had. She touched his arm and gently asked how long he had been caring for his wife in this condition. He looked surprised but answered, "seventeen years." "And who," she asked, "takes care of you?" Breaking into tears the man said quietly, "No one." Suddenly someone had accepted him. This nurse manager's compassion opened a door and the man responded with a remarkable mellowing.

Some patients and family members are also afraid that if the staff disapproves of them, they will not receive good care. This fear is not uncommon. If the NCM or the staff cannot connect with the family, perhaps a minister, rabbi, or psychologist may be able to do so. In the final evaluation, assess whether the NCM was instrumental in helping the family to feel accepted and welcome.

14. To Have Directions as to What to Do at the Bedside. Families are often afraid to touch the ill family member, especially if there are many tubes and machines around. Neonatal intensive care nurses routinely show parents how to handle the "preemies" and sick newborns. Parents of older pediatric patients are also routinely given directions for safe handling of the child. Many family members, especially spouses, would like to do more for the patient but aren't sure what is allowed. The staff nurse and NCM can explain any invasive lines, assess the extent to which the family member would like to help with basic care and help dispel any fears. Assess family satisfaction in this area.

15. To Talk About the Possibility of the Patient's Death. Some people have a great need to talk about their loved one's possible death; it is almost as if, by rehearsing it, they might be better prepared when it happens. Others will not verbalize the possibility, as if, by talking about it, they might bring it on. Sensitivity to the family's needs on this point is critical, and some prefer to speak to a member of the clergy. In the final evaluation (if this is applicable), assess whether the family's needs had been met.

Case Evaluation

In general, families want reassurance that their loved one is well cared for, that they have access to the patient, and that they have all the information they can handle. If these points are addressed, the family is usually satisfied. Overall, how well did the patient/family unit respond to the case plan? The following are some other general questions to ask in case evaluation and follow-up:

- Were the goals and objectives met?
- Were all the essential needs of the patient identified and addressed?
- Were the interventions effective and efficient, or are revisions needed during the postdischarge stage?
- Were all services delivered as planned?
- Were there any problems with the home care agencies or durable medical equipment companies?
- Are new needs surfacing postdischarge, which are serious enough to destabilize the whole plan?

Some cases do not go smoothly and the NCM is not surprised. Perhaps the patient wanted more than insurance would pay for and refused other options that were offered. Or, perhaps the patient's needs and the available resources were a poor match.

What if the discharge appeared to go fairly routinely, yet postdischarge the patient or family expresses disappointment or resentment? The following are some possible questions to ask:

- Did the patient and family really agree to the plan, or were they pressured or coerced or did they simply lack understanding?
- Was the family or patient unrealistic or in denial about the options?
- Did the patient's medical status change after discharge or transfer, necessitating revisions?

- Was poor or inadequate planning responsible for the postdischarge disappointment?
- Was the suboptimal discharge due to the fact that the patient had virtually no resources (socially or financially [insurance]) and refused other available assistance (shelters, community assistance)?
- Was the supervisory facility less than adequate, or was poor "chemistry" with the staff to blame?

There are as many reasons for discharges to falter (in whole or in part) as there are details to a particular discharge; each detail, if improperly evaluated and executed, can destabilize the whole plan. The case management process is not an easy one. But a skilled and experienced NCM can usually overcome obstacles, regardless of what they are or when they occur, and most clients and families are very appreciative of the case management process and the guidance and support extended to them. The final question, the answer to which will test the efficacy of the whole NCM process, is: Did case management efforts improve or at least optimize the quality of life for this person and the family unit? Within this question, lies the heart of case management.

References

Bouley, G., Von Hofe, K., & Blatt, L. (1994). Holistic care of the critically ill: Meeting both patient and family needs. *Dimensions of Critical Care Nursing, 13*(4), 218–223.

Hickey, M. (1990). What are the needs of families of critically ill patients? A review of the literature since 1979. *Heart & Lung, 19*(4), 401–415.

Kleinpell, R. M. (1990). Needs of families of critically ill patients: A literature review. *Critical Care Nurse, 11*(8), 34–40.

Kupferschmid, B. (1987). Families of critically ill patients. *Critical Care Nursing Currents, 5*(2), 7–12.

Mathis, M. (1984). Personal needs of family members of critically ill patients with and without acute brain injury. *Journal of Neurosurgical Nursing, 16*(1), 36–44.

Molter, N. (1979). Needs of relatives of critically ill patients: A descriptive study. *Heart & Lung, 8*(2), 332–339.

PART III
Study Questions

1. How does the NCM process differ from the traditional nursing process? How is it similar?

2. Self-assess your strengths and weaknesses in the area of communication and interpersonal skills. Discuss ways to turn weaknesses into strengths.

3. Cite an example of a case that was not selected for case management but should have been. How did this case fall through the cracks?

4. Discuss the importance of a thorough assessment. What are some barriers to a thorough assessment?

5. Discuss the steps needed to coordinate and develop a treatment or discharge plan. What are some barriers to this stage of the case management process?

6. Develop a list of community agencies in your area.

7. Discuss changes that must be monitored in the case management stage of continuous assessment and monitoring. Evaluate how one change can affect the structure of the whole case plan.

8. Cite a case example in which a discharge was held up because all services were not evaluated and set up by the day that the client was ready for discharge. What could have been set up the day before discharge? Would this have allowed the discharge to go on as scheduled?

9. Discuss the important issues cited by families. How can an NCM help meet those needs?

10. Consider a case that you managed. Were all the steps and stages included? What would you do differently?

PART IV

Practical Applications

To laugh often and much, to win the respect of intelligent people and the affection of children; to earn the appreciation of honest critics and endure the betrayal of false friends; to appreciate beauty, to find the best in others; to leave the world a bit better, whether by a healthy child, a garden patch or a redeemed social condition; to know even one life has breathed easier because you lived. This is to have succeeded.

RALPH WALDO EMERSON

CHAPTER 18

Job Stress Versus Success Factors for Case Management

All helping professionals can succumb to job stress and burnout, and nurse case managers (NCMs) are certainly not exceptions. This chapter will focus on "success factors," which can reduce stress considerably.

Stress itself is not harmful. Too little stress can leave you listless and apathetic, whereas a small dose of stress can provide an edge, a positive boost to action. Volumes have been written on the havoc stress imposes upon physical, psychological, and mental health. An optimal level of stress is the perfect motivator and is essential for success. Finding this optimal level is an individual matter and entails being able to read your own personal stress meter. Through self-awareness, it is possible to notice when the reading gets close to the "stress-overload" level. The actual red flag indicators are different for various people: poor judgment, bursts of anger or frustration, depression, forgetfulness, preoccupation with worrying, nonproductive time, or an inability to make decisions all are signals. Recognizing these reactions not only in yourself but in others allows you the opportunity to act as their support system. I have a coworker whose voice gets quieter and her handwriting larger when she's approaching "stressed out." That's when I step in and ask if I can help out. This is her response to feeling overloaded.

How one handles the perceived insurmountable stress is also an individual matter. Scarlett O'Hara would affirm, "Fiddle dee-dee. I'll think about it tomorrow." Some call on a peer to help process stress; one of my coworkers gives her problems to God. Others quit and find other nursing positions, as in the following case.

Administrators at a 350 bed, nonteaching hospital in southern California decided to make some changes at their facility. Their goals were to decrease present lengths of stay, improve quality of care, and escalate nursing retention. They felt that instituting nursing case management could best accomplish these goals (Biller, 1992).

Three NCMs were selected and told they would be in charge of decreasing the present length of stay and ensuring that the patients received high-quality care. At first, the nurses felt privileged and excited in their new role. But within 2 months, they felt overworked, unprepared, unheard, and unsupported. They all abandoned their NCM roles because of unrelieved frustration and burnout (1992). That the administration goals were positive really didn't matter. Because these nurses were essentially thrown into their new roles with little preparation, education, or support from staff or management, they were doomed to failure.

No matter how much clinical expertise a new NCM has, the role of the NCM includes many new skills and learning curves. It is essential that a NCM have support from the facility's upper management, the nursing staff, and fellow NCMs. It is also imperative that the novice NCM get some training. This hospital learned the hard way that case management support and training are important. This chapter offers usable suggestions that will assist in a successful nursing case management career.

An Understanding of Case Management and Managed Care

The nonteaching hospital in southern California finally came to the conclusion that "preparation is the key to success" (Biller, 1992, p. 146). To understand the ramifications of a DRG (diagnosis-related group) reimbursement compared with a per diem reimbursement; to know the utilization modalities; to grasp the goal of holistic, quality care for an ill human being and his or her family—all that is covered in this book. And the unique knowledge and skills needed for your type of case management are essential for you to be a confident and successful NCM.

Maintaining the most current knowledge base in your area of clinical expertise allows intelligent discussion with the physician, which increases the NCM's credibility. The mental preparation also ensures a proper case plan for the patient. It may take some homework time to do this but, as former stellar UCLA basketball coach John Wooden says, "It's what you learn after you know it all that counts."

Ideally, you will be service-based and working with clients in your area of clinical expertise. Knowledge of standard treatments and expected outcomes allows the NCM to predict the patient's length of stay. This gives the NCM a handle on how much time is needed to manage the case. Keeping current on ever-changing tests, medications, and medical breakthroughs gives the NCM the sharp edge.

At times, NCMs may cover for other types of patients. An adult medical–surgical case manager may feel a little stressed if asked to cover the neonatal intensive care unit. Sincere questions to specialty nurses or attending physicians usually elicit enough information to allow the NCM to speak to families and insurance company representatives and to plan alternative levels of care. If you are routinely asked to cover the stressful area, time spent in learning more about it will be time saved in apprehension and questions.

An at-your-fingertips knowledge of resources available to your clients is a good confidence builder. Visiting the facilities firsthand to actually see the layout and what is offered often allows a better match for the client's needs. A vast world of different services is offered among various extended care facilities, rehabilitation units, hospices, and acute care hospitals.

Perhaps the best resource that a NCM can have is a knowledgeable social worker. Social workers are trained to match the social issues with the community resources available. An up-to-date resource book specifically written for your community or state may be an added comfort for the NCM's office in case a social worker is unavailable.

Take some time to identify your individual case management assets and limitations. Accept both while you turn your limitations into strengths.

Early Intervention

Early intervention in each case has been emphasized repeatedly throughout this book. This is because it is so important to the formulation of a good case plan and to the mental health of a nurse case manager. If you were the type in high school who waited until the day before the term paper was due to start it and are still a last-minute type of person, use caution. "Crisis case management"—cases that need intervention NOW—occur all too frequently anyway. With too many of these, you run the risk of stress overload, poor judgment and possibly suboptimal case plans. Avoid procrastination.

During this early phase you are free to assess a possible discharge or transfer plan without pressure and time constrictions. Unless a case is very strong for the first plan assessed, I usually "try on" a Plan B. Although this is not in vogue in the 90s I do this by thinking negatively. I evaluate Plan A looking for possible areas of failure and solve problems in advance. If Plan A does fail—as in my "worry" scenario—then Plan B is already considered and ready to be put into action; 98% of the time one of these plans, or a modification, is usable. This alleviates scrambling for ideas on the day before or the day of discharge.

Early medical coordination is an important NCM responsibility. With complicated surgical or trauma patients, this may mean fewer surgical procedures, tests, or delays. This coordination makes the doctors happy and the insurance companies happy, and usually the patient is more satisfied with the overall hospital experience. For those using Clinical Pathways, they should be initiated as early as possible and followed daily.

Early intervention and communication with the insurance company are also useful. First, you prove to be a good contact person; this makes your facility or the company you are working for more user-friendly than places where it is sometimes difficult to elicit information about their members for authorization purposes. Second, the NCM can find out what outpatient services are covered early in the illness process. This is essential before Plan A or Plan B can be truly considered. It is a real sore spot (and stressor) when a NCM puts together a wonderful case plan only to find out that there is no pay source. If the patient or family has already agreed to the case plan, this can leave them feeling disappointed and less than confident in your abilities. It is best to know the strengths and limitations in the case as early as possible.

Develop and Maintain a Support System

Maintaining a positive and healthy attitude is not always easy when working with difficult or tragic human predicaments each day. Add to that an insurance atmosphere that is squeezing us tighter with every new idea or criteria that managed care can throw at us—sometimes it feels downright unmanageable.

Remember the three case managers in the beginning of this chapter? They were placed in the role of NCM lacking more than knowledge about managed care and the case management process; they lacked support from upper management and their peers. Upper management gave them no specific role definition to work with. And hard feelings emerged between the NCMs and the other primary nurses on the units, because the staff felt as if they were losing their autonomy (Biller, 1992). No one in the organization acted as support or mentors for these fledgling NCMs, and this hospital's initial attempt at nursing case management failed swiftly and miserably.

There are few case managers, no matter how new, who do not have an area of expertise worthy of being called "mentor" to one less knowledgeable in that area. Each one of us came to the nurse case management profession with a pocketful of information that others may lack. I call in my peers for ideas on cases in which I'm insufficiently knowledgeable about clinical areas or resources, and I am grateful that there is someone I can turn to. Sometimes I just need a sounding board to vent frustration. Reciprocally, I am a mentor to others in my areas of expertise. This mutual support system is a fortunate and effective means of reducing stress and enhancing a positive attitude.

Problem-Solving Techniques

There are times when a case seems to be "stuck," and no amount of rational thinking produces the magic answer to the tenacious problem. When a case has a serious variance from the clinical pathway, a case conference may be indicated. The conference can include any or all of the multidisciplinary staff working on the case. The family or even the patient may be a necessary part of the conference, depending on the problem being addressed. The conference should be planned at as convenient a time as possible, with a time limit specified—15 to 20 minutes is usually sufficient. Guidelines for problem solving include the following steps: (1) variance analysis, (2) focusing on desired outcomes, (3) brainstorming, (4) finding the next intervention, and (5) evaluating the plan (Zander, 1989).

Step 1: Variance Analysis

The first step is to identify the problem. It is important to have a clear idea of *what* you are solving before you can solve it. If possible, break it down into smaller problems. When more than one problem is identified, assess whether there may be a common denominator at the root of the problem or problems.

Step 2: Focus on the Desired Outcomes

What do you, as a group, feel would be the best end result to the problem or problems assessed in step 1? What short-term goals are possible? What long-term goals are possible to achieve? Are there limitations that must be overcome? For example, limited social, financial, or insurance support, limited desire from the patient to manage the illness or limited mental capacity to learn. Can the limitations be successfully overcome or at least diminished?

Step 3: Brainstorming

Anything goes during brainstorming sessions. Participants are encouraged to be as creative as possible in order to explore new ideas and ways of looking at the problem, potential resources, and possible interventions (Zander, 1989). The primary rule during a brainstorming session is that all suggestions are acceptable and all judgment is withheld until all suggestions are squeezed out (the stage of brainstorming that my peers refer to as "brainstemming"!). Judgment often arrests the creative flow, and many potentially useful suggestions may never be spoken.

When all the participants have brainstemmed (ie, have no further suggestions), the ideas can be listed in order of feasibility. Those that may provide the solution are discussed first.

Step 4: Finding the Next Intervention

Often the brainstorming session elicits potentially workable interventions that may be attempted. This intervention must be realistic and take into consideration all the strengths and weakness of the individual case. If no promising intervention is found, ask whether the problem needs to be redefined (Zander, 1989).

Step 5: Evaluation of the New Plan

At the close of the case conference, it is hoped that a new, realistic, individualized plan for the problem case has been defined. This plan compensates for weakness and fills in needed gaps. The case's strengths are assessed and used to their fullest capacity. Occasionally, a case comes along that remains tenaciously difficult; the solutions to the problems remain elusive. Then the case conference may serve as a support system for the dejected NCM, realizing that he or she is not alone, uncreative, or incompetent. The good news is that although some cases seem basically unresolvable, I have never had a case that didn't eventually come to closure. Or, as Will Rogers said, "Things will get better despite our efforts to improve them." The support system is essential; no case is worth burning out a good NCM; too many other patients need our expertise.

Time Management

There is a story about a strapping young man who wanted to be a lumberjack. On his 18th birthday, he set out to get a job in the logging industry. Being young, strong, and healthy, he quickly got his wish. He was given his axe and set out to work. On the first day, he single-handedly felled 12 trees. The boss was very pleased and commended him on his energy and strength. On the second day, the young man seemed to work just as diligently but cut down only 10 trees. On the third day, he cut 7 and on the fourth day, still trying very hard, only 3 trees came down. By the fifth day, with all the effort he could muster, no trees were cut.

The boy went to his boss, feeling terrible, and explained he had not cut one tree today. The boss asked why. "I am working as hard as I can. I'm really trying, sir," was the reply. Then the boss asked, "Have you taken the time to sharpen your axe?" The boy had not. He had been working so hard he didn't take the time to work smart.

Sharpening your axe or your time management skills saves in time and effort. Time is a limited commodity and NCMs usually have a lot to do in their allotted time frame. Some people seem to be naturally disorganized, but, like any skill, time management can be learned. There are articles, books, seminars, and community college courses available on the subject. The time spent sharpening the axe—learning organizational skills—will be rewarded in multiples in reduced stress and frustration. Here are some work efficiency tips.

Assess the Time Robbers

The time robbers include anything that stops us from reaching our objectives most efficiently (Charlesworth & Nathan, 1984). Each person has individualized "robbers" that they allow, ranging from minor distractions and problems with attitudes to the inability to make basic decisions in a reasonable time frame. Once these problem areas have been recognized, the next step is to work to make them strengths.

Make Lists

I love lists. They are my security blanket. After a task goes on my list, I don't waste energy worrying that I might be forgetting something. And lists are the perfect tool for the essential time management skill of prioritizing. They can be labeled, starred, numbered, and crossed out, and details can be added to the main subject—whatever works for the individual NCM.

Sharpen Prioritizing Skills

Establish clear-cut goals, both short-term and long-term. Ask what has to be done this hour, this morning, this afternoon, this day. Do those first (in that order). "This hour" may include a meeting, finalizing a priority case that will be picked up very soon, or the unexpected "now" situation that suddenly occurs. A code blue on one of your patients is a priority; other priorities fall a step below."This day" priorities may include insurance calls or finding resources for clients who will need them in a few days.

Making my priority list is the first thing I do in the morning; it is how I plan my day. I rarely assign item numbers because I find that too rigid. Stars are put on the most pressing cases, but often new situations arise and cases not on the original list are put on and starred. This may include situations such as a new client who needs attention immediately or an unexpected need for a family meeting or case conference.

Be Succinct

If you ask certain people what time it is, they will tell you how to make a watch. Rambling and being tangential are major time wasters and are annoying to the busy recipient of the verbosity. This is not the same as small talk, which in measured doses adds to comradery and job satisfaction.

Be Efficient

One way to be efficient is to plan ahead. NCMs spend a lot of time on the phone and on hold. In this instance, you can make a choice: (A) bring something to do in case you are placed on "eternal hold." This might be a case to review or your list to go over and possibly reprioritize. Or, (B) use the time to take a breath and recharge. A eliminates the frustration of wasting valuable time when so much needs to get done. B is useful and necessary for reduced stress and increased production. The important point is that by planning ahead you have made a conscious choice of how you will use your time; you were in control of the situation. No "terminal hold" stress reaction was initiated.

Efficient use of time also includes not wasting time pursuing avenues that have been closed or are in need of major reconstruction work. For example, if you feel a client needs a special piece of equipment that you cannot negotiate from the insurance company, take another route. Know when persistence may work or when to look elsewhere. Know the limitations of a case early on, and use your time and energy on more viable possibilities.

Delegate

Some people try to be all things to all people. Not only is this impossible, it is a time robber and is often not in the best interests of your client. If the client needs a minister, rabbi, social worker, or any variety of ancillary services, provide that person. Initial processing may be needed to ascertain what is needed, then it is time to delegate. Some people see delegation as of loss of power and control (Charlesworth & Nathan, 1984). Be conscious of this possibility and put your client's needs first. Others simply don't trust others to do the job correctly (1984); they live by the credo that if you want something done correctly, do it yourself. If this is true and back-up people cannot be relied on to do a good job, then that issue should be addressed. It is important to distinguish your own job responsibilities, which are the NCM's responsibilities, from those responsibilities that can or should be delegated. The best interests of the client should always be the deciding factor.

Trust Your Hunches

Let's move from the left, logical side of the brain to the right side for a moment. Balancing the brain can prevent all types of headaches. Nurses have cultivated "nurses intuition" since the days of Florence Nightingale. As staff nurses, we sensed that a patient was going to deteriorate. That intuition should still be used when negotiating an additional hospital day from an insurance company. You are there with the client and can see subtle changes that sound alarms in your nursing data bank. Once, I didn't listen to my intuitive feeling, and the patient was back in the emergency room in 3 hours with a pulmonary emboli.

Perhaps your hunch says that the discharge plan may fail in whole or in part. Try to put your finger on the disconcerting feeling and have a modified Plan B available for use.

Sometimes it behooves the NCM to listen to the patient's intuitions and not waste valuable time making elaborate discharge plans that will never come to pass. Do not underestimate the power of a client to predict the timing of his or her death. One 92-year-old asked for help to the bedside commode early one morning, then promptly said, "Oh, please help me back to bed. I'm going to die now." Within minutes, she was unresponsive; within 30 minutes she had died.

It is surprising how often these hunches become reality. Listening to that small voice called intuition can be a truly efficient time management ally.

Be efficient. Work smarter, not harder. Keep your case management tools sharpened.

Changes

We seem to be living in an age of instability. The face of healthcare is changing so rapidly that in a few years we may scarcely recognize it. Although some people embrace change, most find it intimidating. Nursing case management is more important than ever before in order to *manage these changes* in the best interests of the clients. New and fast-changing financial constraints must also be managed in order to keep necessary institutions fiscally healthy. Staff nurses feel squeezed from unrelenting downsizing, and many physicians can't play by the new rules; they want the "good old days" back. The situation will not go back to the way it was. We cannot change that. But "strangely enough, this is the past that somebody in the future is longing to go back to" (Ashleigh Brilliant). Looking at the changes from that future perspective, perhaps the state of healthcare in the 90s is worthy of another assessment. Compare your job duties to the nurses of 1887 (see Figure 18–1).

Everything changes—even death and taxes; 50 years ago we did not have the technology to hold human beings on the threshold of death, and taxes change every year. We cannot do much about the fact that change happens. We can do a lot about our response to change. Because of the unpredictable nature of change, some people respond to it with fear. Others, realizing that inherent in change is need to give up something (exchange one thing for another), react with anger. More positively, still others choose to reframe the situation. Changing how you mentally look

Nurses' Duties in 1887

In addition to caring for your fifty patients, each nurse will follow these regulations:

1. Daily sweep and mop the floors of your ward, dust the patient's furniture and window sills.

2. Maintain an even temperature in your ward by bringing in a scuttle of coal for the day's business.

3. Light is important to observe the patient's condition. Therefore, each day fill kerosene lamps, clean chimneys, and trim wicks. Wash the windows once a week.

4. The nurse's notes are important in aiding the physician's work. Make your pens carefully; you may whittle nibs to your individual taste.

5. Each nurse on day duty will report every day at 7 A.M. and leave at 8 P.M., except on the Sabbath, on which day you will be off from 12 noon to 2 P.M.

6. Graduate nurses in good standing with the director of nurses will be given an evening off each week for courting purposes or two evenings a week if you go regularly to church.

7. Each nurse should lay aside from each payday a goodly sum of her earnings for her benefits during her declining years so that she will not become a burden. For example, if you earn $30 a month, you should set aside $15.

8. Any nurse who smokes, uses liquor in any form, gets her hair done at a beauty shop, or frequents dance halls will give the director of nurses good reason to suspect her worth, intentions, and integrity.

9. The nurse who performs her labors and serves her patients and doctors faithfully and without fault for a period of five years will be given an increase by the hospital administration of five cents a day, providing there are no hospital debts that are outstanding.

Figure 18-1. Nurses' duties in 1887. (Source: Cobb Memorial Hospital, Pheonix City, AL.)

at the situation often changes how you respond to it. Here are some attitudes to try on when changes occur that may have you feeling frustrated or off-balance.

Sometimes the Dragon Wins. You've worked hard with the case and used the clinical pathways. Then it seems the case is falling off the path at every turn, and variances (or dragons) are winning. The magnetic resonance imaging (MRI) machine breaks down; there's still barium in the patient's colon necessitating another bowel prep before proceeding with the test; the family refuses to pick up Mom after she's been discharged (why didn't they mention anything on the phone this morning!); the patient refuses every other test and there is still no definitive diagnosis; the patient who insisted on going home rather than to an extended care facility is back in the emergency room within 24 hours. Every NCM can add his or her own story. There is no shortage of dragons. First, assess whether you could have done anything differently for a better outcome. If so, learn from it. If not, realize that sometimes the dragon wins.

Choose Your Battles. Once, during an extremely frustrating case, a wise physician counseled me with this pearl of wisdom. Many aspects of nursing case management are completely out of the NCM's realm of control. Assess whether the problem is something that you can make an impact on. If not, save your "battle energy" for more productive endeavors.

Remember This Wise Adage. Dr. Robert Eliot, a cardiologist at the University of Nebraska, had developed two rules for keeping things in perspective (Charlesworth & Nathan, 1984):

1. Don't sweat the small stuff.
2. It's all small stuff.

Although this is not meant for us to take our responsibilities lightly, from a cardiologist's perspective the present problem is probably not worth having a coronary over. Then *you* are in the hospital with a NCM managing you!

Anticipate Changes. Don't wait for changes to happen. This has been said in many different ways. Be proactive. Have Plan B ready when change in the patient's condition or the family's attitude occurs. By anticipating changes, you remain poised and alert for them. This allows you to refocus quickly—often without missing a step—rather than becoming flustered. This rapid refocusing necessitates a certain degree of flexibility and spontaneity. Here you stand at the crossroads between what is and is not in your control. You could not control the change in plans, but you could quickly redirect the case in a new direction.

> We cannot direct the wind . . .
> But we can adjust the sails.
> (Unknown)

Judgment Daze

Critical thinking and use of critical judgment are essential when matching lab data, radiology, and the patient's symptoms to the case plan. No nurse should leave home without them. But being critically judgmental when it refers to a client's life choices has little place in the nursing profession. A large number of hospitalized patients or clients in rehab are there because of their life choices: alcohol, poor diet, noncompliance (watch judgment on this one!), illegal drugs, high-risk sexual practices, and smoking. I have seen excellent clinical nurses, utilization review nurses, and case managers burn out through excessive condemning and sitting in judgment. They became so miserable (and made others miserable) that they felt they needed a change of jobs. I watched one particularly critical nurse go through four job changes; unfortunately, she took her judgmental attitude with her and was no happier for the changes.

Being judgmental seems to be a universal human habit. But when I find myself criticizing someone else I remind myself that I have no right to do so because I have no way of knowing the whole story. Someone wrote to Ann Landers once, angry that taxpayers' dollars in the form of food stamps were being used frivolously. It seems this writer was a cashier at a grocery when she observed another woman purchasing a $32 bag of shrimp and a $17 birthday cake with her food stamps. The grocery clerk railed against this use of food stamps for luxury items, and in support of her stance an onslaught of angry letters ensued applauding the courageous complainer. Then came another letter from the "perpetrator of the crime." The shrimp and cake purchaser remembered the withering look of the store clerk. But what the clerk didn't know was that the expensive birthday cake and the shrimp (a favorite food) was for her little girl who had terminal bone cancer. She was not expected to live out the year; this birthday would be her last. I cut out this letter and I keep it in my daily planner as a reminder.

I, too, have found myself dazed and unobjective at times. What is worse is when a healthcare professional makes an unkind comment only to find the patient or a family member within earshot. Minimizing judgmental behavior will definitely lower the incidence of foot-in-the-mouth disease—and burnout.

Humor

Not far from the Ann Landers column, I have a picture of a disgruntled-looking little guy saying, "God put me on this earth to accomplish a certain number of things. Right now I am so far behind I will never die." I suspect most NCMs will live a long, long time. Taking oneself lightly certainly lifts burdens, but what about the use of humor with patients, families, physicians, and peers? Are "needling" patients and going for the "jocular" vein in good taste?

Like other treatments, humor can be assessed using the rights learned in nursing school; assess the right timing, the right recipient, and the right dose (not too much). Some patients and families relish a lighter perspective, a break in the focus on illness and anxiety.

Mrs. Farris' esophageal cancer had progressed to the point where she needed a permanent feeding tube. After an 8-day hospitalization with a variety of medical complications, she had become quite confused. Because this was her third visit on the same unit, the staff and family had become well acquainted with each other. As yet another day ended with Mrs. Farris still confused, her husband pleaded with the charge nurse to give her something for sleep so that he could get some rest. "She's been calling me every 15 minutes from Las Vegas asking for money," he related. The charge nurse, deadpan, asked, "Tell me something, Mr. Farris, has she won anything?" "No!" he responded. "That's why she keeps calling me for money!"

After the mutual laughter, the walls tumbled down. The laughter allowed Mr. Farris a moment of release, and he was able to share his fear about his wife being so ill and explained that in 50 years of marriage he had never seen her in such a state. The ability to laugh during bleak times sends a message that life is tolerable, even now. Often the family needs that healing message as much as the patient.

Studies have shown that humor and that universal means of communication, laughter, have a wonderful array of positive benefits when used judiciously. Humor and laughter can:

- Help keep stressful situations in perspective.
- Reduce stress and tension. Some nurse educators rely on humor during the teaching process, feeling it allays fear and anxiety related to serious diseases (White & Howse, 1993).
- Help facilitate more serious communication and in some situations, neutralize conflicts (1993).
- Build and maintain group morale and bonding by promoting a sense of affiliation and cohesion (1993).
- Provide a catharsis and release pent up energy (1993).
- Increase heart rate, increase oxygenation to rates seen in aerobic activity, release endorphins (the morphinelike biochemical responsible for "runner's high"), and exercise hundreds of muscles throughout the body (Braverman, 1993).

The Norman Cousins story about how he managed a rare disease with vitamin C and laughter is common knowledge. A lesser-known study shows what happened in a burn unit. An enterprising physician created a humor room and filled it with comedy tapes, funny books, and funny toys. The burn patients were encouraged to recall humorous moments in their lives and to laugh as often as possible. The result: a 13% to 33% increase in cell regeneration over the average (Braverman, 1993).

The Hawaiian Hunas have a saying: "Where your attention goes, energy flows." In essence, this is because joy and sadness pathways cannot operate simultaneously (White & Howse, 1993). Humor and anger, for example, are antithetical; try holding onto anger during a prolonged belly laugh!

Although some nurses have difficulty with the use of lightheartedness when it comes to patients, consider the following story about a young mother of four who was dying of cancer. Once, in a workshop she was attending, the woman asked the group how they felt about a 28-year-old mother with four young children who was dying of cancer. The participants responded with a barrage of joylessness, anger, pity, sadness, and horror. Then she asked, "How would you feel if you were that 28-year-old mother and everyone who came to visit you felt that way?" (Braverman, 1993).

For everyone to constantly focus on the illness does not always serve that person. As a patient advocate, and a human being, try to maintain a balanced perspective that includes joy, hope, support and, whenever possible, the gift of laughter.

References

Biller, A. M. (1992). Implementing nursing case management. *Rehabilitation Nursing, 17*(3), 144–146.

Braverman, T. (1993). Warning: Humor may be hazardous to your health. *The Arizona Light*, August 1993, 14.

Charlesworth, E., & Nathan, R. (1984). *Stress management: A comprehensive guide to wellness.* New York: Atheneum.

White, C., & Howse. (1993) Managing humor: When is it funny—and when is it not? *Nursing Management, 24* (4), 80–92.

Zander, K. (1989). Case consultation: Determines the next action. *Definition, 4* (1), 38–41.

CHAPTER 19

A Day in the Life of a Nurse Case Manager

Several years ago, I attended a case management seminar given by one of the pioneer case management teams in the southwestern United States. When the speakers asked for audience questions, I asked each speaker to describe a typical workday. Their stories were interesting and educational, but what surprised me was how varied their individual experiences were. Only one case manager's day resembled my own! After some reflection, I realized that even my own tasks differ dramatically from day to day. As I listened, I realized that there are many forms of case management, with different managers putting emphasis on different facets of the case management system. To some, discharge planning is a priority. Others act as utilization review nurses. One nurse case manager appeared to be involved with basic staff nursing (direct patient care) but had strong ties to the multidisciplinary team. No singular set of role definitions could describe this group. Soon I realized the reason: case management is in its adolescence, complete with identity crisis and a growing, awkward form. Case managers attempt to do everything for everyone—an impossible task—while insurance regulations, state laws, and professional standards are ever changing.

I believe our identity as nurse case managers will arise out of our own field. Certification examinations are already a reality, and standards on case management practice as well as legal and ethical guidelines will be written to guide us through life as case managers.

I am a hospital case manager. My patient population is a medical mix, with some surgical patients. My patients are all ages and may have multisystem failure, pulmonary disease, HIV, suicide gestures, gastrointestinal bleeding, cancer, pancreatitis—in other words, almost any medical problem. When other units are full, orthopedic, neurologic, obstetric, cardiac, surgical, or even older pediatric patients may appear in my ward and need case managing.

An Ideal Day in the Life of a Nurse Case Manager

An "ideal day in the life" for me would be to use the morning to review patient charts; input utilization review data; check on any quality of care issues; set up transfers and equipment needs; elicit plans from doctors during their morning rounds, then pass these on to insurance company liaisons and others who are part of the plans. After these preliminaries are handled and as needs arise, I would visit patient rooms and catch family members for brief consultations. Then an "ideal" ½-hour lunch without shop talk.

The afternoon would be the time to tie up loose ends, finish utilization review from the morning, complete transfers to other facilities, and do patient rounds. Patient rounds are room-to-room visits designed for introduction, initial assessment of possible discharge needs or further plans for discharge, patient education on various topics, emotional support for impending invasive procedures or surgeries, assessment of patient satisfaction, and handling the many different issues that pop up unexpectedly. This is my ideal day, not my "typical" day.

An Actual Day in the Life of a Nurse Case Manager

I have picked a day to share that is without long meetings because such a day would not provide the educational intent of this section, which is to draw a clear picture of the nurse case manager serving on the front lines. However, long meetings are often a vexing reality; therefore, setting daily priorities is essential.

6:30 AM. I pick up my laptop computer and patient census. I delete discharged patients from the computer and make sure all new admissions are programmed in. I quickly look at new admissions for ages and admitting diagnoses and log in necessary social service referrals. Then, I attend to the notes taped to my door!

7:00 AM. Shift report. I set my first priority list for the day—which frequently changes. Today's list looks like this:

- Mrs. Adams—Speak to physicians about a "do not resuscitate" order—impending code!
- Visit Mr. Innes—Multicomplaints to staff.
- Transfer Mr. Block to extended care facility (ECF) today. Dr. T to follow.
- Mrs. Cohn to ECF today. Find a doctor to follow.
- Ms. Diamond—Call mental health agency—Is it possible involuntary transfer today. Make sure psychiatric sitters are available.
- Mrs. Elliot—Possible ECF transfer tomorrow. Finish plans.
- Mr. Frank—Review arterial blood gas values. Does patient need home oxygen?
- Mrs. Garrett and Mr. Harris—Put in for social referrals.
- Talk with physical therapist about Mr. Harris—Is it safe for him to go home?
- Mr. Johns—Probable discharge today or tomorrow. Arrange for home IV antibiotics; get authorization from insurance company.

7:45 AM. I leave hurriedly to attend a short daily NCM meeting. I ask the charge RN to *please* make a notation to ask Mrs. Adams' doctors (if they come by) about a "do not resuscitate" order. (If the doctors don't show up by the time I get back, I'll call them.)

8:10 AM. Back on the unit. The physicians called Mrs. Adams' daughter. She wants "everything done." I expect the worst in this case (ie, that she will code shortly) but privately hope that my gut feelings are wrong.

I am moving along on my priority list:

- I look at Mr. Block's chart. His temperature spiked last night. Doctors wish to hold patient transfer and culture blood and urine. This will take at least 48 hours. The following calls need to be made about change of plans:

  1. Patient/family
  2. Social worker
  3. ECF—Will they hold bed? (Yes, thanks!)
  4. Transportation—Cancel stretcher van.
  5. Insurance company—Need authorization for additional hospital days.

- I document all of the above in the computer or on the chart.

The psychiatric RN phones me. The mental health agency has completed the paperwork for an involuntary admission to a mental health facility for Ms. Diamond. The sheriff should be arriving to pick her up around 9:30 AM. (Not much time!) Ms. Diamond is unaware of the plan. Her doctors feel it is not in her best interest to tell her beforehand because she has a history of suicide attempts and adamantly refuses help. The psychiatric RN will be there but recommends a call to security, since this procedure sometimes gets ugly. I alert security and the attending and resident physicians of plans. All are relieved that after 4 days in this hospital Ms. Diamond will finally be in a proper setting for her problems.

The unit secretary gives me Mr. Frank's arterial blood gas results, which show a PO$_2$ of 49. I call the doctor for a verbal order for home oxygen, then the durable medical equipment company for delivery of two portable oxygen tanks to the hospital for Mr. Frank's ride home, since the patient lives 50 miles away. I coordinate the home oxygen setup with the company and the patient's family.

Better check to see whether Mrs. Cohn is stable for transfer. Yes. I haven't found a doctor yet to follow her up at the nursing home. *Priority*: Find one!

Now facing me are four large men in civilian clothes. They're here to "escort" Ms. Diamond to the mental health facility. They've come early. Why four? They explain that two are in training. Ms. Diamond is a fragile, petite woman; I don't want her to be frightened. I ask "the boys" to be patient, then call the psychiatric RN, who arrives to speak with Ms. Diamond about the plan. I call security. Ms. Diamond is visibly upset, crying. She is making loud accusations, heard throughout the ward, toward the staff and her significant other. I comfort the significant other, realizing that he has tried to do what is best. Meanwhile, the psychiatric nurse works magic in calming the patient. Finally, Ms. Diamond, escorted by the four deputies, leaves peaceably, quietly crying. We are all left with a little sadness. Ms. Diamond is a pretty, intelligent young woman in a lot of emotional pain. I document each detail into the computer.

Back to Mrs. Cohn. Which doctor goes to the ECF? I look in my files and pick one whom I often have success with.

EMERGENCY! Before I have a chance to make the call, I hear a "Code Blue." It is for Mrs. Adams! I run to her room. Compressions have already started. I cut open the code cart while the code team rushes in. I begin recording. We get a fleeting heartbeat 5 and 8 minutes, then lose it. Every ACLS medication is used. The chaplain, already alerted, has called Mrs. Adams' daughter, who is already on her way to the hospital. I ask the chaplain to try to stop the daughter before she arrives at the room. At 20 minutes, the heartbeat is erratic, but she's intubated. A bed in the ICU is available. (Thank goodness the daughter didn't walk in on this.) Mrs. Adams is transferred to ICU. I look up to see the doctor speaking to Mrs. Adams' daughter. In tears, she accompanies him to the ICU. I document the transfer into the computer.

Back to the nurses' station. I hear someone say, "Is this a full moon?"

Another answers, "It looked full last night."

A resident physician turns his head skyward and howls like a wolf. Laughter breaks some of the tension.

10:30 AM. Back to finding a doctor for Mrs. Cohn. I page the doctor I have chosen. He calls back and agrees to follow up Mrs. Cohn at the nursing home. Relief! (Sometimes finding a doctor to follow up at an ECF is an all-day task.) I call the resident to write transfer orders and dictate the discharge summary. I call the family; they are pleased with the transfer news. The ECF is close to home, making visiting easy. Mrs. Cohn also is happy to be "graduating" from the hospital. The social worker sets up transportation; I inform the ECF of the doctor's name and phone number, Mrs. Cohn's health status today, and her time of departure. The charge nurse and staff nurses are told of the transfer and time. I document.

I am starting to feel pressured because I haven't yet done any utilization review or looked at my new patient charts.

Mr. Johns' doctor tells me he can leave the hospital today if I can set up twice-daily intravenous ceftriaxone at home. The physician has already spoken with his patient about leaving today, and Mr. Johns won't take "tomorrow" for an answer! Okay. I can do that! I check the facesheet for the name of the insurance company and call them. The insurance representative likes the idea of sending him home; it saves 5 hospital days. I am also given the okay to use our hospital's home health agency. I call the home health agency and the agency's coordinator does the rest. I enter Mr. Johns' room and tell him to be patient and that we'll get him out as soon as possible. Does he have transportation home? No problem. I document.

I look at my list again—social service referrals. These will take only a few minutes so I get them done.

Finally, I have time to do some "admission" reviews on my new patients. I add a few thoughts to my priority list: one patient may not be able to return to independent living; another is being worked up for probable new diagnosis of cancer, with possible referrals to chaplain services and oncology life enrichment; another patient is a 19-year-old new admission, entering for diabetic ketoacidosis. I make a note to call the diabetic nurse educator to start teaching. I document everything.

The charge RN lets me know Mr. Frank's oxygen hasn't arrived. I make another call; it's in the truck, on its way.

From overhead, I hear: "Any trauma surgeon—to medical ICU." I call to see whether this is about Mrs. Adams. Yes. She "coded" again in the ICU. She has one chest tube inserted and needs another. The daughter still wants every effort made. It looks grim.

12:00 PM. Phone call for me. Lunch, already! Ready in 15 minutes. I want to squeeze in some admission reviews; then a quick lunch. The luncheon rule is no shop talk allowed. It seeps through at times, anyway. I sit down and take a deep breath. Whoo! At what time this morning did I stop breathing?

12:30 PM. Back to the front lines. I had better see to Mr. Innes' "multicomplaints" while I'm refreshed. Mr. Innes has chronic obstructive pulmonary disease, and the staff knows him from previous recent admits. Usually a pleasant patient, this time he is different. He also has a new diagnosis—severe anemia. I review Mr. Innes' chart for updates: upon admission, his hemoglobin and hematocrit were very low. He received 3 units of blood and is fairly stable now. After several procedures and tests, no source of bleeding can be identified. Mr. Innes recognizes me when I enter. I tell him that I hear he's unhappy with some aspects of his care and suggest that perhaps I can help. Mr. Innes has many concerns, ranging from the wrong diet on his meal trays to too much noise from the nearby nurses' station. But other, more important, clues to his discontent emerge subtly as we continue our talk. He is concerned about how his debilitated wife is getting along, with his being so often in the hospital. And after so many tests, "Why won't they tell me what's wrong?" We take each issue one at a time. A call to dietary department (actually, three calls to dietary) fixes the dietary problem.

I suggest a room change (if available) to a quieter part of the unit. He is pleased with this idea. Together, we call his wife, and they agree to have home nurse and social worker visits. With the approval of their family physician, I set this in motion. The next major hurdle is Mr. Innes' health concerns. I ask him if he feels that no one is telling him the truth. He answers "yes," and expresses fear that bad news is on the way. I know that his tests are negative. I explain that it may *feel* that he is not being told the truth, but the tests truly don't show a bleeding source anywhere. I also explain that his lab test values are stable; he's doing well. He agrees to allow me to discuss his concern with his doctor, which I do. The doctor then spends time with him, showing him the written test results and making plans for further workups if his hematocrit and hemoglobin drop again. The complaints stop; Mr. Innes seems more relaxed and remains so way for the remainder of his stay.

1:00-2:00 PM. Weekly multidisciplinary patient rounds. Each patient on the unit is discussed. The focus is on the entire range of needs for each patient and how well we (as a team) are meeting these needs.

I call back down to the ICU. Mrs. Adams has a grim prognosis, with three chest tubes now in place. There are no family members present at this time.

I recheck Mr. Frank's oxygen. It has arrived and he's departed.

I recheck Mrs. Cohn's transfer. The transport team is in the room now.

I recheck Mr. Johns. Home health IV antibiotics are set up and he's a happy guy.

I review Mrs. Elliot's chart; she is scheduled for possible transfer to ECF tomorrow. Her chart looks good. I call the ECF; her bed is available. Social service can call for transportation tomorrow. Taxi is appropriate, relevant to discussions with physician, patient, and family. I document and proceed to the next priority.

I check Mr. Harris' chart; Is it safe for him to go home? I look at the physical therapist's notes—excellent progress today. Perhaps one more day of physical therapy. I didn't think Mr. Harris would do this well. He is spunky, though!

A family member finds me and needs to talk. We go into the family room. Dad is deteriorating more each month. He has Parkinson's disease and the family is feeling overwhelmed with the care. This family feels guilty about putting Dad in a nursing home. What other options do they have? We explore insurance benefits, financial ability to get home health aide care, increase in respite care time, and family/neighbor/church support. I ask the social worker to speak to this family about possible community resources. We plan to have a family meeting the next day with the social worker to explore options further. This gives me time to find out more about insurance benefit possibilities. I add this patient to my priority list.

I review more charts until time for my 3:00 PM monthly case managers' meeting.

Discussion

The nature of the written word necessitates telling a story in a linear fashion. However, I can attest to the fact that many of these events actually occur simultaneously during a busy "day in the life."

What this account *doesn't* depict are the many other interactions: support for staff members, answering phone calls and pagers, discussing patient plans with dozens of physicians, social service personnel, physical therapists, home health professionals, and more. Each day, there are reports to and negotiations with insurance companies regarding length of stay and patient needs. Education of patients in areas pertaining to their own individual needs is a key component. Also, many individual problems and concerns arise, which are unique to an individual patient's diagnosis and life supports.

The pace is often breakneck. Boredom isn't even in a nurse case manager's dictionary. I frequently look at the clock and wonder what happened to the day.

This type of case management is not for everyone and could leave some on the ragged edge. I once overheard a job description in which the employee appeared to be able to do one activity at a time. Discussing it with the charge RN on the unit, I said that it was a unique concept, doing one thing at a time. She smiled at me and said, "Don't get any ideas. You love this pace." She was right.

CHAPTER 20

A Case Study With and Without Case Management

The following case study is an example of how nursing case management intervention can change the course of a person's illness curve. This case was selected for case management for the following reasons:

1. The patient was readmitted into the acute hospital level of care within 2 weeks.
2. The condition of the patient on admission indicated poor care at home.
3. The home health agency liaison reported that the patient's significant other felt exhausted and totally overwhelmed with the care required.
4. The diagnosis included a recent tracheostomy with a fistula formation, pneumonia, and malnutrition—all red-flag indicators.

Case Study

Fifty-eight-year old Mr. Travers was admitted to a medical floor with a primary diagnosis of cancer of the larynx (squamous cell) with metastases to the lymph nodes and neck. His admitting diagnoses included right lower lobe pneumonia, a fistula leaking into his tracheobronchial tree, extreme swelling of the neck, and malnutrition.

On hospital day 2, the home health liaison referred this case for case management, stating that Mr. Travers' mate was exhausted and overwhelmed with his care. Afraid of "causing more damage," she wanted the patient placed in an extended care facility. However, Mr. Travers, being alert and oriented, did not want to be placed in a nursing home; he wanted to maintain his independence.

A review of the patient's history revealed that about 3 weeks before this admission, Mr. Travers had gone to the doctor's office with a 2-month history of hoarseness. A massive tumor was found; he was scoped and a tracheostomy was immediately placed to relieve airway compromise. The following day the surgeons performed a total laryngectomy, partial pharyngectomy, and a left radical neck dissection. His postoperative course included fever and major swelling of the neck after the removal of two Jackson-Pratt drains, necessitating a reopening of the neck wound and reinsertion of one drain.

Mr. Travers remained in the hospital for 10 days. During this time, a home health agency was consulted and met with him and his mate. A speech therapist referred him to the American Cancer Society for support and a "loaner" electrolarynx; she also conducted a brief session on stoma care and recommended one or two speech therapy visits at home. However, the electrolarynx was not obtained and insurance would not pay for home speech therapy visits.

During the first hospitalization, nurses performed all stoma care, changing of inner cannulas, and tube feeding care. The day before discharge, a nurse reported that Mr. Travers' mate refused to learn tracheostomy care. This was the first time anyone had broached the subject, and the mate was fearful, stating that she preferred an extended care facility stay. On the day of discharge, the physician's orders were the following:

- Discharge home with Jackson-Pratt bulb suction
- Discharge to home health or extended care facility
- Needs: tracheostomy care, tube feeding, empty Jackson-Pratt bulb each day, and office visit in 4 to 5 days

On the *day of discharge*, the discharge nurse instructed the patient and his mate in the following:

1. Various aspects of tracheostomy care
2. How to change the inner cannula
3. How to cleanse the stoma
4. How to redress the stoma
5. How to flush the feeding tube with water
6. How to empty the Jackson-Pratt drain

Written instructions were given and a home health nurse was authorized for two to three visits for tube feeding purposes. No equipment other than a feeding pump and oxygen was obtained for this patient, and no social services were requested.

Mr. Travers received no teaching. He did not know how to suction himself, clean and dress his tracheostomy, or set up his tube feedings and pump. He did not even know how to cough correctly; he covered his mouth (as was his habit since childhood), and sputum was expelled out of his tracheostomy. Although the mate was very supportive, she was unsure of herself and needed more help.

Mr. Travers was readmitted to the hospital with the tracheostomy grossly infected; suctioning revealed significant amounts of bloody sputum with clots. Treatment included intravenous antibiotics, frequent suctioning every 2 to 4 hours, intravenous fluids, chest percussion therapy and small volume nebulizer (SVN) treatments every 2 to 4 hours, and tube feedings for malnutrition. A social service consult was placed.

This time the nurse case manager assessed Mr. Travers' needs and self-care capabilities with the medical staff, the social worker, the patient, and the patient's mate. They came to agreement that the hospital days would be used for intensive teaching in addition to healing the fistula and treating the pneumonia. If Mr. Travers could become independent in self-care, his mate might not feel so overwhelmed.

After the infection started subsiding, orders were written for respiratory therapists to teach all aspects of self-suctioning. Mr. Travers quickly became proficient at suctioning, along with tracheostomy cleaning and redressing. Another order was written for nurses to teach the patient to administer his own tube feeding independently; again, Mr. Travers quickly learned to do this.

The speech therapist requested that a barium swallow study be performed near the day of discharge, which showed only one questionable, tiny fistula remaining and little or no aspiration. Puréed foods were added, which the patient had no difficulty swallowing. The dietary department helped him by teaching nutritious combinations and incorporated some of his favorite foods in puréed form. Because Mr. Travers had lost about 30 pounds before his initial surgery, the physician chose to continue tube feedings at 75 mL/hour from 9:00 PM to 7:00 AM each day, in addition to his puréed diet. Again, Mr. Travers was encouraged to get the electrolarynx from the American Cancer Society, since his Medicaid plan would not cover the cost of one for him. Home health visits were reinstated.

During the hospitalization, a catheter was inserted into the fistula and placed to suction. The fistula gradually closed, allowing the discontinuation of that catheter prior to discharge. Mr. Travers' pneumonia cleared up, and he was discharged with liquid antibiotics. The following items were set up or ordered for Mr. Travers upon discharge:

- A hospital bed
- A bedside commode (from American Cancer Society)
- A shower chair (from American Cancer Society)
- Feeding bags, tubing, and feeding solution was ordered. Mr. Travers was given his new feeding schedule. A tube feeding pump was already in the home.
- A portable oxygen tank to allow more mobility and an aerosol set-up for the tracheotomy wound to reduce the chance of infection and bleeding from dryness. (Oxygen was already in the home.)
- A suction machine and catheters were ordered because Mr. Travers still required intermittent suctioning.
- Tracheostomy and stoma supplies including dressings, tracheostomy ties, peroxide and normal saline solutions, and cleaning brushes. (Mr. Travers' type of tracheostomy was changed during this admission, and he no longer required inner cannulas.)

This time, when Mr. Travers was discharged, both he and his mate were comfortable doing the tasks required. Because Mr. Travers was independent in his self-care, his mate did not feel solely responsible. In addition, Mr. Travers felt more in control of his situation and less depressed.

At a certain point in Mr. Travers' disease process, a short stay in an extended care facility was needed for strengthening and finishing up a course of IV antibiotics. At this point, a hospice referral was initiated because of his advanced stage of cancer. Through the care of the hospice attendants, Mr. Travers was able to return home, as was his wish. He died shortly after with hospice and loved ones present.

Discussion

Without case management, Mr. Travers and his family experienced exhaustion, frustration, and a preventably deteriorating condition. Case management added the element of self-care and independence to his life, allowing the remainder of his life to be lived at home, which was his wish. This patient received quality care. Because the family and patient provided the remainder of his care at home with intermittent home health and finally hospice visits, his care was also cost-effective.

I have seen many patients who were not provided the skills of a nurse case manager. In general, these patients stay in the hospital too long because the diagnostic and treatment portions of their care were drawn out; they often contract nosocomial infections, which further extend their stay.

Examples of poorly managed care—in hospitals and extended care facilities or in the community—are common. For example, patients may be subjected to two operations (one for a foot and bone debridement and one for a long-term intravenous access) when one operation may suffice. Or, perhaps home health is ordered when the skills and emotional support of hospice case management are more appropriate. Conversely, perhaps more support is ordered than was required merely because a thorough psychosocial assessment was not performed. This assessment might reveal a strong formal and informal patient support system, which could easily have met all the unskilled needs that the client required. Subjecting the client to professional agencies, often at a high premium for the patient, may not be in the client's best interests.

An analysis of cases that received nursing case management compared with those that have been poorly managed reveals that quality care *is* cost-efficient care. A case that has been skillfully assessed and creatively planned should translate into the two main goals of case management and managed care: quality of client care and the wise use of healthcare resources.

CHAPTER 21

Case Studies

The following case studies reflect real life situations and dilemmas. In case management, answers are neither right nor wrong; the case management field is a fluid, creative process tailored to the immediate and changing needs of the patient. No two patient situations are alike; each patient is a kaleidoscope of medical and psychosocial components. Therefore, no "answers" will be given at the back of this chapter. The cases herein are included for the purpose of discussion, teaching, and practicing case management "by proxy."

Not a day goes by in which I lack interesting or challenging cases. Sometimes the outcomes are so well orchestrated that everyone is satisfied. At other times, my hands have been so tied by the magnitude of the needs and lack of financial, social, or insurance support that the outcomes cause sleepless nights. Although these instances are rare, most NCMs with any longevity have had their share of them.

I remember a particularly poignant case that was mine not so long ago. All the nurses were fond of Chuck, nicknamed Chuckles because of his bright and positive attitude. Chuck, in his 20s, suffered from a form of leukemia that seemed intractable to all therapies attempted. The only hope for his survival was a bone marrow transplantation.

In the mid-1980s, his state's Medicaid plan did not include bone marrow transplantation in its list of covered services. Nonetheless I delivered a barrage of phone calls over a 6-month period, and physicians wrote several letters to Medicaid on Chuck's behalf. But Medicaid's stance was firm—no bone marrow transplantations.

Suddenly a letter was received from Medicaid stating that in 3 months' time, autologous bone marrow transplantations would be added to their list of covered services. I quickly made all arrangements and scheduled Chuck's appointment so that on the first "allowable" day Chuck would be ready to go.

On the day preceding his appointment, Chuck went into *grand mal* seizures. His disease had spread, and he had central nervous system involvement. The transplantation procedure was postponed. An Ommaya reservoir, chemotherapy, and two further bone marrow transplantations were planned, but each time Chuck was too ill to attempt the surgery. He died a short time later.

My experience with Chuck was my first big revelation about the inequities in the healthcare system, and for a time I felt somewhat bitter that Chuck was denied timely access to a procedure for a possible cure.

The NCM can have an impact—positively—on a case-by-case basis. Although it was too late for Chuck, I can't help feeling that all our calls and letters helped to identify a major problem and eventually to change Medicaid policy.

Therefore, as these practice cases are being applied, broaden your scope and look for ways that NCMs can effect future changes in the healthcare system.

While reading the following case studies, keep these considerations in mind and add other facets to resolve difficulties that occur to you:

Look at Role Definitions

1. What might the NCM do in this situation?
2. What value might the social worker be in this circumstance?
3. What might both the NCM–social worker team share?

Assess Strengths in Each Case Study

1. Is there a strong support system? This may include family, significant others, friends, neighbors, and any informal support that can be tapped into.
2. Does the patient or family have the financial ability to provide the patient with the optimal circumstances?
3. Is the insurance policy adequate to meet the needs assessed for medical care and discharge planning?
4. Are the patient's own emotional, mental, and spiritual resources positive?

Consider the Limitations in Each Case

1. Assess any knowledge deficits, both in the patient and in any caretakers.
2. Assess the limitations of insurance coverage.
3. Assess limitation or lack of social support.
4. Assess housing or homelessness.
5. Assess limitations due to poor medical status that cannot be changed or improved.
6. Consider the limitations resulting from noncompliance.
7. Assess limitations from poor financial status.
8. Assess which limitations might be improved and how it can be accomplished.

During Hospitalization

1. Actualize a tight medical plan.
2. Determine appropriate utilization of resources.
3. Assess for quality of care and use of standardized medical guidelines.
4. Assess the status of advance medical directives.

For Posthospital Care

1. Determine placement and discharge needs.
2. Assess availability of insurance coverage, either private insurance or Medicaid/Medicare.
3. Assess availability of public community resources.
4. Determine level of rehabilitation needed. This may range in scope from in-home physical, speech, or occupational therapies to acute (inpatient) rehabilitation.
5. Assess the home environment for safety.

Miscellaneous Issues

1. Are there any psychological issues such as competency, gravely disabled, danger to self, and danger to others?
2. Are there any substance abuse issues?
3. Are there any adult or child abuse issues?
4. Assess the need for ethics committee involvement.
5. Determine any legal issues that need attention.

Finally, ask: Is this a case in which everything that could be done was attempted but still failed? If so, don't get discouraged. Remember that sometimes the dragon wins.

Case Study 1: Mrs. Brownell

Mrs. Brownell, aged 77 and widowed, lives in a supervisory care setting where she has her own room and bathroom. The minimum requirement for living in this setting is the ability to get to and from the bathroom and dining room independently. Prior to this admission, Mrs. Brownell was alert and oriented and able to ambulate independently with a walker.

Mrs. Brownell's past history includes gastrointestinal bleeding from ulcers, non–insulin-dependent diabetes mellitus, hypertension, breast cancer with bilateral mastectomies 12 years earlier, atrial fibrillation, a cerebral vascular accident 5 years earlier, and alcohol abuse with hepatic cirrhosis and hepatic encephalopathy. She now presents to the hospital with a cough with brown sputum, diarrhea, mental status changes, and a decreased ability to ambulate because of weakness, falling at home, and anorexia. A left facial drop and right-sided weakness are also noted.

Mrs. Brownell was admitted with bilateral pleural effusions noted on chest x-ray, specifically *Klebsiella* pneumonia found by sputum culture. Her blood urea nitrogen (BUN) was 50 and her white blood cell count was 19.5 TH/UL. She was immediately hydrated and placed on IV antibiotics. A computed tomography (CT) scan of the head revealed nothing except for some ischemic small vessel disease. X-rays revealed the possibility of metastases; therefore, a bone scan was ordered. Uptake was noted in the thoracic and lumbar areas, but these findings were more consistent with degenerative or osteoarthritic changes.

During the course of hospitalization, Mrs. Brownell's mental state and weakness improved. Physical therapy was instituted.

It is the anticipated day of discharge, since all antibiotics are oral and Mrs. Brownell's temperature has remained normal for 24 hours. She is eating 100% of her diet, and her lab values are within normal limits. She can walk 20 to 40 feet with a minimum of assistance but cannot get up and out of bed independently, secondary to severe back pain.

Case Study 2: Mr. Collins

Mr. Collins, aged 52, has been a diabetic since 1973. In 1989, he had a left below-knee amputation at ankle level. His history includes retinal macular degeneration, which has rendered him nearly blind. He also has pulmonary edema from severe valvular insufficiency.

Mr. Collins is admitted with multiple bilateral leg ulcers; one of them is huge with foul-smelling drainage. He states that this condition, along with a steadily increasing abdominal girth, has been ongoing for nearly 4 months. A physical examination reveals anasarca. Bilateral above-knee amputations may also be necessary.

Mr. Collins has several nonmedical problems: a recent nasty divorce, impending loss of his private insurance, and current unemployment. He also recently lost his home. Mr. Collins has five sons, none of whom he feels he can turn to for help.

Although Mr. Collins is very ill and facing the possibility of losing both legs, he is fixated on nonhealth matters. His physician feels that this patient is in maximum denial of his illness (as evidenced by his waiting 4 months to seek medical assistance) and has some "paranoid ideation."

Case 3: Mr. Luber

Mr. Luber, aged 31, disappeared from his girlfriend's home 4 days prior to admission. On his return he was shaking, seemed disoriented, and then fell in a parking lot. Paramedics were called. Emergency room doctors found Mr. Luber to be agitated, combative, and inappropriate. The emergency room assessment showed blood pressure 130/86, pulse 130, respirations 40, and temperature 103.3°F (39.6° C). A toxic screen was positive for cocaine and marijuana. This patient also has a history of alcohol abuse.

A chest x-ray revealed a left lobe infiltrate; Mr. Luber was admitted for pneumonia (probable aspiration), fever, and confusion and to rule out meningitis. The lumbar puncture proved unremarkable, and the patient was placed on appropriate IV antibiotic therapy for pneumonia.

Mr. Luber claims he has had amnesia for the past 2 years; doctors have conflicting opinions about this. Mr. Luber says he remembers driving a truck cross-country 3 years ago but doesn't remember that he has lived with his girlfriend for the past 18 months. The neurologist on the case feels his amnesia is "fictitious," whereas the psychologist feels that it is a possible dissociative state or psychoactive substance-induced organic mental disorder.

Mr. Luber's girlfriend says that he currently makes a living making bottles at a manufacturing plant. Mr. Luber lost both parents when he was 12; they died 6 months apart. His mother may have had amnesiac states. He has two children who live 800 miles away. He has served several jail sentences for "driving under the influence" and assault and battery. Mr. Luber has no support system other than his girlfriend, and he has no medical insurance.

Case 4: Mr. Quinlan

This is the third admission in 6 weeks for 46-year-old Mr. Quinlan, who is developmentally delayed and living in a training center. Each admission diagnosis has been for dehydration, acute renal failure (BUN 50, creatinine greater than 3.0), thrombocytopenia, anemia, and mental status changes. His history also includes seizures.

During the first two admissions, dehydration, renal failure, and mental status changes returned to normalcy by the time of discharge. It was felt that his seizure medication was causing the thrombocytopenia, and it was changed to another agent. Still, his problems returned and compounded.

Mr. Quinlan had been independent in self-care and had been living in a cottage on the center's grounds with other "high-functioning" persons. Because his condition began to deteriorate, he was moved to the center itself, where more care could be provided. The training center attendants reported that Mr. Quinlan's condition had been going downhill for the past 4 months. Recently, he started refusing food and was losing considerable weight. When questioned, the attendants said they believed this behavior to be related to a temper tantrum reaction.

The patient had many bruises on admission. The caretaker told us that the patient had fallen against a railing. The staff nurses were aware of Mr. Quinlan's thrombocytopenia and knew that he bruised easily. But also, the staff nurses reported fearful cries of "don't hit me" when the patient was incontinent. When asked who was hitting him, Mr. Quinlan consistently named the training center attendants.

This time, the hospital course has been very complex and without clear answers as to a cause of his symptoms. It started much like the previous two hospitalizations, with the symptoms of renal failure and dehydration resolving quickly.

Intravenous medications were needed, but no IV access could be obtained because of the patient's poor vein status. Since a percutaneous endoscopic gastrostomy (PEG) feeding tube placement was felt to be in the patient's best interests, a central line was be inserted at the same time. The patient was at times wildly agitated, so the procedures were obtained under general anesthesia. Mr. Quinlan did not resume spontaneous breathing and a postoperative chest x-ray showed right-sided "whiteout" with questionable pleural effusions versus aspiration. Two IV antibiotics were initiated while the patient remained ventilated. A nasogastric tube insertion produced a heme-positive return, and his anemia deteriorated to a hemoglobin of 6.7 and a hematocrit of 19.0, requiring transfusions. Three days later, Mr. Quinlan masterfully extubated himself and was able to resume spontaneous respirations.

Mr. Quinlan was sent to floor status with IV antibiotics, a nasogastric tube (still draining bile colored secretions), and orders to start physical therapy. Tube feedings were initiated after 5 days of attempts because of intolerance and vomiting of the formulas. Several competent physicians including pulmonary, gastrointestinal, and neurology specialists are still unsure of the cause of the patient's diagnosis.

Case 5: *Mr. Vaquero*

Mr. Vaquero, aged 26, has a history of insulin-dependent diabetes mellitus. Consistently noncompliant with his medical care for most of his life, Mr. Vaquero, developed retinopathy, neuropathies, several diabetic foot ulcers, and chronic renal failure. He is now legally blind. A year ago, Mr. Vaquero's renal function became so impaired that hemodialysis was initiated.

Mr. Vaquero lives in the country, almost 50 miles from the nearest hemodialysis unit. His parents live next door, but his mother is also blind and his father has advanced Alzheimer's disease. He has only one friend, and this friend is unable to help. There is no public or volunteer transportation to help him get to and from hemodialysis three times each week, and no other social support is acknowledged.

Mr. Vaquero has been in the acute care setting many times in diabetic ketoacidosis (DKA) and, with a dangerously elevated BUN, creatinine, phosphorus, and potassium from being inadequately dialyzed. He also has been hospitalized for several foot problems, resulting from carelessness and not wearing shoes. His injuries include nonhealing cuts and cellulitis and second-degree burns from a hot pavement. Mr. Vaquero, has private insurance, but the policy has no long-term care or extended care facility (ECF) benefits.

Case 6: *Mrs. Oliver*

Mrs. Oliver is 58 years old. She has a medical history that includes lupus erythematosus, insulin-dependent diabetes mellitus, diabetic neuropathies, neurogenic bladder requiring an indwelling Foley catheter, chronic yeast bladder infections, chronic renal failure, congestive heart failure with cor pulmonale, and frequent episodes of shortness of breath resulting in frequent emergency room visits. Mrs. Oliver also has gained hundreds of pounds over the past several years, making her morbidly obese. She now weighs about 550 pounds. This raises the question of pickwickian episodes. The abdominal skin folds frequently break down, making abdominal cellulitis another recurring problem.

Two months previous, Mrs. Oliver was able to get out of bed and use her walker to get to a bedside commode or chair. Now she is totally bedbound and requires a maximum assistance of two physical therapists to "stand" her for 5 seconds.

Mrs. Oliver habitually requires a lengthy hospitalization every few months, often on a telemetry unit. Her first hospitalization of the current year was in February for congestive heart failure and pneumonia in addition to her other chronic problems. Her husband, aged 70 and 135 pounds, is very supportive but is finding it almost impossible to care for his wife at home any longer. Nevertheless, each time the issue of an ECF is broached, Mrs. Oliver bursts into tears and begs her husband to take her home. To complicate matters, at the last stage of one hospital stay after discharge orders are written, the home health agency previously helping with her care, declined her case on the grounds of serious safety issues. No other home health agency could be found to take on the case.

There seems to be only one alternative now, and Mr. Oliver convinces a protesting and teary Mrs. Oliver to go to an ECF for physical therapy in an effort to get her back to baseline.

Two weeks later, Mr. Oliver is calling the NCM. He said that Mrs. Oliver insisted on leaving the ECF. A home health agency was found to take her case. Unfortunately, the agency is not providing enough help. Mrs. Oliver is on a waiting list for an ECF with an excellent reputation for rehab/physical therapy, but while waiting for a bed to become available, Mr. Oliver finds himself at his outermost limits. He doesn't feel he can handle his wife's care any longer.

The bed in the ECF did not manifest soon enough. After two more emergency room visits for shortness of breath, Mrs. Oliver was readmitted with pneumonia. The long-awaited ECF bed became available, and Mrs. Oliver was transferred while finishing her last days of IV antibiotics.

Six weeks later, Mrs. Oliver is still not making progress in physical therapy at the ECF. Her insurance company will pay for up to 50 skilled home health nurse visits and 100 days of ECF skilled care for 1 year. Mr. Oliver has too many assets to qualify for the state's long-term care and too few assets to privately pay for all the care she requires. No one else in Mr. Oliver's family will help.

By June, Mrs. Oliver has been bounced from the ECF to the hospital several times with severe respiratory distress, congestive heart failure, and pulmonary edema. Her CO_2 has reached the middle 70s and bipap ventilation has been tried. She now has 3 weeks of ECF coverage remaining.

Case 7: Ms. Simms

Seventy-two-year-old Ms. Simms has a history of schizophrenia and chronic obstructive pulmonary disease. The emergency room report states that she has been extremely schizophrenic, delusional, and paranoid for the past week. Her chief complaint is shortness of breath. Her physical exam reveals some expiratory wheezes after a small-volume nebulizer treatment, but no respiratory distress, rales, or rhonchi and no use of accessory muscles. She is speaking in full sentences. Ms. Simms is afebrile; blood pressure 143/90; pulse 96; respirations 26. The emergency room diagnoses are rule out paranoid schizophrenia and chronic obstructive pulmonary disease. She is admitted to a medical floor.

Ms. Simms is very frightened. She feels the Vietnamese, the Chinese, and the Germans are out to get her and her family. She believes she is not safe anywhere and will not make it out of the hospital alive. The Asian resident assigned to the case had to make himself scarce because Ms. Simms exhibited severe fright, accusing him of following her and planning to transfer her out of town to be tortured.

Ms. Simms wishes to go to the state hospital, although she is sure the staff will rape her and put her into a machine that will crush her.

Ms. Simms never married. She lived in a convent many years ago, but her bizarre behaviors made it impossible for her to become a nun. She trusts the Catholic priests and states that God has talked to her.

Ms. Simms has a twin. When her sister is out of town, as she is during this admission, the schizophrenic exacerbations intensify. Her niece and grandnephew are sympathetic and willing to help, but when they visit they are physically attacked by their aunt.

Ms. Simms has been on appropriate psychotropic medication, but there is some question about her compliance. A transfer to an inpatient mental health unit has been arranged, but she refuses to voluntarily sign the "conditions of admission" forms.

Case 8: Mrs. Ling

Seven years ago, Mrs. Ling, who was on hemodialysis, received a kidney from her son, one of her 10 children. The kidney transplantation was a success, and for many years under the meticulous care of her husband, she maintained a serum creatinine level of 0.8. Mr. Ling closely monitored his wife's complicated medical requirements for diabetes, chronic urinary tract infections, anemia, coronary artery disease, hypertension, and medications to maintain the kidney. She also had a history of a left cerebral vascular accident and underwent laser surgery to her eyes from diabetic complications.

About 6 months ago. Mr. Ling suffered a cerebral vascular accident and was no longer able to care for his wife. The adult children took over the care of both parents, but their care proved to be haphazard. Cyclosporine was not listed among Mrs. Ling's medications, and azathioprine was being given incorrectly.

Mrs. Ling was admitted to the hospital with intractable nausea and vomiting, unable to keep down food and was intolerant of any medications. Her critical admission lab values included the following:

BUN 178 (normal 5–25)

Creatinine 17.5 (normal 0.7–1.5)

Potassium 7.8 (normal 3.5–5.5)

Phosphorus 12.3 (normal 2.5–4.5)

The degree of kidney failure indicated that the rejection was not acute. Mrs. Ling's physicians had not seen her in more than 6 months; this was in contrast to the careful way Mr. Ling made and kept physician appointments. It is difficult to say how long the rejection had been going on. After 10 days on heavy IV methylprednisolone (Solu-Medrol), doses and frequent hemodialysis, the creatinine was still around 6.5. Outpatient hemodialysis was set up. The patient has Medicaid and although only 61 years of age will soon be eligible for Medicare because of hemodialysis.

Case 9: Ms. Johnson

Ms. Johnson is a 36-year-old divorced woman with a long history of multiple hospital admissions for medical and psychiatric problems. She lives with her 15-year-old daughter. Her mother had bipolar disorder, and her father was schizophrenic. Her insurance coverage is Medicare and Medicaid. She is unemployed and on disability.

She also hospital-hops, so that it is difficult to assess true hospital admission numbers. In 1 year, Ms. Johnson entered one hospital 18 times—six in 1 month's time. It is not known how many times she was also admitted to various other hospitals during the same time period.

Medically, Ms. Johnson's history includes asthma with frequent exacerbations, bowel obstructions, seizures, and bladder incontinence, and an appendectomy. Psychiatrically, Ms. Johnson meets criteria for chronically mentally ill, with the diagnoses of borderline personality and psychotic depression. She has had several inpatient hospital stays at five different mental health facilities.

Ms. Johnson's behaviors include superficially slashing her wrists—at one point three times in 1 week—overdosing on carbamazepine and other pills, hallucinating, excessive alcohol consumption, and manipulation. Her "usual" admission can be psychiatric, medical, or a combination of both, and it is very short. If presented with a plan that Ms. Johnson finds distasteful she leaves against medical advice (AMA). Often, she shows up in an emergency room within 1 or 2 days of the AMA episode.

After several such events, one psychiatrist deemed Ms. Johnson severely mentally ill, and a petitioning process was initiated. She was court-ordered into treatment (she fired that particular psychiatrist), but after her court-ordered "incarceration," she resumed her previous behaviors of multiple suicide gestures, asthma exacerbation admissions, and leaving AMA.

Ms. Johnson has learned that it is easier to leave AMA when she "voluntarily" agrees to a psychiatric admission than when the involuntary "court order" is initiated, so now she rarely, if ever, refuses a psychiatric admission.

Case 10: Ms.Cole

Ms. Cole is a 29-year-old cachectic female with recurrent hospitalizations. Almost 10 years ago, Ms. Cole was diagnosed with metastatic ovarian cancer. After an extensive pelvic resection was performed, she was given high-dose radiation. The cancer never returned, but the radiation left Ms. Cole with severe radiation gastroenteritis, necessitating several bowel resections. She has a colostomy and for many years required chronic total parenteral nutrition (TPN) for severe short bowel syndrome and malnutrition.

Over the years, Ms. Cole has required numerous hospitalizations. Her diagnoses have included *Pseudomonas* and herpes pneumonia, disseminated candidiasis, cholecystectomy, persistently elevated liver function tests (her bilirubin stays in the 14 to 17 range), recurrent gastrointestinal bleeding episodes, and multiple central line problems. The latter two are her most critical problems. Throughout the years, the gastrointestinal bleeding has included etiologies from esophageal varices, Mallory-Weiss tears, gastritis, esophagitis, and peptic and duodenal ulcers.

Recently, Ms. Cole needed more extensive resections in two separate operations from intractable gastrointestinal bleeding. The last surgery, preceded by 8 units of red blood cells, resulted in removal of the remaining duodenum and a large portion of the stomach. Very little bowel remains.

Ms. Cole has endured multiple revisions of her central venous access (needed for the TPN dependence). She has had several episodes of line sepsis and chronic superior vena cava syndrome. Her multiple lines and severe thrombotic disease have made finding a place for an access all but impossible. Her present central line extends into the inferior vena cava; no other venous access can be obtained and she is again in the hospital with central line sepsis.

Much of the problem with venous lines throughout the years has been due to Ms. Cole's habit of accessing her catheters for IV cocaine. Many were clogged, secondary to poor flushing and the cocaine was very caustic to the veins. She now realizes that this may be perhaps her last chance at a venous access and has switched to smoking crack cocaine.

Ms. Cole is alert and oriented. She is intermittently noncompliant with her TPN, and the home health nurses often found a closet full of TPN bags unused. She does not keep outpatient clinic visits for IV antibiotics or for physician checkups. She (sometimes) lives with her mother; until recently, she had her own apartment. The insurance plans are Medicare and Medicaid, and she has used up most of her Medicare lifetime reserve days.

Case 11: Ms. Paine

Thirty-two-year-old Ms. Paine was diagnosed with HIV 5 years ago. Three of her eight children have died of AIDS. The remaining five children, the youngest of whom is 3 months old, live with relatives or are in foster care. Ms. Paine earns her living through prostitution. This supports her polysubstance abuse habit, which includes the use of cocaine (inhaled and injected), alcohol, and whatever else will keep her "drugged out." She practices no regular birth control and does not practice "safe sex" protocol. She is presently homeless. Her mental status is assessed as lethargic, alert, and oriented, but she is inconsistent in her answers to different examiners. For example, she changes her occupation from prostitute to burglar when broached with the issue of "safe sex."

Ms. Paine has a history of being admitted to hospitals and leaving AMA—she actually "disappears" when specific issues are raised. She is savvy about the system and knows she cannot be deemed incompetent or incarcerated involuntarily in a mental health unit unless she "threatens her own life or the life of someone else in this state."

On her first admission to a particular local hospital, Ms. Paine appeared cachectic, ill-kempt, and disheveled. She had not had anything to eat or drink for 3 days, secondary to frequent smoking of crack during this time. Her left foot had obvious cellulitis. She was admitted for dehydration, cellulitis (rule out osteomyelitis), and electrocardiographic T-wave abnormalities and bradycardia. She has a history of severe oral thrush and pneumonia. On this admission, Ms. Paine's thrush was severe and her chest x-ray was clear, but she had a persistent dry cough. IV antibiotics, IV fluids, and supportive care were initiated.

In addition to treating Ms. Paine's obvious physical problems and checking her toxic screen (positive for cocaine *during* the hospitalization) and pregnancy test (negative), the attending physician used the time to address the many psychosocial needs and issues of this case. The attending physician felt that Ms. Paines was definitely a public health concern and ordered a psychiatric evaluation.

The psychiatrist deemed Ms. Paine competent with antisocial tendencies. The recommendation was to explore petitioning on the grounds that she showed definite judgment impairment, that she was "acutely and persistently disabled," and that she was unable to safely care for herself. But this psychiatric status could not be court-ordered, since the patient knew of alternative options for taking care of herself (she can live with relatives) and she has no previous documented psychiatric history.

Hint: Ethical and legal issues define and also limit the possibilities and probable outcomes for this case.

Case 12: Mr. Jensen

Mr. Jensen was a pleasant but persistently noncompliant patient known to every hospital emergency room in the metropolitan area. He was a brittle diabetic (even during hospital admissions) with a lifetime of poor diabetic control. His sugars would routinely register "HHH" or "LLL" on the glucose monitors, and yet he was able to sit up and carry on a full conversation with a blood sugar level of 18. It is no surprise that Mr. Jensen suffered from every diabetic "opathy" in medical literature.

In his late 30s, Mr. Jensen underwent several angioplasties to his lower extremities for severe coronary artery disease. He had chronic, extensive leg ulcers and partial foot amputations, but he managed to maintain self-care with the use of a wheelchair.

Mr. Jensen had an impressive IV drug abuse habit, and after injecting a large amount of cocaine one day, suffered a myocardial infarction, necessitating a four-vessel coronary artery bypass. Mr. Jensen's drug use did not decrease, and many more hospital emergency room visits and admissions were needed to treat congestive heart failure, chest pain, diabetic ketoacidosis, pneumonia, endocarditis, and out-of-control diabetes. Most emergency room visits included the complaint of chest pain. Although Mr. Jensen's assessment revealed drug-seeking behaviors, it is also likely that he did have pain and that his tolerance for pain medications was high.

Mr. Jensen's insurance coverage was fairly thorough; he had both Medicare and Medicaid. But with all his extensive hospital utilization, he was dipping heavily into his Medicare lifetime reserve days. When not residing in the hospital, emergency room visits would range from daily to several times per week.

Mr. Jensen has lived with his girlfriend for many years. She is much healthier than he physically, but several times she had to be escorted off hospital units for abusive behavior to the staff. She was also an "aider and abettor" during several episodes when Mr. Jensen went "downstairs for a smoke." A two-pack-a-day guy, Mr. Jensen often returned to the floor glassy-eyed and with positive toxic screens.

Mr. Jensen received maximum social service, psychiatric, and nurse case management attention but never followed through on medical or community suggestions and referrals.

Discharge planning was complicated by several factors. Although home IV therapy would have shortened hospital length of stays, no physician could safely send Mr. Jensen home with an easy IV access because of his IV drug abuse. Home nurses were ruled out because those who visited him at home refused to go back, scared because of all the drug paraphernalia and hard-core addicts hanging around his apartment. Eventually, no home health agency would touch his case.

Extended care facilities soon became out of the question, too. When sent to an ECF for endocarditis, which required several weeks of IV antibiotics, Mr. Jensen would (as in the hospital) go outside where someone would meet him and come back "stoned." He was even caught trying to sell drugs to other nursing home residents. Nips of alcohol would be supplied freely to these residents. ECFs, like home health agencies, are no longer an option for Mr. Jensen.

Appendices

A P P E N D I X   A

The Medicare DRGs

DRG	MDC 1	Diseases & Disorders of the Nervous System	*GM LOS
1	1 SURG	Craniotomy age >17 except for trauma	10.5
2	1 SURG	Craniotomy for trauma age >17	10.4
3	1 SURG	* Craniotomy age 0–17	12.7
4	1 SURG	Spinal procedures	8.1
5	1 SURG	Extracranial vascular procedures	4.8
6	1 SURG	Carpal tunnel release	2.1
7	1 SURG	Periph + cranial nerve + other nerv syst proc with CC	10.7
8	1 SURG	Periph + cranial nerve + other nerv sys proc w/o CC	2.9
9	1 MED	Spinal disorders + injuries	6.7
10	1 MED	Nervous system neoplasms with CC	7.1
11	1 MED	Nervous system neoplasms w/o CC	4.2
12	1 MED	Degenerative nervous system disorders	6.6
13	1 MED	Multiple sclerosis + cerebellar ataxia	6.2
14	1 MED	Specific cerebrovascular disorders except TIA	6.7
15	1 MED	Transient ischemic attack and precerebral occlusions	4.0
16	1 MED	Nonspecific cerebrovascular disorders with CC	6.5
17	1 MED	Nonspecific cerebrovascular disorders w/o CC	4.3
18	1 MED	Cranial + peripheral nerve disorders with CC	5.6
19	1 MED	Cranial + peripheral nerve disorders w/o CC	3.8
20	1 MED	Nervous system infection except viral meningitis	8.4
21	1 MED	Viral meningitis	6.8
22	1 MED	Hypertensive encephalopathy	4.1
23	1 MED	Nontraumatic stupor + coma	4.1
24	1 MED	Seizure + headache age >17 with CC	5.1
25	1 MED	Seizure + headache age >17 w/o CC	3.3
26	1 MED	Seizure + headache age 0–17	3.6
27	1 MED	Traumatic stupor + coma, coma >1 hr	4.0
28	1 MED	Traumatic stupor + coma, coma <1 hr age >17 w/ CC	5.8
29	1 MED	Traumatic stupor + coma, coma <1 hr age >17 w/o CC	3.3
30	1 MED	* Traumatic stupor + coma, coma <1 hr age 0–17	2.0
31	1 MED	Concussion age >17 with CC	4.2
32	1 MED	Concussion age >17 w/o CC	2.5
33	1 MED	* Concussion age 0–17	1.6
34	1 MED	Other disorders of nervous system with CC	5.6
35	1 MED	Other disorders of nervous system w/o CC	3.6

(Continued)

DRG	MDC 2	Diseases & Disorders of the Eye	GM LOS
36	2 SURG	Retinal procedures	1.7
37	2 SURG	Orbital procedures	2.6
38	2 SURG	Primary iris procedures	2.1
39	2 SURG	Lens procedures with or without vitrectomy	1.5
40	2 SURG	Extraocular procedures except orbit age >17	2.1
41	2 SURG	* Extraocular procedures except orbit age 0–17	1.6
42	2 SURG	Intraocular procedures except retina, iris & lens	1.8
43	2 MED	Hyphema	3.4
44	2 MED	Acute major eye infections	5.2
45	2 MED	Neurological eye disorders	3.4
46	2 MED	Other disorders of the eye age >17 with CC	3.4
47	2 MED	Other disorders of the eye >17 w/o CC	2.8
48	2 MED	* Other disorders of the eye age 0–17	2.9

DRG	MDC 3	Diseases & Disorders of the Ear, Nose & Throat	GM LOS
49	3 SURG	Major head + neck procedures	5.3
50	3 SURG	Sialoadenectomy	2.0
51	3 SURG	Salivary gland procedures except sialoadenectomy	2.0
52	3 SURG	Cleft lip + palate repair	2.2
53	3 SURG	Sinus + mastoid procedures age >17	2.0
54	3 SURG	* Sinus + mastoid procedures 0–17	3.2
55	3 SURG	Miscellaneous ear, nose, mouth + throat proc	1.7
56	3 SURG	Rhinoplasty	1.9
57	3 SURG	T + A proc, except tonsillectomy +/or adenoidectomy only, age >17	3.3
58	3 SURG	* T + A proc, except tonsillectomy +/or adenoidectomy only, age 0–17	1.5
59	3 SURG	Tonsillectomy and/or adenoidectomy only, age >17	1.6
60	3 SURG	* Tonsillectomy and/or adenoidectomy only, age 0–17	1.5
61	3 SURG	Myringotomy with tube insertion age >17	2.8
62	3 SURG	* Myringotomy with tube insertion age 0–17	1.3
63	3 SURG	Other ear, nose, mouth + throat O.R. proc	3.6
64	3 MED	Ear, nose, mouth + throat malignancy	5.3
65	3 MED	Dysequilibrium	3.1
66	3 MED	Epistaxis	3.2
67	3 MED	Epiglottitis	3.9
68	3 MED	Otitis media + URI age >17 with CC	4.7
69	3 MED	Otitis media + URI age >17 w/o CC	3.6
70	3 MED	Otitis media + URI age 0–17	2.5
71	3 MED	Laryngotracheitis	3.8
72	3 MED	Nasal trauma + deformity	3.4
73	3 MED	Other ear, nose, mouth + throat diag age >17	4.2
74	3 MED	* Other ear, nose, mouth + throat age 0–17	2.1

DRG	MDC 4	Diseases & Disorders of the Respiratory System	GM LOS
75	4 SURG	Major chest procedures	10.6
76	4 SURG	Other respiratory system O.R. procedures with CC	10.4
77	4 SURG	Other respiratory system O.R. procedures w/o CC	4.1
78	4 MED	Pulmonary embolism	8.2
79	4 MED	Respiratory infections + inflammations age >17 with CC	8.7
80	4 MED	Respiratory infections + inflammations age 17 w/o CC	6.1
81	4 MED	* Respiratory infections + inflammations age 0–17	6.1
82	4 MED	Respiratory neoplasms	6.6
83	4 MED	Major chest trauma with CC	5.7
84	4 MED	Major chest trauma w/o CC	3.3
85	4 MED	Pleural effusion with CC	6.6
86	4 MED	Pleural effusion w/o CC	3.9
87	4 MED	Pulmonary edema + respitory failure	5.6
88	4 MED	Chronic obstructive pulmonary disease	5.8
89	4 MED	Simple pneumonia + pleurisy age >17 with CC	6.8
90	4 MED	Simple pneumonia + pleurisy age 17 w/o CC	5.1
91	4 MED	Simple pneumonia + pleurisy age 0–17	3.8
92	4 MED	Interstitial lung disease with CC	6.6
93	4 MED	Interstitial lung disease w/o CC	4.6
94	4 MED	Pneumothorax with CC	6.7
95	4 MED	Pneumothorax w/o CC	4.1
96	4 MED	Bronchitis + asthma age >17 with CC	5.5
97	4 MED	Bronchitis + asthma age 17 w/o CC	4.2
98	4 MED	Bronchitis + asthma age 0–17	3.5
99	4 MED	Respiratory signs + symptoms with CC	3.4
100	4 MED	Respiratory signs + symptoms w/o CC	2.4
101	4 MED	Other respiratory system diagnoses with CC	4.8
102	4 MED	Other respiratory system diagnoses w/o CC	3.1

DRG	MDC 5	Diseases & Disorders of the Circulatory System	GM LOS
103	5 SURG	Heart transplant	25.9
104	5 SURG	Cardiac valve procedure with pump + with cardiac cath	16.5
105	5 SURG	Cardiac valve proc. with pump + w/o cardiac cath	11.6
106	5 SURG	Coronary bypass with cardiac cath	12.9
107	5 SURG	Coronary bypass w/o cardiac cath	9.8
108	5 SURG	Other cardiothoracic or vascular proc, with pump	11.5
109	5 SURG	Other cardiothoracic proc w/o pump no longer valid	0.0
110	5 SURG	Major reconstructive vascular proc w/o pump with CC	9.5
111	5 SURG	Major reconstructive vascular proc w/o pump w/o CC	6.9
112	5 SURG	Percutaneous cardiovascular procedures	4.2
113	5 SURG	Amputation for circ system disorders except upper limb + toe	13.5
114	5 SURG	Upper limb + toe amputation for circ system disorders	8.3

(Continued)

115	5 SURG	Perm cardiac pacemaker implant with AMI, heart failure or shock	10.9
116	5 SURG	Perm cardiac pacemaker implant w/o AMI, heart failure or shock	5.0
117	5 SURG	Cardiac pacemaker replace + revis exc device replacement	3.3
118	5 SURG	Cardiac pacemaker device replacement	2.4
119	5 SURG	Vein ligation + stripping	3.5
120	5 SURG	Other circulatory system O.R. procedures	6.6
121	5 MED	Circulatory disorders with AMI + C.V. comp. disch. alive	7.4
122	5 MED	Circulatory disorders with AMI w/o C.V. comp. disch. alive	5.2
123	5 MED	Circulatory disorders with AMI, expired	2.9
124	5 MED	Circulatory disorders exc AMI, with card cath + complex diag	4.2
125	5 MED	Circulatory disorders exc AMI, with card cath w/o complex diag	2.3
126	5 MED	Acute + subacute endocarditis	14.6
127	5 MED	Heart failure + shock	5.7
128	5 MED	Deep vein thrombophlebitis	7.0
129	5 MED	Cardiac Arrest, unexplained	2.2
130	5 MED	Peripheral vascular disorders with CC	6.0
131	5 MED	Peripheral vascular disorders w/o CC	4.6
132	5 MED	Atherosclerosis with CC	3.8
133	5 MED	Atherosclerosis w/o CC	2.8
134	5 MED	Hypertension	3.6
135	5 MED	Cardiac congenital + valvular disorders age >17 with CC	4.5
136	5 MED	Cardiac congenital + valvular disorders age >17 w/o CC	3.0
137	5 MED	* Cardiac congenital + valvular disorders age 0–17	3.3
138	5 MED	Cardiac arrhythmia + conduction disorders with CC	4.2
139	5 MED	Cardiac arrhythmia + conduction disorders w/o CC	2.8
140	5 MED	Angina pectoris	3.4
141	5 MED	Syncope + collapse with CC	4.1
142	5 MED	Syncope + collapse w/o CC	3.0
143	5 MED	Chest pain	2.6
144	5 MED	Other circulatory system diagnoses with CC	4.7
145	5 MED	Other circulatory system diagnoses w/o CC	3.0

DRG	MDC 6	Diseases & Disorders of the Digestive System	GM LOS
146	6 SURG	Rectal resection with CC	11.3
147	6 SURG	Rectal resection w/o CC	8.0
148	6 SURG	Major small + large bowel procedures with CC	12.7
149	6 SURG	Major small + large bowel procedures w/o CC	8.0
150	6 SURG	Peritoneal adhesiolysis with CC	10.9
151	6 SURG	Peritoneal adhesiolysis w/o CC	5.7
152	6 SURG	Minor small + large bowel procedures with CC	8.6
153	6 SURG	Minor small + large bowel procedures w/o CC	6.3
154	6 SURG	Stomach, esophageal + duodenal procedures age >17 with CC	13.9
155	6 SURG	Stomach, esophageal + duodenal procedures age >17 w/o CC	6.5
156	6 SURG	* Stomach, esophageal + duodenal procedures age 0–17	6.0

157	6 SURG	Anal + stomal procedures with CC	4.5
158	6 SURG	Anal + stomal procedures w/o CC	2.3
159	6 SURG	Hernia procedures except inguinal + femoral age >17 with CC	4.5
160	6 SURG	Hernia procedures except inguinal + femoral age >27 w/o CC	2.6
161	6 SURG	Inguinal + femoral hernia procedures age >17 with CC	3.2
162	6 SURG	Inguinal + femoral hernia procedures age >17 w/o CC	1.7
163	6 SURG	Hernia procedures age 0–17	3.2
164	6 SURG	Appendectomy with complicated princ. diag with CC	9.2
165	6 SURG	Appendectomy with complicated princ. diag w/o CC	5.9
166	6 SURG	Appendectomy w/o complicated princ. diag with CC	5.5
167	6 SURG	Appendectomy w/o complicated princ. w/o CC	3.4
168	6 SURG	Mouth procedures with CC	3.5
169	6 SURG	Mouth procedures w/o CC	2.0
170	6 SURG	Other digestive system O.R. procedures with CC	10.5
171	6 SURV	Other digestive system O.R. procedures w/o CC	4.6
172	6 MED	Digestive malignancy with CC	6.8
173	6 MED	Digestive malignancy w/o CC	3.4
174	6 MED	G.I. hemorrhage with CC	5.2
175	6 MED	G.I. hemorrhage w/o CC	3.5
176	6 MED	Complicated peptic ulcer	5.6
177	6 MED	Uncomplicated peptic ulcer with CC	4.8
178	6 MED	Uncomplicated peptic ulcer w/o CC	3.5
179	6 MED	Inflammatory bowel disease	6.8
180	6 MED	G.I. obstruction with CC	5.5
181	6 MED	G.I. obstruction w/o CC	3.6
182	6 MED	Esophagitis, gastroent. + misc. digest. dis age >17 with CC	4.6
183	6 MED	Esophagitis, gastroent. + misc. digest. dis age >17 w/o CC	3.2
184	6 MED	Esophagitis, gastroenteritis + misc. digest. disorders age 0–17	2.8
185	6 MED	Dental + oral dis. exc extractions + restorations, age >17	4.2
186	6 MED	* Dental + oral dis. exc extractions + restorations age 0–17	2.9
187	6 MED	Dental extractions + restorations	2.6
188	6 MED	Other digestive system diagnoses age >17 with CC	5.1
189	6 MED	Other digestive system diagnoses age >17 w/o CC	2.7
190	6 MED	Other digestive system diagnoses age 0–17	4.2

DRG	MDC 7	Diseases & Disorders of the Hepatobiliary System and Pancreas	GM LOS
191	7 SURG	Major pancreas, liver + shunt procedures w/o CC	14.3
192	7 SURG	Minor pancreas, liver + shunt procedures w/o CC	7.4
193	7 SURG	Biliary tract proc w/o CC exc only cholecystectomy with or without CDE	13.2
194	7 SURG	Biliary tract proc w/o CC exc only cholecyst with or w/o CC	7.7
195	7 SURG	Total cholecystectomy with C.D.E. with CC	10.2
196	7 SURG	Total cholecystectomy with C.D.E. w/o CC	6.9
197	7 SURG	Cholecyst ex by laparoscope w/o C.D.E. with CC	8.2

(Continued)

198	7 SURG	Cholecyst ex by laparoscope w/o C.D.E. w/o CC	4.5
199	7 SURG	Hepatobiliary diagnostic procedure for malignancy	10.3
200	7 SURG	Hepatobiliary diagnostic procedure for non-malignancy	8.7
201	7 SURG	Other hepatobiliary or pancreas O.R. procedures	12.2
202	7 MED	Cirrhosis + alcoholic hepatitis	6.7
203	7 MED	Malignancy of hepatobiliary system or pancreas	6.5
204	7 MED	Disorders of pancreas except malignancy	5.9
205	7 MED	Disorders of liver exc malig, cirr, alc hepa with CC	6.4
206	7 MED	Disorders of liver exc malig, cirr, alc hepa w/o CC	3.6
207	7 MED	Disorders of the biliary tract with CC	5.1
208	7 MED	Disorders of the biliary tract w/o CC	2.9

DRG	MDC 8	Diseases of the Musculoskeletal System & Connective Tissue	GM LOS
209	8 SURG	Major joint and limb reattachment pros lower ex	8.6
210	8 SURG	Hip + femur procedures except major joint age >17 with CC	10.0
211	8 SURG	Hip + femur procedures except major joint age >17 w/o CC	7.6
212	8 SURG	Hip + femur procedures major joint age 0–17	4.3
213	8 SURG	Amputations for musculoskeletal system + conn. tissue disorders	8.9
214	8 SURG	Back + neck procedures with CC	7.3
215	8 SURG	Back + neck procedures w/o CC	4.4
216	8 SURG	Biopsies of musculoskeletal system + connective tissue	9.6
217	8 SURG	Wnd debrid + skin graft exc hand, for musculoskeletal + conn. tiss. dis	13.1
218	8 SURG	Lower extrem + humer proc exc hip, foot, femur age >17 with CC	6.3
219	8 SURG	Lower extrem + humer proc exc hip, foot, femur age >17 w/o CC	3.9
220	8 SURG	* Lower extrem + humer proc exc hip, foot, femur age 0–17	5.3
221	8 SURG	Knee procedures with CC	7.1
222	8 SURG	Knee procedures w/o CC	3.6
223	8 SURG	Major shoulder/elbow proc, or other upper extremity proc with CC	2.8
224	8 SURG	Shoulder, elbow or forearm proc, exc major joint proc, w/o CC	2.3
225	8 SURG	Foot procedures	3.3
226	8 SURG	Soft tissue procedures with CC	5.4
227	8 SURG	Soft tissue procedures w/o CC	2.6
228	8 SURG	Major thumb or joint proc, or oth hand or wrist proc with CC	2.6
229	8 SURG	Hand or wrist proc, except major joint proc, w/o CC	1.8
230	8 SURG	Local excision + removal of int fix devices of hip + femur	3.8
231	8 SURG	Local excision + removal of int fix devices except hip + femur	3.7
232	8 SURG	Athroscopy	3.1
233	8 SURG	Other musculoskelet sys + conn tiss O.R. procedure with CC	7.9
234	8 SURG	Other musculoskelet sys + conn tiss O.R. proc w/o CC	3.7
235	8 MED	Fractures of femur	6.4
236	8 MED	Fractures of hip + pelvis	5.9

237	8 MED	Sprains, strains + dislocations of hip, pelvis + thigh	4.0
238	8 MED	Osteomyelitis	9.7
239	8 MED	Pathological fractures + musculoskeletal + conn. tiss. malignancy	7.2
240	8 MED	Connective tissue disorders with CC	6.5
241	8 MED	Connective tissue disorders w/o CC	4.1
242	8 MED	Septic arthritis	7.5
243	8 MED	Medical back problems	5.0
244	8 MED	Bone diseases + specific arthropathies with CC	5.2
245	8 MED	Bone diseases + specific arthropathies w/o CC	3.6
246	8 MED	Non-specific arthropathies	4.2
247	8 MED	Signs + symptoms of musculoskeletal system + conn tissue	3.5
248	8 MED	Tendonitis, myositis + bursitis	4.5
249	8 MED	Aftercare, musculoskeletal system + connective tissue	3.7
250	8 MED	Fx, sprns, strns + disl of forearm, hand, foot age >17 with CC	4.4
251	8 MED	Fx, sprns, strns + disl of forearm, hand, foot age >17 w/o CC	2.7
252	8 MED	Fx, sprns, strns + disl of forearm, hand, foot age 0–17	1.8
253	8 MED	Fx, sprns, strns + disl of uparm, lowleg ex foot age >17 with CC	5.4
254	8 MED	Fx, sprns, strns + disl of uparm, lowleg ex foot age >17 w/o CC	3.3
255	8 MED	Fx, sprns, strns + disl of uparm, lowleg ex foot age 0–17	2.9
256	8 MED	Other diagnoses of musculoskeletal system + connective tissue	3.6

DRG	MDC 9	Diseases of the Skin, Subcutaneous Tissue & Breast	GM LOS
257	9 SURG	Total mastectomy for malignancy with CC	3.8
258	9 SURG	Total mastectomy for malignancy w/o CC	3.0
259	9 SURG	Subtltal mastectomy for malignancy with CC	3.1
260	9 SURG	Subtotal mastectomy for malignancy w/o CC	2.0
261	9 SURG	Breast proc for non-malig except biopsy + loc exc	2.1
262	9 SURG	Breast biopsy + local excision for non-malignancy	2.3
263	9 SURG	Skin-grafts +/or debrid for skin ulcer or cellulitis with CC	13.5
264	9 SURG	Skin-grafts +/or debrid for skin ulcer or cellulitis w/o CC	7.8
265	9 SURG	Skin-graft +/or debrid exc for skin ulcer or cellulitis with CC	5.8
266	9 SURG	Skin-graft +/or debrid exc for skin ulcer or cellulitis w/o CC	2.9
267	9 SURG	Perianal + pilonidal procedures	2.6
268	9 SURG	Skin, subcutaneous tissue + breast plastic procedures	2.7
269	9 SURG	Other skin, subcut tiss + breast O.R. proc with CC	7.8
270	9 SURG	Other skin, subcut tiss + breast O.R. proc w/o CC	2.7
271	9 MED	Skin ulcers	8.1
272	9 MED	Major skin disorders with CC	6.8
273	9 MED	Major skin disorders w/o CC	4.8
274	9 MED	Malignant breast disorders with CC	6.3
275	9 MED	Malignant breast disorders w/o CC	2.7
276	9 MED	Non-malignant breast disorders	4.4
277	9 MED	Cellulitis age >17 with CC	6.6

(Continued)

278	9 MED	Cellulitis age >17 w/o CC	5.0
279	9 MED	* Cellulitis age 0–17	4.2
280	9 MED	Trauma to the skin, subcut tiss + breast age >17 with CC	4.4
281	9 MED	Trauma to the skin, subcut tiss + breast age >17 w/o CC	3.0
282	9 MED	* Trauma to the skin, subcut tiss + breast age 0–17	2.2
283	9 MED	Minor skin disorders with CC	5.0
284	9 MED	Minor skin disorders w/o CC	3.4

DRG	MDC 10	Endocrine, Nutritional & Metabolic Diseases	GM LOS
285	10 SURG	Amputation of lower limb for endocrine, nutritional + metabolic dis.	13.3
286	10 SURG	Adrenal + pituitary procedures	8.2
287	10 SURG	Skin grafts + wound debride for endoc, nutrit + metab disorders	12.4
288	10 SURG	O.R. procedures for obesity	6.9
289	10 SURG	Parathyroid procedures	3.4
290	10 SURG	Thyroid procedures	2.5
291	10 SURG	Thyroglossal procedures	1.7
292	10 SURG	Other endocrine, nutrit + metab O.R. proc with CC	11.1
293	10 SURG	Other endocrine, nutrit + metab O.R. proc w/o CC	4.7
294	10 MED	Diabetes age >35	5.4
295	10 MED	Diabetes age 0–35	4.2
296	10 MED	Nutritional + misc. metabolic disorders age >17 with CC	5.6
297	10 MED	Nutritional + misc. metabolic disorders age >17 w/o CC	3.8
298	10 MED	Nutritional + misc. metabolic disorders age 0–17	3.2
299	10 MED	Inborn errors of metabolism	4.4
300	10 MED	Endocrine disorders with CC	6.6
301	10 MED	Endocrine disorders w/o CC	3.8

DRG	MDC 11	Diseases & Disorders of the Kidney and Urinary Tract	GM LOS
302	11 SURG	Kidney transplant	12.9
303	11 SURG	Kidney, ureter + major bladder procedure for neoplasm	10.3
304	11 SURG	Kidney, ureter + maj bldr proc for non-neopl with CC	9.4
305	11 SURG	Kidney, ureter + maj bldr proc for non-neopl w/o CC	4.7
306	11 SURG	Prostatectomy with CC	6.1
307	11 SURG	Prostatectomy w/o CC	3.3
308	11 SURG	Minor bladder procedures with CC	5.8
309	11 SURG	Minor bladder procedures w/o CC	2.8
310	11 SURG	Transurethral procedures with CC	3.7
311	11 SURG	Transurethral procedures w/o CC	2.0
312	11 SURG	Urethral procedures, age >17 with CC	3.6
313	11 SURG	Urethral procedures, age >17 w/o CC	2.0
314	11 SURG	* Urethral procedures, age 0–17	2.3
315	11 SURG	Other kidney + urinary tract O.R. procedures	6.5
316	11 MED	Renal failure	6.2

317	11 MED	Admit for renal dialysis	2.8
318	11 MED	Kidney + urinary tract neoplasms with CC	5.8
319	11 MED	Kidney + urinary tract neoplasms w/o CC	2.5
320	11 MED	Kidney + urinary tract infections age >17 with CC	6.3
321	11 MED	Kidney + urinary tract infections age >17 w/o CC	4.6
322	11 MED	Kidney + urinary tract infections age 0–17	3.9
323	11 MED	Urinary stones with CC, and/or ESW lithotripsy	3.0
324	11 MED	Urinary stones w/o CC	2.0
325	11 MED	Kidney + urinary tract signs + symptoms age >17 with CC	4.1
326	11 MED	Kidney + urinary tract signs + symptoms age >17 w/o CC	2.7
327	11 MED	Kidney + urinary tract signs + symptoms age 0–17	3.1
328	11 MED	Urethral stricture age >17 with CC	3.6
329	11 MED	Urethral stricture age >17 w/o CC	1.9
330	11 MED	* Urethral stricture age 0–17	1.6
331	11 MED	Other kidney + urinary tract diagnoses age >17 with CC	5.2
332	11 MED	Other kidney + urinary tract diagnoses age >17 w/o CC	2.9
333	11 MED	Other kidney + urinary tract diagnoses age 0–17	5.0

DRG	MDC 12	Diseases & Disorders of the Male Reproductive System	GM LOS
334	12 SURG	Major male pelvic procedures with CC	7.4
335	12 SURG	Major male pelvic procedures w/o CC	6.2
336	12 SURG	Transurethral prostatectomy with CC	4.3
337	12 SURG	Transurethral prostatectomy w/o CC	3.2
338	12 SURG	Testes procedures, for malignancy	3.8
339	12 SURG	Testes procedures, non-malignancy age >17	3.1
340	12 SURG	* Testes procedures, non-malignancy age 0–17	2.4
341	12 SURG	Penis procedures	3.1
342	12 SURG	Circumcision age >17	2.6
343	12 SURG	* Circumcision age 0–17	1.7
344	12 SURG	Other male reproductive system O.R. procedures for malignancy	3.1
345	12 SURG	Other male reproductive system O.R. proc except for malig	3.2
346	12 MED	Malignancy, male reproductive system, with CC	5.3
347	12 MED	Malignancy, male reproductive system, w/o CC	2.5
348	12 MED	Benign prostatic hypertrophy, with CC	3.9
349	12 MED	Benign prostatic hypertrophy, w/o CC	2.3
350	12 MED	Inflammation of the male reproductive system	4.6
351	12 MED	Sterilization, male	1.3
351	12 MED	Other male reproductive system diagnoses	3.1

DRG	MDC 13	Diseases & Disorders of the Female Reproductive System	GM LOS
353	13 SURG	Pelvic evisceration, radical hysterectomy + radical vulvectomy	8.8
354	13 SURG	Uterine, adnexa proc for non-ovarian/adnexal malign with CC	6.5

(Continued)

355	13 SURG	Uterine, adnexa proc for non-ovarian/adnexal malign w/o CC	4.4
356	13 SURG	Female reproductive system reconstructive procedures	3.5
357	13 SURG	Uterine + adnexa procedures, for ovarian or adnexal malignancy	19.4
358	13 SURG	Uterine + adnexa proc for non-malignancy, with CC	5.2
359	13 SURG	Uterine + adnexa proc for non-malignancy, w/o CC	3.9
360	13 SURG	Vagina, cervix + vulva procedures	3.8
361	13 SURG	Laparoscopy + incisional tubal interruption	3.2
362	13 SURG	Endoscopic tubal interruption	1.4
363	13 SURG	D + C, conization + radio-implant, for malignancy	2.9
364	13 SURG	D + C, conization except for malignancy	2.6
365	13 SURG	Other female reproductive system O.R. procedures	6.6
366	13 MED	Malignancy, female reproductive system, with CC	6.1
367	13 MED	Malignancy, female reproductive system w/o CC	2.6
368	13 MED	Infections, female reproductive system	5.8
369	13 MED	Menstrual + other female reproductive system disorders	3.0

DRG	MDC 14	Pregnancy, Childbirth & Puerperium	GM LOS
370	14 SURG	Cesarean section with CC	4.9
371	14 SURG	Cesarean section w/o CC	3.8
372	14 SURG	Vaginal delivery with complicating diagnoses	3.1
373	14 SURG	Vaginal delivery w/o complicating diagnoses	2.0
374	14 SURG	Vaginal delivery with sterilization +/or D + C	2.6
375	14 SURG	* Vaginal delivery with O.R. proc except steril +/or D + C	4.4
376	14 MED	Postpartum and post abortion diagnoses w/o O.R. procedure	2.6
377	14 SURG	Postpartum and post abortion diagnoses with O.R. procedure	3.0
378	14 MED	Ectopic pregnancy	3.1
379	14 MED	Threatened abortion	2.4
380	14 MED	Abortion w/o D + C	1.6
381	14 MED	Abortion with D + C, aspiration curretage, or hysterotomy	1.6
382	14 MED	False labor	1.2
383	14 MED	Other antepartum diagnoses with medical complications	3.1
384	14 MED	Other antepartum diagnoses w/o medical complications	2.1

DRG	MDC 15	Normal Newborns & Other Neonates with Certain Conditions Originating in the Perinatal Period	GM LOS
385	15	* Neonates, died or transferred to another acute care facility	1.8
386	15	* Extreme immaturity or respiratory distress syndrome, neonate	17.9
387	15	* Prematurity with major problems	13.3
388	15	* Prematurity w/o major problems	8.5
389	15	* Full term neonate with major problems	5.3
390	15	* Neonates with other significant problems	4.4
391	15	* Normal newborns	3.1

DRG	MDC 16	Diseases & Disorders of the Blood and Blood-Forming DRG Organs and Immunity	GM LOS
392	16 SURG	Splenectomy age >17	10.6
393	16 SURG	* Splenectomy age 0–17	9.1
394	16 SURG	Other O.R. procedures of the blood + blood forming organs	5.3
395	16 MED	Red blood cell disorders age >17	4.5
396	16 MED	Red blood cell disorders age 0–17	1.8
397	16 MED	Coagulation disorders	7.3
398	16 MED	Reticuloendothelial + immunity disorders with CC	6.1
399	16 MED	Reticuloendothelial + immunity disorders w/o CC	4.0

DRG	MDC 17	Myeloproliferative Disorders and Poorly Differentiated Malignancy, and Other Neoplasms NEC	GM LOS
400	17 SURG	Lymphoma + leukemia with major O.R. procedure	8.1
401	17 SURG	Lymphoma + non-acute leukemia with other O.R. proc with CC	10.0
402	17 SURG	Lymphoma + non-acute leukemia with other O.R. proc w/o CC	3.3
403	17 MED	Lymphoma + non-acute leukemia with CC	7.8
404	17 MED	Lymphoma + non-acute leukemia w/o CC	3.8
405	17 MED	* Acute leukemia without major O.R. procedure age 0–17	4.9
406	17 MED	Myeloprolif disord or poorly diff neoplasm w major O.R. proc with CC	9.9
407	17 MED	Myeloprolif disord or poorly diff neopl w maj O.R. proc w/o CC	4.5
408	17 MED	Myeloprolif disord or poorly diff neopl with other O.R. proc	4.9
409	17 MED	Radiotherapy	5.8
410	17 MED	Chemotherapy w/o acute leukemia	2.9
411	17 MED	History of malignancy w/o endoscopy	2.2
412	17 MED	History of malignancy with endoscopy	2.1
413	17 MED	Other myeloprolif dis or poorly diff neopl Dx with CC	7.2
414	17 MED	Other myeloprolif dis or poorly diff neopl Dx w/o CC	4.1

DRG	MDC 18	Infections and Parasitic Diseases (systemic)	GM LOS
415	18 SURG	O.R. procedure for infections + parasitic disease	14.2
416	18 MED	Septicemia age >17	7.2
417	18 MED	Septicemia age 0–17	4.9
418	18 MED	Postoperative + post-traumatic infections	6.2
419	18 MED	Fever of unknown origin age >17 with CC	5.5
420	18 MED	Fever of unknown origin age >17 w/o CC	4.2
421	18 MED	Viral illness age >17	4.2
422	18 MED	Viral illness + fever of unknown origin age 0–17	3.5
423	18 MED	Other infectious + parasitic diseases + diagnoses	7.7

DRG	MDC 19	Mental Illness	GM LOS
424	19 SURG	O.R. procedures with principal diagnosis of mental illness	13.9
425	19 MED	Acute adjust react + disturbances of psychosocial dysfunction	4.3

(Continued)

426	19 MED	Depressive neuroses	5.0
427	19 MED	Neuroses except depressive	4.9
428	19 MED	Disorders of personality + impulse control	5.7
429	19 MED	Organic disturbances + mental retardation	7.4
430	19 MED	Psychoses	8.4
431	19 MED	Childhood mental disorders	5.8
432	19 MED	Other diagnoses of mental disorders	4.5

DRG	MDC 20	Substance Use and Substance Induced Organic Mental Disorders	GM LOS
433	20	Alcohol/drug use and induced organic mental disorders, left AMA	2.8
434	20	Alc/drug abuse or dependence, detox or other sympt trt with CC	5.1
435	20	Alcohol/drug dependence, detox +/or other sympt trt w/o CC	4.2
436	20	Alcohol/drug dependence with rehabilitation therapy	15.1
437	20	Alcohol/drug dependence, rehabilitation + detox therapy	142.8
438		No longer valid	0.0

DRG	MDC 21	Injury, Poisoning, and Toxic Effects of Drugs	GM LOS
439	21 SURG	Skin grafts for injuries	6.1
440	21 SURG	Wound debridements for injuries	7.6
441	21 SURG	Hand procedures for injuries	2.2
442	21 SURG	Other O.R. procedures for injuries with CC	5.8
443	21 SURG	Other O.R. procedures for injuries w/o CC	2.4
444	21 MED	Multiple trauma age >17 with CC	4.9
445	21 MED	Multiple trauma age >17 w/o CC	3.2
446	21 MED	* Multiple trauma age 0–17	2.4
447	21 MED	Allergic reactions age >17	2.5
448	21 MED	* Allergic reactions age 0–17	2.9
449	21 MED	Poisoning and toxic effects of drugs age >17 with CC	3.8
450	21 MED	Poisoning and toxic effects of drugs age >17 w/o CC	2.2
451	21 MED	Poisoning and toxic effects of drugs age 0–17	4.2
452	21 MED	Complications of treatment with CC	4.0
453	21 MED	Complications of treatment w/o CC	2.6
454	21 MED	Other injuries, poisonings + toxic eff diag with CC	4.3
455	21 MED	Other injuries, poisonings + toxic eff diag w/o CC	2.3

DRG	MDC 22	Burns	GM LOS
456	22 MED	Burns, transferred to another acute care facility	5.1
457	22 MED	˜ Extensive burns w/o O.R. procedure	2.6
458	22 SURG	Non-extensive burns with skin grafts	15.2
459	22 SURG	Non-extensive burns with wound debridement or other O.R. procedure	10.7
460	22 MED	Non-extensive burns w/o O.R. procedure	6.0

DRG	MDC -23	Selected Factors Influencing Health Status and Contact with Health Services	GM LOS
461	23 SURG	O.R. proc with diagnoses of other contact with health services	2.4
462	23 MED	Rehabilitation	13.3
463	23 MED	Signs + symptoms with CC	4.7
464	23 MED	Signs + symptoms w/o CC	2.9
465	23 MED	Aftercare with history of malignancy as secondary Dx	1.9
466	23 MED	Aftercare w/o history of malignancy as secondary Dx	2.4
467	23 MED	Other factors influencing health status	2.5
468		Unrelated O.R. procedures	12.9
469		** PDX invalid as discharge diagnosis	
470		** Ungroupable	
471	8 SURG	Bilateral or major joint procedures of the lower extremities	10.6
472	22 SURG	Extensive burns with O.R. procedure	17.8
473	17 MED	Acute leukemia w/o major O.R. procedures age >17	9.6
474	4	No longer valid	0.0
475	4 MED	Respiratory system diagnosis with ventilator support	9.8
476		Prostatic OR Procedures unrelated to principal diagnosis	13.4
477		Non-extensive OR procedure unrelated to principal diagnosis	6.0
478	5 SURG	Other vascular procedures with CC	6.6
479	5 SURG	Other vascular procedures w/o CC	4.0
480	SURG	Liver transplant	27.6
481	SURG	Bone marrow transplant	36.2
482	SURG	Trach with mouth, larynz or pharynx disorder	13.3
483	SURG	Trach except for mouth, larynx or pharynx disorder	43.9
484	24 SURG	Craniotomy for multiple significant trauma	13.3
485	24 SURG	Limb reattachment, hip & femur procedures for multiple significant trauma	12.5
486	24 SURG	Other O.R. procedures for multiple significant trauma	10.2
487	24 MED	Other multiple significant trauma	7.3
488	25 SURG	HIV with extensive O.R. procedure	15.8
489	25 MED	HIV with major related condition	8.8
490	25 MED	HIV with or without other related condition	5.3
491	8 SURG	Major joint and limb reattachment procedures U.E.	5.0
492	17 MED	Chemotherapy with acute leukemia as secondary diagnosis	10.9
493	7 SURG	Laparoscopic cholecystectomy w/o CDE w/CC	4.3
494	7 Surg	Laparoscopic cholecystectomy w/o CDE w/o CC	1.7

* GM LOS is Geometric Mean Length of Stay.
46390 Federal Register/Vol. 58, No. 168/Wednesday, September 1, 1993/Rules and Regulations

APPENDIX B

Important Addresses and Phone Numbers

Case Management Society of America (CMSA)
8201 Cantrell, Suite 230
Little Rock, AR 72227
(501) 225-2229, FAX (501) 221-9068

Individual Case Management Association (ICMA)
10809 Executive Center Drive—Suite 310
Little Rock, AR 72211
(501) 223-5204, FAX (501) 223-0519, Member services 1-800-664-2620

For more information on the ten Medigap policies:
1994 Medicare and Medigap Update from the United Seniors Health Cooperative
131 H Street NW—Suite 500
Washington, DC 20005
(enclose $1 to cover postage and handling)

Medigap Insurance or for general Medicare information
1-800-432-4040
Social Security Administration (for Medicare applications or information
on Medicare)
1-800-234-5772

Where to call for Medicare Handbook
(aka Guide to Health Insurance for People with Medicare)
1-800-772-1213
or write:
Medicare Publications
Health Care Financing Administration
6325 Security Blvd
Baltimore, Maryland 21207-5187
(Publication No. HCFA 10050)

Length of stay (by diagnosis and operations)
HCIA, Inc.
300 E. Lombard Street
Baltimore, MD 21202
1-800-521-6210
(1993 copy = $164)

CCM (Certification for Case Manager) Exam
Write:
Certification for Case Manager
1835 Rohlwing Road–Suite D
Rolling Meadows, IL 60008
(708) 818-0292

Milliman & Robertson, Inc.
1301 Fifth Avenue–Suite 3800
Seattle, WA 98101-2605
(206) 340-0607
(Note: There are approximately 25 offices. Call for a list or for the one nearest to you.)

InterQual, Inc.
44 Lafayette Road
North Hampton, NH 03862-0988
(603) 964-7255
or InterQual, Inc.
293 Boston Post Road West–Suite 180
Marlborough, MA 01752
(508) 481-1181

HCFA Hotline (for questions about Medicare or Medicaid)
1-800-638-6833

Clinical Guideline Manuals
Center for Research Dissemination and Liaison
AHCPR Clearinghouse
PO Box 8547
Silver Spring, MD 20907
1-800-358-9295 or (301) 495-3453

Bibliography

Bibliography

Acute Pain Management Guideline Panel. *Acute pain management: Operative or medical procedures and training* (AHCPR Pub. No. 92-0032). Rockville, MD: Agency for Health Care Policy and Research, Public Health Service, US Department of Health and Human Services.

Adams, R. (1987). The impact of utilization review on nursing. *JONA, 17*(9), 44–46.

AHA Council Report. (1987). *Case management: An aid to quality and continuity of care.* American Hospital Association. Chicago: Author.

Alfaro, R. (1986). *Application of the nursing process: A step by step guide.* Philadelphia: J. B. Lippincott.

American Nurses Association. (1985). *Code for nurses with interpretive statements.* Kansas City: Author.

American Nurses Association. (1988). *Nursing case management.* Kansas City: Author.

American Nurses Association. (1991). *CHN communique* (Council of Community Health Nursing). Washington, DC: Author.

American Nurses Association. (1991). *Nursing case management.* Kansas City: Author.

American Nurses Association. (1992). *Nursing case management.* Kansas City: Author.

Anonymous. (1990). Medical records access: Practical legal tips for the 1990s. *AGG Notes, 4*(2), 1–4.

Anonymous. (1991). CMs find innovative options for clients between the ICU and the acute care bed. *Case Management Advisor, 2*(8), 113–117.

Anonymous. (1992). Case management opportunities grow as Medicare explores managed care. *Case Management Advisor, 3*(8), 101–4.

Anonymous. (1993). Comparing case management styles. *Journal of Nursing Administration, 23*(1), 6, 38, 59.

Anonymous. (1994). Acute pain management in adults: Operative procedures—Quick reference guide for clinicians. *MEDSURG Nursing, 3*(2), 99–107.

Anonymous. (1994). Case managers increase attention to HIV pain management. *AIDS Alert, 9*(1), 9–11.

Anonymous. (1994). Collaboration—and trust—save four hospitals $896,000 on CABG patients. *Hospital Case Management, 2*(5), 73–5.

Anonymous. (1994). CMSA Standards of Practice. *The Case Manager, 5*(1), 59–71.

Anonymous. (1994). Emergency departments visits mostly non-urgent. *Arizona Hospital Association Weekly Newsletter, 8*(33), 1.

Anonymous. (1994). Hospital laser center institutes critical paths. *Hospital Case Management, 2*(5), 83–5.

Anonymous. (1994). Hospital system saves $501,000 with maternity case management. *Hospital Case Management, 2*(5), 85–7.

Anonymous. (1994). How decision trees can simplify patient triaging, CM role. *Hospital Case Management, 2*(5), 83.

Anonymous. (1987, Fall). Managing your risk—A primer on contractual liability. 149–151.

Austin, C. D. (1983). Case management in long-term care: Options and opportunities. *Health and Social Work, 8*(1), 16–30.

Bair, N., Griswold, J., & Head, J. (1989). Clinical RN involvement in bedside-centered case management. *Nursing Economics, 7*(3), 150–154.

Bergen, A. (1992). Case management in community care: Concepts, practices, and implications for nursing. *Journal of Advanced Nursing, 17*(9), 1106–13.

Bilella, R. J., Somogyi, A., Bach, A., & Mazie, J. (1994). Implementing a case managment program in a large city hospital. *Strategies for health care excellence, 7*(4), 1–6.

Biller, A. M. (1992). Implementing nursing case management. *Rehabilitation Nursing, 17*(3), 144–146.

Blodgett, C. (1992). HMO case management: Medical group model. *The Case Manager, 3*(3), 35–38.

Bokos, P. J., Mejta, C. L., Mickenberg, J. H., Monks, R. L. (1992). Case management: An alternataive approach to working with intravenous drug users. *NIDA Research Monograph*, 127, 92–111.

Boland, P. (1991). *Making managed health care work: Practical guide to strategies and solutions.* New York: McGraw Hill.

Boling, J. (1991, July). Profile—John Banja. *The Case Manager*, 76–81.

Boling, J. (1993, Aug/Sept). Conflict with case management...The ethical agenda. *The Case Manager*, 6.

Bookin, L. (1994). Effects of capitation on home health care. *Geriatric Nursing, 15*(3), 167–168.

Borgford-Parnell, D., & Hope, K. R. (1994). A homeless teen pregnancy project: An intensive team case management model. *American Journal of Public Health, 84*(6), 1029–30.

Bosek, M. (1994). Ethics from the other side of the bed: A daughter's perspective. *MEDSURG Nursing, 3*(4), 316–318, 334.

Bosek, M. S. D., & Fitzpatrick, J. (1992). A nursing perspective on advance directives. *MED-SURG Nursing, 1*(1), 33–38.

Bouley, G., Von Hofe, K., & Blatt, L. (1994). Holistic care of the critically ill: Meeting both patient and family needs. *Dimensions of Critical Care Nursing, 13*(4), 218–223.

Bower, K. (1988). *Case management by nurses.* Kansas City: American Nurses Publishing.

Bower, K. (1988). Case management: Meeting the challenge. *Definition, 3*(1), 1–3.

Bradley, J. C., & Edinberg, M. A. (1986). *Communication in the nursing context.* Norwalk, Connecticutt: Appleton-Century-Crofts.

Braverman, T. (1993, August). Warning: Humor may be hazardous to your health. *The Arizona Light*, p. 14.

Bricker, P., et al. (1988). Team approach enables frail elderly to stay home. *Health Progress, 60*(6), 46–49.

Brockopp, D. Y., Porter, M., Kinnaird, S., & Silberman, S. (1992). Fiscal and clinical evaluation of patient care: A case management model for the future. *JONA, 22*(9), 23–27.

Browdie, R. (1992). Ethical issues in case management from a political and systems perspective. *Journal of Case Management, 1*(3), 87–89.

Brown, B. J., & Heg Yvary, S. (1993). Population-based care systems. *Nursing Administration Quarterly, 17*(3), vi–91.

Brucker, J. M. (1992). Developing a pediatric neuro-oncology case manager. *Journal of Pediatric Nursing, 7*(1), 77–78.

Bueno, M. M., & Hwang, R. F. (1993). Understanding variances in hospital stay. *Nursing Management, 24*(11), 51–57.

California Medical Review, Inc. (CMRI). (1990). *Utilization Review Seminar Workbook.* San Francisco: Author.

Cancer care may cost more than it's worth, study says. (1993, February 11). *The Phoenix Gazette,* p. B8.

Cave, D. G., & Tucker, L. J. (1990). Optimizing the effectiveness of your case management program. *Employee Benefits Journal,* September, 4–9.

Cesta, T. G. (1993). The link between continuous quality improvement and case management. *Journal of Nursing Administration, 23*(6), 55–61.

Charlesworth, E., & Nathan, R. (1984). *Stress management: A comprehensive guide to wellness.* New York: Atheneum.

Chenevert, M. (1988). *STAT-Special techniques in assertiveness training for women in the health professions* (3rd ed.). St. Louis: C. V. Mosby.

Cline, B. G. (1990). Case management: Organizational models and administrative methods. *Caring, 9*(7), 14–18.

Clough, J., & Thomas K. (1992). Health promotion/illness prevention through wellness clinics and nursing case management. *Arizona Nurse, 45*(3), 1.

Coffey, R. J., Richards, J. S., Remmert, C. S., LeRoy S. S., Schoville, R. R., & Baldwin, P. J. (1992). An introduction to critical paths. *Quality Management in Health Care, 1*(1), 45–54.

Cohen, E. L. (1991). Nursing case management: Does it pay? *JONA, 21*(4), 20–26.

Coker, E. B., & Schreiber, R. (1990). The nurse's role in a team conference. *Nursing Management, 21*(3), 46–48.

Coleman, J. (1994). The managed care organization evolution. *The Case Manager, 5*(1), 75–82.

Coleman, J. R. (1991). HMOs and individual case management. *The Case Manager, 1*(3), 55–61.

Coleman, J. R., & Hagen E. (1991). Collaborative practice: Case managers and homecare agency nurses. *The Case Manager, 2*(4), 64–72.

Collins, L. (1989). Case management reduces high-risk pregnancy cost. *Business Insurance, 23* (8), 70–73.

Cooper, R. G., & Leja, J. A. (1990). An investigation of managed health care case management. *Journal of Allied Health, 19*(3), 219–225.

Corkery, E. (1989). Discharge planning and home health care: What every staff nurse should know. *Orthopoedic Nursing, 8*(6), 18–26.

Cronin, C., & Makelbust, J. (1989). Case-managed care: Capitalizing on the clinical nurse specialist. *Nursing Management, 20*(3), 38–47.

Crummer, M. B., & Carter, V. (1993). Critical pathways—The pivotal tool. *Journal of Cardiovascular Nursing, 7*(4), 30–7.

Cruzan vs. Director. (1990). Missouri Department of Health, 110 S. Ct. 2841.

Curtin, L. (1992). On writing a column on ethics. *Nursing Management, 23*(7), 18–20.

Curtin, L. L. (1993). Informed consent: Cautious, calculated candor. *Nursing Management, 24*(4), 18–19.

Curtin, L. L. (1993). Patient privacy in a public institution. *Nursing Management, 24*(6), 26–27.

Curtin, L. L. (1994). Ethical concerns of nutritional life support. *Nursing Management, 25*(1), 14–16.

Cwiek, M. A., Hervey, D., & Mortland, C. (1992, December). Improving utilization and patient care. *Health Progress,* 35–37, 58.

Dees, J., & Taylor, J. (1990). Health care management, A tool for the future. *AAOHN Journal, 38*(2), 52–58.

Del Bueno, D., & Leulanc, D. (1989). Nursing managed care: One approach. *JONA, 19*(11), 24–27.

Del Togono-Armanasco, V., Olivas, G. S. & Harter, S. (1989). Developing an integrated case management model. *Nursing Management, 20*(10) 26–29.

Desimone, B. (1988, July). The case for case management. *Continuing Care,* 22–23.

Dinerman, M. (1992). Managing the maze: Case management and service delivery. *Administration in Social Work, 16*(1), 1–9.

Doughery, C., Kizer, W., & O'Brien, R. (1990). Covering America's uninsured: Who has the answer to rising health care costs. *Creighton University Window, 6*(3), 16–21.

Dubler, N. N. (1992). Individual advocacy as a governing principle. *Journal of Case Management, 1*(3), 82–86.

Emmanuel, E. J. (1992). Proxy decision making for incompetent patients. *Journal of the American Medical Association,* p. 2067.

Erkel, E. A. (1993). The impact of case management in preventive services. *Journal of Nursing Administration, 23* (1), 27–32.

Etheredge, M. L. (Ed.). (1987). Critical paths. *Definition, 2*(3), 1–4.

Etheredge, M. L. (Ed.). (1988). Why managed care "works." *Definition, 3*(4), 1–4.

Etheredge, M. L. S. (Ed.). (1986). The maps for managed care. *Definition, 1*(3), 1–3.

Etheredge, M. L. S. (Ed.). (1989). *Collaborative care: Nursing case management.* Chicago: American Hospital Publishing.

Ethridge, P. (1988–89). Nursing innovation cuts hospital costs. *New Mexico Nurse, 23*(4), 6.

Ethridge, P., & Lamb, G. (1990). Professional nursing case management improves quality, access and costs. *Nursing Management,* 20(3), 30–35.

Evers, C., Odon, S., Latulip-Gardner, J., & Paul, S. (1994). Developing a critical pathway for orientation. *American Journal of Critical Care, 3*(3), 217–223.

Faaoso, N. (1992). Automated patient care systems: The ethical impact. *Nursing Management, 23*(7), 46–48.

Fanucci, D., Hammil, M., Johannson, P., Leggett, J., & Smith, M. J. (1993). Quantum leap into continuous quality improvement. *Nursing Management, 24*(6), 28–30.

Feldman, C., Olberding, L., Shortridge, L., Toole, K., & Zappin, P. (1993). Decision making in case management of home health care clients. *Journal of Nursing Administration, 23*(1), 33–38.

Feltes, M., Wetle, T., Clemens, E., Crabtree, B., Dubitzky, D., & Kerr, M. (1994). Case managers and physicians: Communication and perceived problems. *Journal of the American Geriatric Society, 42,* 5–10.

Ferrell, B., & Rhiner, M. (1994). Managing cancer pain: A three-step approach. *Nursing 94, 24*(7), 57–59.

Feutz-Harter, S. A. (1991). *Nursing and the law.* Eau Claire, Wisconsin: Professional Education Systems.

Fiesta, J. (1992). Refusal of treatment. *Nursing Management, 23*(11), 14–18.

Fisher, K. (1987, August). QA update: Case management. *Quality Review Bulletin,* 287–290.

Flynn, A. M., & Kilgallen, M. B. (1993). Case management: A multidisciplinary approach to the evaluation of cost and quality standards. *Journal of Nursing Care Quality, 8*(1), 58–66.

Fondiller, S. H. (1991). How case management is changing the picture. *American Journal of Nursing, 91*(1), 64–80.

Ford, R., & Ryan, P. (1992). Meeting needs with case management. *Nursing Standard, 39*(6), 29–32.

Gibson, S. J., Martin, S. M., Johnson, M. B., Blue, R., & Miller, D. S. (1994). CNS-directed case management. Cost and quality in harmony. *Journal of Nursing administration, 24*(6), 45–51.

Goodwin, D. R. (1992). Critical pathways in home healthcare. *Journal of Nursing Administration, 22*(2), 35–40.

Gordon, M. L. (1992). Case management: Professional excellence and quality care. *Ohio Nurses Review, 67*(3), 10.

Graybeal, K. B., Gheen, M., & McKenna, B. (1993). Clinical pathway development: The overlake model. *Nursing Management, 24*(4), 42–45.

Grimaldi, P. (1992). Medigap insurance policies standardized. *Nursing Management, 23*(11), 20, 22, 24.

Guilano, K., & Poirier, C. (1991). Nursing case management: Critical pathways to desirable outcomes. *Nursing Management, 22*(3), 52–57.

Hagin, D. C. (1989, April 4). Case management system cuts costs, reduces stays. *Health Care Strategic Management.*

Health Care Financing Administration. (1994). *The Medicare 1994 Handbook.* DHHS Publication No. HCFA 10050, Baltimore, MD.

Healthcare Knowledge Resources. (1991). *Length of stay by diagnosis and operation.* Ann Arbor: Author.

Hegyvary, S. T. (1993). Population-oriented care systems. *Nursing Administration Quarterly, 17*(3), viii–ix.

Hein, E. C., & Nicholson, M. J. (1994). *Contemporary leadership behavior.* Philadelphia: J. B. Lippincott.

Hembree, W. E. (1985, July/August). Getting involved: Employers as case managers. *Business and Health,* 11–14.

Henderson, M. G., & Collard, A. (1988, February). Measuring quality in medical case management programs. *Quality Review Bulletin.*

Henkelman, W. (1994). Inadequate pain management: Ethical considerations. *Nursing Management-Critical care edition, 25*(1), 48A–48D.

Hickey, M. (1990). What are the needs of families of critically ill patients? A review of the literature since 1979. *Heart & Lung, 19*(4), 401–415.

Hicks, L., Stallmeyer, J. M., & Coleman, J. R. (1992). Nursing challenges in managed care. *Nursing Economics, 10*(4), 265–276.

Holloway, C. M., & Pokorny, M. E. (1994). Early hospital discharge and independence: What happens to the elderly? *Geriatric Nursing, 15*(1), 24–27.

Holzemer, W. L. (1992). Linking primary health care and self-care through case management. *International Nursing Review, 39*(3), 83–89.

InterQual, & Tennant, T. (Ed.). (1993). *The ISD-A (TM) review system with Adult ISD (TM) criteria.* North Hampton: Author.

InterQual, & Tennant, T. (Ed.). (1993). *Utilization review and management training manual.* North Hampton: Author.

Jackson, B., Finkler, D., & Robinson, C. (1992). A case management system for infants with chronic illnesses and developmental disabilities. *Childrens Health Care, 21*(4), 224–232.

Johnson, K., & Morrison, E. F. (1993). Control or negotiation: A health care challenge. *Nursing Administration Quarterly, 17*(3), 27–33.

Joint Commission on Accreditation of Health Care Organizations. (1994). *Accreditations Manual for Hospitals: Volume 1—Standards.* Oakbrock Terrace, IL: Author.

Kane, R. A. (1988). Case management: Ethical pitfalls on the road to high-quality managed care. *Quality Review Bulletin,* pp. 161–166.

Kantor, J. (1989). Clinical case management: Definition, principles, and components. *Hospital and Community Psychiatry, 40*(4), 361–368.

Karls, J., & Wandrei, K. E. (1992). The Person-in-environment system for classifying client problems: A new tool for more effective case management. *Journal of Case Management, 1*(3), 90–95.

Kelly, M. P., Bacon, G. T., & Mitchell, J. A. (1994). Glossary of managed care terms. *Journal of Ambulatory Care Management, 17*(1), 70–6.

Kerr, M. H., & Birk, J. M. (1988). A client centered case management model. *Quarterly Review Bulletin, 14*(9), 279–283.

Kleinsell, R. M. (1990). Needs of families of critically ill patients: A literature review. *Critical Care Nurse, 11*(8), 34–40.

Knollmueller, R. (1989). Case management: What's in a name? *Nursing Management, 20* (10), 38–42.

Kolodner, D. E. (1992). Advance medical directives after Cruzan. *MEDSURG Nursing, 1*(1), 56–59.

Kongstvedt, P. R. (1993). *The managed health care handbook.* Gaithersburg: Aspen Publishers.

Knox, R. (1994, May 27). Noted deaths reflect attitude shift: Most patients and families oppose resuscitation efforts, study finds. *The Phoenix Gazette,* A26.

Kortbawi, P. A. (1993). An orientation plan for hospital-based case managers. *Journal of Continuing Education in Nursing, 24*(2), 69–73.

Kreiger, G., & Sullivan, J. (1987). The case for case management. *Occupational Health and Safety, 56*(5), 92.

Krmpotic, D. (1992). Successful implementation of case management. *Nursing Connections, 5*(2), 49–55.

Kupferschmid, B. (1987). Families of critically ill patients. *Critical Care Nursing Currents, 5*(2), 7–12.

Kurtz, L., Badarozzi, D., & Pollane, L. (1984). Case management in mental health. *Health and Social Work, 9*(3), 201–211.

Ladden, M. (1991). On-site perinatal case management: An HMO model. *Journal of Perinatal Neonatal Nursing, 5*(1), 27–32.

Lajeunesse, D. (1990). Case management: A primary nursing approach. *Caring, 9*(8), 13–15.

Lamb, G. S., & Stempel, J. E. (1994). Nurse case management from the client's view: Growing as insider-expert. *Nursing Outlook, 42*(1), 7–13.

Landsberg, G., & Rock, M. (1994). County mental health directors' evaluation of statewide intensive case management program: The New York experience. *Journal of Mental Health Administration, 21*(2), 193–200.

Latini, E. E., & Foote, W. (1992). Obtaining consistent quality patient care for the trauma patient by using a critical pathway. *Critical Case Nursing Quarterly, 15*(3), 51–55.

LeClair, C. L. (1991). Introducing and accounting for RN case management. *Nursing Management, 22*(3), 44–49.

Leddy, S., & Pepper, M. (1989). *Conceptual bases of professional nursing.* Philadelphia: J. B. Lippincott.

Levenson, J., & Pettrey, L. (1994). Controversial decisions regarding treatment and DNR: An algorithmic guide for the uncertain in decision-making ethics (GUIDE). *American Journal of Critical Care, 3*(2), 87–91.

Like, R. C. (1988). Primary care case management: A family physician's perspective. *Quarterly Review Bulletin, 14*(6), 175–178.

Lowery, S. L. (1992, Oct-Dec). Qualifications for the successful case manager. *The Case Manager,* 66–72.

Luluage, A. (1991). RN-LPN teams: Toward unit case management. *Nursing Management, 22*(3), 44–49.

Mahn, V. A. (1993). Clinical nurse case management: A service line approach. *Nursing Management, 24*(9), 48–50.

Mann, A. H., Hazel, C., Geer, C., Hurley, C. M., & Podrapovic, T. (1993). Development of an orthopaedic case manager. *Orthopaedic Nursing, 12*(4), 23–27.

Marr, J. A., & Reid, B. (1992). Implementing managed care and case management: The neuroscience experience. *Journal of Neuroscience Nursing, 24*(5), 281–5.

Martin, D., & Redland, A. (1988). Legal and ethical issues in resuscitation and withholding of treatment. *Critical Care Nursing Quarterly, 10*(4), 1–8.

Mathis, M. (1984). Personal needs of family members of critically ill patients with and without acute brain injury. *Journal of Neurosurgical Nursing, 16*(1), 36–44.

Mayer, G. G., Madden, M. J., & Lawrenz, E. (Eds.). (1990). *Patient care delivery models.* Rockville, MD: Aspen Publishers.

Mazzola, M. (1991, January). Effectiveness of case management: Cost savings methodology. *The Case Manager,* 56–59.

McBride, S. M. (1992). Rehabilitation case managers: Ahead of their time. *Holistic Nursing Practice, 6*(2), 67–75.

McCaffery, M., & Ferrell, B. (1994). How to use the new AHCPR cancer pain guidelines. *American Journal of Nursing, 94,* 42–46.

McGuire, L. (1994). The nurse's role in pain relief. *MEDSURG Nursing, 3*(2), 94–98.

McIntosh, L. (1987). Hospital base case management. *Nursing Economics, 5*(5), 232–236.

McKenzie, C. B., Torkelson, N. G., & Holt, M. A. (1989). Care and cost: Nursing case management improves both. *Nursing Management, 20*(10), 30–34.

Merrill, J. (1985, July/August). Defining case management. *Business and Health,* pp. 5–9.

Michaels, C. (1992). Carondelet St. Mary's nursing enterprise. *Nursing Clinics of North America, 27*(1), 77–85.

Miller, L. L., & Miller, J. (1989). Selecting medical case management programs: The employer's/purchaser's perspective. *Quality Review Bulletin,* pp. 121–126.

Miller, M. E., & Gengler, D. J. (1993). Medicaid case managment: Kentucky's patient access and care program. *Health Care Financing Review, 15*(1), 55–69.

Milliman & Robertson. (1992). *Healthcare management guidelines.* Seattle: Author.

Moin, L., & Stumpf, N. (1994). Use of physical restraints in the hospital setting: Implications for the nurse. *Geriatric Nursing, 15*(3), 127–131.

Molter, N. (1979). Needs of relatives of critically ill patients: A descriptive study. *Heart & Lung, 8*(2), 332–339.

Mosher, C., Cronk, P., Kidd, A., McCormick, P., Stockton, S., & Sulla, C. (1992). Upgrading practice with critical pathways. *American Journal of Nursing,* January, 41–44.

Moss, M. T. (1994). Nursing tools: A global perspective . . . three tools form a triangular analytical instrument, outcomes management, case management and critical pathways. *Nursing Management, 25*(6), 64A–B.

Mullahy, C. (1992). Case managers and physicians-working associates not adversaries. *The Case Manager, 3*(3), 62–68.

Mullahy, C. (1992). Empowering the case manager. *Continuing Care,* pp. 15–30.

Murphy-Berman, V. (1994). A conceptual framework for thinking about risk assessment and case management in child protective service. *Child Abuse and Neglect, 18*(2), 193–201.

Neidig, J. R. (1992). The critical path: An evaluation of the applicability of nursing case managment in the NICU. *Neonatal Network-Journal of Neonatal Nursing, 11*(5), 45–52.

Netting, F., & Williams, F. (1989). Ethical decision-making in case management programs for the elderly. *Health Values, 13*(3), 3–8.

Newald, J. (1986). Diversifying: Better think case management. *Hospitals, 60* (16), 84.

Newman, M., Lamb, G., & Michaels, C. (1991). Nursing case management: The coming together of theory and practice. *Nursing & Health Care, 12*(9), 484–488.

Northrop, C. E., & Kelly, M. E. (1987). *Legal issues in nursing.* St. Louis: C. V. Mosby.

O'Connor, C. T. (1990). Patient education with a purpose. *Journal of Nursing Staff Development, 6*(3), 145–147.

Olivas, G. S., Del Togno-Armanasco, V., Erickson, J. R. & Harter, S. (1989). Case management—A botttom-line care delivery model. Part I: The concept. *JONA, 19*(11), 16–20.

Olivas, G. S., et al. (1989). Case management—A bottom-line care delivery model. Part II: Adoption of the model. JONA, *19* (12), 12–17.

Ovretveit, J. (1992). Fulfilling the need for a coordinated approach: Case management and community nursing. *Professional Nurse, 7*(4), 264–269.

Parker, M., & Secord, L. J. (1988). Case managers: Guiding the elderly through the health care maze. *American Journal of Nursing, 88* (12), 1674–1676.

Parker, M., & Secord, L. J. (1988). Private geriatric case management: Current trends and future direction. *Health Care Supervisor, 7* (1), 68–75.

Parker, M., Quinn, J., Viehl, M., McKinley, A. H., Polich, C. L., Hartwell, S., Van Hook, R., & Detzner, D. F. (1992). Issues in rural case management. *Family & Community Health, 14*(4), 40–60.

Pavalovich, M. (1994). Pediatric case management. *The Case Manager, 5*(1), 87–92.

Payne, F. J., Sharrett, C. S., Poretz, D. N. Eron, L. J., Stage, T., Foroobar, R., Bowman, C., & Miller, R. K. (1992). Community-based case management of HIV disease. *American Journal of Public Health, 82*(6), 893–894.

Perin, R. L. (1992). *Arizona statutes affecting nursing practice.* Eau Claire, Wisconsin: Professional Education Systems.

Petryshen, P. R., & Petryshen, P. M. (1992). The case management model: An innovative approach to delivery of patient care. *Journal of Advanced Nursing, 17*(10), 1188–1194.

Pierce, P. M., & Freedman, S. A. (1988). The teach project: Training in case management. *Quality Review Bulletin,* .

Pierini, S. (1988). Case managing the elderly: Best bet for the future. *Health Progress, 69* (11), 42–45.

Possin, B. (1991). A consortium introduces RN case management regionwide. *Nursing Management, 22*(3), 62–64.

President's Commission for the Study of Ethical Problems in Medicine and Biomedical and Behavioral Research. (1983). *Deciding to forego life- sustaining treatment.* Washington, DC: US Government Printing Office.

Prins, M. M. (1992). Patient advocacy: The role of nursing leadership. *Nursing Management, 23*(7), 78–80.

Quinn, J. (1992). Case management: A crucial part of our long term care system. *Journal of Case Management, 1*(1), 4.

Redford, L. J. (1992). Case management: The wave of the future. *Journal of Case Management, 1*(1), 5–8.

Rehr, H. (1986). Discharge planning: An ongoing function of quality care. *Quality Review Bulletin, 12*(2), 47–50.

Reinhard, S. C. (1988). Case managing community services for hip fractured elders. *Orthopaedic Nursing, 7*(5), 42–49.

Resnick, R. (1992, Sept). Case management evolves into a quality care program. *Business & Health,* 51–56.

Riley, P. A., & Fortinsky, R. H. (1992). Developing consumer-centered quality assurance strategies for home care: A case management model. *Journal of Case Management, 1*(2), 39–48.

Riley, T. A. (1992). HIV-infected client care: Case management and the HIV team. *Clinical Nurse Specialist*, 6(3), 136–141.

Ritter, J., Fralic, M. F., Tonges, M. C., & McCormac, M. (1992). Redesigning nursing practice: A case management model for critical care. *Nursing Clinics of North America*, 27(1), 119–128.

Rogers, M., Riordan, J., & Swindle, D. (1991). Community-based nursing case management pays off. *Nursing Management*, 22(3), 30–34.

Sabin, J., Forrow, L., & Daniels, N. (1991). Clarifying the concept of medical necessity. *Medical Interface*, December, 35–42.

Salladay, S., & McDonnell, Sr. M. (1989). Spiritual care, ethical choices, and patient advocacy. *Nursing Clinics of North America*, 24(2), 543–548.

Saue, J. M. (1988, August). Legal issues related to case management. *Quality Review Bulletin*, 80–85.

Schmidt, T. (1992). Case management problems and home care. *Journal of the Association of Nurses in AIDS Care*, 3(3), 37–44.

Schueman, S. A. (1987, September). A model of case management for mental health services. *Quality Review Bulletin*.

Scott, M. P., & Packard, K. P. *Telephone assessment with protocols for nursing practice*. Philadelphia: W. B. Saunders.

Scully, G. L. & Nichols, A. O. (1990). Case management compilation of definitions. *The Case Manager*, 212–45.

Sederer, L. I. (1987). Utilization review and quality assurance: Staying in the black and working with the blues. *General Hospital Psychiatry*, 9, 210–19.

Simmons, F. M. (1992). Developing the trauma nurse case manager role. *Dimensions of Critical Care Nursing*, 11(3), 164–170.

Simmons, W. J., & White, M. (1989). Hospital sponsored case management services. *CAHHS Insight*, 13(1).

Sinnen, M., & Schifalacqua, M. (1991). Coordinated care in a community hospital. *Nursing Management*, 22(3), 38–42.

Smith, M. C. (1993). Case management & nursing theory-based practices. *Nursing Science Quarterly*, 6(1), 8–9.

Smith, P., Pass, C. M., Stream, C. P., & Jones, B. (1992). Implementing nurse case management in a community hospital. *MEDSURG Nursing*, 1(1), 47–52.

Smith, R. (1988). Quality assurance in equipment ordering for the spinal cord-injured client. *American Journal of Occupational Therapy*, 42(1), 36–39.

Solomon, P., & Draine, J. (1994). Family perceptions of consumers as case managers. *Community Mental Health Journal*, 30(2), 165–176.

Stillwagon, C. A. (1989). The impact of nurse managed care on the cost of nurse practice and nurse satisfaction. *Journal of Nursing Administration*, 19(11), 21–27.

Stone, C. L., & Krebs, K. (1990). The use of utilization review nurses to decrease reimbursement denials. *Home Healthcare Nurse*, 8(3), 13–17.

Strong, A. G. (1992). Case management and the CNS. *Clinical Nurse Specialist*, 6(2), 64.

Taban, H. (1993). The nurse case manager in acute care settings. *JONA*, 23(10), 53–61.

Tassel, M. V. (1994). Case managers use entrepreneurial skills. *Hospital Case Management*, August, 143.

Theis, E. C. (1990). Lifesustaining technologies—Ordinary or extraordinary? *Focus on Critical Care—AACN*, 17(6), 445–450.

Trella, R. S. (1993). A multidisciplinary approach to case management of frail, hospitalized older adults. *Journal of Nursing Administration*, 23(2), 20–26.

Wadas, T. M. (1993). Case management and caring behavior. *Nursing Management, 24*(9), 40–46.

Wahlstedt, P., & Blaser, W. (1987). Nurse case management for the frail elderly: A curriculum to prepare nurses for that role. *Home Health Care Nurse, 4*(2), 30–35.

Wallace, M. (1994). Assessment and management of pain in the elderly. *MEDSURG Nursing, 3*(4), 293–298.

Westhoff, L. J. (1992). Care management: Quelling the confusion. *Health Progress, 73*(5), 43–58.

Wetle, T. (1992). A taxonomy of ethical issues in case management of the frail older person. *Journal of Case Management, 1*(3), 71–75.

White, C., & Howse. (1993). Managing humor: When is it funny—and when is it not? *Nursing Management, 24*(4), 80–92.

Williams, L. R., & Cooper, M. K. (1993). Nurse-managed postpartum home care. *Journal of Obstetric, Gynecologic, & Neonatal Nursing, 22*(1), 25–31.

Williams, S. J., & Torrens, P. R. (1993). *Introduction to health services.* New York: Delmar.

Wiseman, S. J. (1990). Patient advocacy: The essence of perioperative nursing in ambulatory surgery. *AORN Journal, 51*(3), 754–762.

Witek, J. R., & Hostage, J. L. (1994). Medicaid managed care: Problems and promise. *Journal of ambulatory Care Management, 17*(91), 61–9.

Woldum, K. (1987). Critical paths: Marking the course. *Definition, 2*(3), 1–4.

Wong, S. (1993, March 17). Hospital resuscitation brings cost "avalanche": Price of reviving patients put at $161,000. *The Phoenix Gazette.*

Wright, R. A. (1987). *Human values in healthcare: The practice of ethics.* New York: McGraw-Hill.

Yee, D. L. (1990, July). Developing a quality assurance program in case management service settings. *Caring Magazine*, pp. 30–35.

Zander, K. (1988). Nursing case management: Strategic management of cost and quality outcomes. *JONA, 18*(5), 23–30.

Zander, K. (1988). Nursing case management: Resolving the DRG paradox. *Nursing Clinics of North America, 23*(3), 503–520.

Zander, K. (1988). Revising the production process: When "more" is not the solution. *Healthcare Supervisor, 3*(3), 44–54.

Zander, K. (1989). Case consultation: Determines the next action. *Definition, 4*(1), 38–41.

Zander, K. (1989). Second generation critical paths. *Definition, 4*(4), 1-back page.

Zander, K. (1990). Differentiating managed care and case management. *Definition, 5*(2), 1.

Zander, K. (1990). Case management: A golden opportunity for whom? McClosky & Grace (Eds.). *Current issues in nursing* (3rd ed.). St. Louis: C. V. Mosby.

Zander, K. (1990). *Estimating and tracking the financial impact of critical paths. 5*(4), 1–2.

Zander, K. (1990). The 1990s: Core values, core change. *Frontiers in Health Services Management, 7*(2), 28–32.

Zander, K. (1991). Case management in acute care: Making the connections. *The Case Manager, 2*(1), 39–43.

Zander, K. (1992). Focusing on patient outcome: Case management in the 90s. *Dimensions of Critical Care Nursing, 11*(3), 127–129.

Zander, K. (1992). Physicians, Care Maps (TM), and collaboration. *Definition, 7*(1), 1–4.

Glossary

Glossary

ABC   Adjusted billed charge

Activities of daily living   Activities necessary for basic self-care such as hygiene, dressing, feeding, sleeping, and social functioning

Acute care   Patient care that takes place at the hospital level. Other facilities such as free standing rehabilitation hospitals or transitional hospitals may have acute levels in their care structure.

ADLs   Activities of daily living

Admission review   A medical review performed within 24 to 48 hours of a patient's hospital admission to determine whether the hospitalization was reasonable and appropriate

Advance Directives   Legally executed documents drawn up while the individual is still competent, used only if that individual becomes incapacitated or incompetent

Adverse patient outcome (APO)   Any adverse patient occurrence which, under optimal conditions, is not a natural consequence of the patient's disease process, or the end result of a procedure

AFDC   Aid to Families with Dependent Children

ALOS   Average length of stay

Alternative level of care   A level of care that can safely be used in place of the current care level. Alternative levels of care for a hospitalized patient may include home, ECF, or ambulatory centers.

APO   adverse patient outcomes

Appropriateness (of care)   Matching the proper level of care and correct treatment to the severity and stability of a client's medical status

APS   Adult Protective Services

Attending physician   The primary physician responsible for a patient's care while in an institution

Cap   Maximum dollar amounts allowed in an insurance policy

Capitation   The amount of dollars per patient per month (rather than dollars per services). A primary care physician, a health plan, or an institution is paid according to the number of members provided for during a specified time period (usually per month).

Case manager   See nurse case manager.

Catastrophic cases   A claim with a large dollar amount

CCM   Certified Case Manager

CHAMPUS   Civilian Health and Medical Program of the Uniformed Services

CISW   Certified Independent Social Worker

Clinical Pathways   A multidisciplinary management tool that proactively depicts important events that should take place on a day-by-day sequence

CM   Case manager

CMPs   Competitive medical plans

Coinsurance   Percentage amount each insurance plan member must pay (often 20% of bill), usually with a ceiling dollar amount

COB   Coordination of benefits

COBRA   Consolidated Omnibus Budget Reconciliation Act

Concurrent review   A medical review for appropriateness and necessity performed while the patient is in the facility

Continued stay review   A medical review that is done at specific time frames within the hospital stay. The length of time between reviews usually depends on the severity of the patient's illness and his medical stability.

Coordination of benefits   Action to prevent double payment for services when a member has coverage from two or more insurance plans

Copayment   A set dollar amount that each insurance plan member must pay at the time services are rendered

Cost containment   A wise and appropriate use of resources, reasonably priced, for a particular case

CPS   Child Protective Services

CPT-4   *Current Procedural Terminology*, 4th edition

CQI   Continuous quality improvement

Critical Pathways   See Clinical Pathways.

Current Procedural Terminology, 4th edition (CPT-4)   Five-digit coding system used for billing purposes

Custodial care (also known as personal care)   Care to aid a client in meeting his or her activities of daily living. Does not require skilled medical attention and is not always covered under insurance coverage.

Days per thousand   Number of hospital days used in 1 year for each 1000 patients

Deductible   The set dollar amount that the insurance plan member must pay before the plan begins paying

Defensive medicine   Excess tests, scans, hospital admissions, or any medical service that is provided to prevent the possibility of a malpractice lawsuit

Deferred liability   Defers the expenses of specific cases for a period of time. This helps a Medicaid plan maintain financial control by receiving some reimbursement for a newly enrolled member who is in the hospital on the day of admission.

Denial   No authorization obtained for services. Reviewer is unable to verify medical necessity and appropriateness of treatment or length of stay. This can occur before services would be performed or during hospitalizations, in which case the middle or end days of hospital stays would be denied (ie, receive no reimbursement).

Diagnosis-related groups (DRG)   A patient classification system based on diagnoses. Each classification is scored according to potential consumption of resources; hospitals may receive a flat rate for a patient based on the DRG assigned to that patient.

Disabled   Inability to return to full employment of the last employment situation due to injury or health conditions

Discharge planning   Posthospital/extended care facility (ECF)/rehabilitation care planned early in the admission. Frequent monitoring may be necessary for a safe, efficient discharge plan.

Disenrollment   The process of termination of coverage

DME   Durable medical equipment

DNR   Do not resuscitate.

DRG   Diagnosis-related groups

Durable Power of Attorney for Healthcare   See Medical Power of Attorney.

EAC   Eligible Assistance Children (also known as "food stamp" children)

ECF   Extended care facility

ELIC   Eligible Low Income Children

ELOS   Estimated length of stay

EPO   Exclusive Provider Organization

EPSDT Services   Early and Periodic Screening, Diagnosis and Treatment Services (preventive services included for those under 18 years of age)

Exclusive Provider Organization   Much like a preferred provider organization (PPO) except that outside physicians are not be reimbursed

Fee-for-service   Traditional payment style whereby services billed to the insurance company are paid by the insurance company

Gatekeeper   A primary care physician who "stands at the gate" of available healthcare services, deciding which services are required for each member. The provider makes referrals to specialists as deemed necessary and continuously monitors patient's care

Grievance   A complaint that stems from an adverse action (eg, hospital may file a grievance for denial of reimbursement)

Group Model   Health maintenance organization (HMO) contracts with a group of physicians who provide care for HMO members

HCBS   Home and community-based services

HCFA   Health Care Financing Administration

Health Care Financing Administration (HCFA)   The federal agency that oversees financing for Medicare

Health Maintenance Organization (HMO) A managed-care style insurance model that uses primary care physicians as gatekeepers and contracted facilities. Five models of HMOs are staff model, group model, direct contract model, network model, and Independent Practice Association (IPA)

HHA Home health agency

HHC Home healthcare

HHN Home health nursing

HMG Healthcare Management Guidelines (from Milliman & Robertson, Inc)

HMO Health Maintenance Organization

Holistic medicine Usually nontraditional forms of medicine that consider the whole person rather than a disease or group of diseased organs; considers the body/mind/emotion/spirit connection

Home healthcare Home-based skilled services to ill, disabled, or convalescing clients who are homebound. Services may include physical/speech/occupational therapies, home nursing and personal care (the latter is not always covered by many insurance companies).

ICD-10 *International Classification of Diseases,* 10th revision

ICF Intermediate care facility

Important aspects of care Aspects of care that occur frequently, affect large numbers of patients, or place patients at risk for serious consequences if not provided for optimally. They are often the target of performance improvement activities.

Incident report A communication tool used to record adverse events or unusual occurrences

Incident An accident or the discovery of a hazardous condition that is inconsistent with standards of care

Indemnity plan The traditional insurance plan before the advent of managed care. Some indemnity plans still exist and offer the most flexibility among all the types of plans.

Indicator A measure that can monitor and assess the quality of important aspects of patient care or services

Informed consent A document signed by a competent patient or surrogate stating that he or she has been reasonably informed of the patient's condition and agrees to the stated procedure

International Classification of Diseases, 10th revision Classifies diseases by diagnosis

IPA Independent Practice Association

IS Intensity of service

ISD-A Criteria (specifically from InterQual) Intensity of Service, Severity of Illness, Discharge Appropriateness

JCAHO Joint Commission for the Accreditation of Health Care Organizations

Joint Commission for the Accreditation of Health Care Organizations   Organization that accredits hospitals, outpatient facilities and other institutions

Length of stay (LOS)   Number of days allowed for a hospitalization or extended care stay

Level of care (LOC)   Terminology referring to the placement needed to match the stability of the patient. Levels of care include home, outpatient clinic, emergency room, intensive care unit, floor, stepdown unit, telemetry, rehab, nursing home, and so on.

Living will   A legal document that directs the healthcare team in holding or withdrawing life support measures

LOC   Level of care

LOS   Length of stay

LTC   Long-term care

MAC   Maximum allowable charge

Malpractice   Unsafe or inappropriate care or treatment; unprofessional, illegal or immoral conduct or unreasonable lack of skill

Managed care organization (MCO)   A generic term that applies to all managed care organizations

Managed care   A healthcare delivery system whereby all aspects of patient care are managed in such a way as to encourage cost-effective, efficient, and quality care, some aspects of which require prior approval

Managed competition   An economic theory that combines the free-market approach with government regulation, in which large groups of consumers purchase health insurance from networks of providers. Business competition among those networks would ideally limit high prices and foster quality of care.

MAO   Medical assistance only

MC   Managed care

MCO   Managed care organization

MDC   Major diagnostic category

Medicaid   A federally funded insurance program that provides health services for the poor

Medical necessity   Comparison of the state of illness with the treatment rendered. Medical necessity asks if the treatment or the level of care is appropriate for this set of medical conditions.

Medical power-of-attorney   A legal document that names a surrogate decision maker in the event that the principle becomes unable to make his or her own decisions about healthcare

Medicare Risk Contract   Agreement in which Medicare pays an HMO on a monthly basis for each member enrolled. The HMO is at risk if the services needed are more costly than the fixed payment. Conversely, if the enrollee does not need services during the period, the HMO benefits.

Medicare   A federally funded insurance program for US citizens over 65 years of age and certain groups classified as disabled

Medigap plans   Insurance plans designed to supplement what Medicare does not cover

MIS   Management Information System   A managed care computer hardware/software system

Mixed model   Managed care plans that mix more than one type of insurance model

MN/MI   Medically needy/medically indigent

MSO   Medical Services Organization, which buy and manage medical practices, then contract out these practices to insurance companies. The owners may be private corporations, hospitals, or other facilities.

NCM   Nurse case manager

Negligence   Failure to take action that a reasonable, professionally guided person would do or taking action that a reasonable, professionally guided person would not do

Network model   A health plan that contracts with multiple groups of physicians to provide healthcare to its members

NH   Nursing home

NHP   Nursing home placement

Notch group   The part of the population whose income is too low to afford medical insurance but too high to be eligible for federally funded insurance programs

Nurse case manager (NCM)   A nurse who uses the multidisciplinary team approach to collaborative care to match a client's healthcare needs with available services and resources. This leads to improved continuity and quality of care and the cost-efficient use of resources.

OBV   Observation

Occupational therapy (OT)   Therapy to bring clients as close as possible to baseline activities to regain independence and coordination (especially ADLs)

Office of Prepaid Health Care   The federal agency that oversees eligibility and compliance of HMOs and CMPs; part of HCFA

Open Enrollment Period   A specified time period wherein a member can change health plans. It is considered an important part of many medical and managed care plans.

OPHC   Office of Prepaid Health Care

OPT   Outpatient

ORG   Optimal Recovery Guidelines (Milliman & Robertson's Healthcare Guidelines)

OT   Occupational therapy

Outcomes   The results and consequences from the care received; outcomes also result from care that was *not* received. Outcome studies look for trends and potentially adverse events. Poor outcomes revealed through outcome studies often lead to policy and procedural changes in an effort to improve the problem.

Outlier   Circumstance when cost or length of stay exceeds that which has been determined for a specific DRG

Overutilization   Use of more resources, services, or care than is required for that patient's medical condition

OWA   Other weird arrangement

PA   Physician advisor

PA   Physician assistant

PAR   Preadmission review

PAS Norms   The Professional Activity Study resulting in a book of average length of stays called *LOS: Length of Stay by Diagnosis*

PAS   Preadmission screening

PCC   Patient care coordinator

PCP   Primary care physician

Peer Review Organization   Groups of doctors in each state who are paid by Medicare to review hospital care for Medicare patients

Personal care   See Custodial care.

PHOs   Physician Hospital Organizations

Physician Hospital Organizations (PHO)   Model that bonds a hospital with an attending physician staff for the purpose of linking with a managed care plan

POA   Power-of-attorney

Point of Service Plans (POS)   Plans in which, when services are needed, the member can choose any physician, but significant differences in reimbursement rates exist between "plan providers" and those outside the plan

POS   Point of Service Plan

Potentially compensable event   A potentially compensable event is one in which the end result could be litigation

PPA   Preferred Provider Arrangements (same as a PPO)

PPO   Preferred Provider Organization

PPS   Prospective Payment System

Preadmission review ([PAR] same as prospective review and precertification)   Authorization of services before services take place. Attempts to determine the appropriateness of a hospital admission.

Precertification   See Preadmission review.

Preexisting condition A condition or illness that was apparent and treated prior to the client being issued an insurance policy

Preferred Provider Organization (PPO) An insurance model using a preferred panel of physicians. Outside physicians may be used but the reimbursement rate is lower, which incurs greater cost to the member.

Prehospital Medical Care Directive A menu of possible aspects of the resuscitation effort. The patient can choose all, some, or none in the event of an arrest.

Premature discharge The discharge of patients before they are deemed medically stable, while still needing continued care or observation

Preventive medicine Care that focuses on the prevention of disease or the prevention of further deterioration of disease through immunizations, early detection, educational programs, and other health-promoting activities

Primary care physician (PCP) The primary physician assigned to a member of a health plan (see gatekeeper)

PRO Peer Review Organization

Prospective payment systems A method of hospital reimbursement in which inpatient hospital stays are based on DRGs and paid in advance of services (see Diagnosis-Related Groups)

Prospective review See Preadmission review.

PT Physical therapy

QA Quality Assurance

QI Quality Improvement (see Quality Assurance)

QM Quality Management (see Quality Assurance)

QR Quality Review

Quality assurance (QA) Activities designed to monitor, prevent, and correct quality deficiencies

Quality of care The quality of excellence of the medical care received; takes into account all medical services, technical competence, humanitarian treatment, and appropriateness

Quality review Quality of medical care evaluated by reviewing a patient's medical record using medical standards for assessment

Reinsurance Insurance purchased by an insurance company to protect itself against extremely expensive cases

Retrospective review Medical review performed after discharge or after services were provided

Risk management (RM) The process of minimizing losses that cannot be prevented through legal methods and public relations

RM Risk management

RN Registered nurse

S.O.B.R.A. Sixth Omnibus Budget Reconciliation Act

SI Severity of illness

Skilled care Patient care that requires a licensed professional such as a registered nurse or physical/occupational/speech therapist

SNAT Suspected nonaccidental trauma (implies child abuse)

SNF Skilled nursing facility

Spend down The process by which a client can financially qualify for Medicaid

SSD Social Security Disability

SSI Supplemental Security Income

ST Speech therapy

Staff Model An HMO that employs the physicians to care for its members. These physicians use HMO facilities.

Standards Professional criteria indicating acceptable performances or outcomes

Subacute care Generally, patient care that takes place at a skilled nursing facility. Other facilities such as rehabilitation or transitional hospitals may have a subacute level in their care structure.

Surrogate A substitute decision maker who acts in the best interests of the patient, closely matching what the patient would have wanted

Third party liability (TPL) Refers to an accident or event that makes a third party liable for the expenses (eg, automobile insurance in the case of a motor vehicle accident)

TPL Third party liability

UM Utilization Management

Unbundling A bill containing multiple fees, in which previously only one fee showed. For example, dressings and instruments were previously lumped in one fee for a minor procedure. Unbundled, these charges are shown separately.

Underutilization Occurs when a patient is not given the necessary services, tests, and therapies (resources) to diagnose or treat a medical condition

UR Utilization Review

Utilization Management Managing the utilization of healthcare resources

Utilization Review (UR) The process whereby medical services are evaluated for efficiency, appropriateness, and necessity

Variances Deviations from expected care. Three types of variances are practitioner, system/institutional, and patient/family variances.

WHO World Health Organization

Wholistic medicine See holistic medicine.

WIC Women, Infants, and Children's Program

Workers' Compensation A program for work-related injuries

Wraparound Plan A supplemental plan that pays for copayments deductibles, and other miscellaneous charges that the primary insurance plan does not cover. Some Medigap plans may be considered wraparound plans.

Index

Powell: Nursing Case Management. © 1996 Lippincott–Raven Publishers

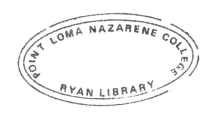